Advanced Approaches in Echocardiography

PRACTICAL ECHOCARDIOGRAPHY SERIES

Look for these other titles in Catherine M. Otto's Practical Echocardiography Series

Donald C. Oxorn
Intraoperative Echocardiography

Mark B. Lewin & Karen Stout
Echocardiography in Congenital Heart Disease

Martin St. John Sutton & Susan E. Wiegers
Echocardiography in Heart Failure

Advanced Approaches in Echocardiography

PRACTICAL ECHOCARDIOGRAPHY SERIES

Linda D. Gillam, MD
Vice Chair of Cardiovascular Medicine
Morristown Medical Center
Atlantic Health System
Morristown, New Jersey
Professor of Clinical Medicine
Columbia University College of Physicians
New York, New York

Catherine M. Otto, MD
J. Ward Kennedy-Hamilton Endowed Chair in Cardiology, Professor of Medicine
Director, Cardiology Fellowship Programs
University of Washington School of Medicine
Associate Director, Echocardiography Laboratory
University of Washington Medical Center
Seattle, Washington

ELSEVIER
SAUNDERS

SAUNDERS

1600 John F. Kennedy Blvd.
Ste 1800
Philadelphia, PA 19103-2899

Notices

Knowledge and best practice in this field are constantly changing. As new research and experience
broaden our understanding, changes in research methods, professional practices, or medical
treatment may become necessary.

Practitioners and researchers must always rely on their own experience and knowledge in
evaluating and using any information, methods, compounds, or experiments described herein. In
using such information or methods they should be mindful of their own safety and the safety of
others, including parties for whom they have a professional responsibility.

With respect to any drug or pharmaceutical products identified, readers are advised to check the
most current information provided (i) on procedures featured or (ii) by the manufacturer of each
product to be administered, to verify the recommended dose or formula, the method and duration of
administration, and contraindications. It is the responsibility of practitioners, relying on their own
experience and knowledge of their patients, to make diagnoses, to determine dosages and the best
treatment for each individual patient, and to take all appropriate safety precautions.

To the fullest extent of the law, neither the Publisher nor the authors, contributors, or editors,
assume any liability for any injury and/or damage to persons or property as a matter of products
liability, negligence or otherwise, or from any use or operation of any methods, products,
instructions, or ideas contained in the material herein.

Library of Congress Cataloging-in-Publication Data
Advanced echocardiographic approaches / [edited by] Linda D. Gillam, Catherine M. Otto.
p. ; cm. — (Practical echocardiography series)
Includes bibliographical references and index.
ISBN 978-1-4377-2697-8 (hardcover : alk. paper)
I. Gillam, Linda D. II. Otto, Catherine M. III. Series: Practical echocardiography series.
[DNLM: 1. Echocardiography—methods—Handbooks. WG 39]
LC classification not assigned
616.1'207543—dc23
                                                          2011033838

Senior Acquisitions Editor: Dolores Meloni
Editional Assistant: Brad McIlwain
Publishing Services Manager: Pat Joiner-Myers
Project Manager: Marlene Weeks
Designer: Steven Stave

Printed in Canada.

Last digit is the print number: 9 8 7 6 5 4 3 2 1

Working together to grow
libraries in developing countries

www.elsevier.com | www.bookaid.org | www.sabre.org

ELSEVIER   BOOK AID International   Sabre Foundation

Contributors

Theodore P. Abraham, MD
Associate Professor, Department of Cardiology, The Johns Hopkins University School of Medicine, Baltimore, Maryland
Echocardiographic Tools for Cardiac Resynchronization Therapy

Ana G. Almeida, MD, PhD
Associate Professor, Department of Medicine/Cardiology, Lisbon University Medical School; Senior Consultant, Cardiology, University Hospital Santa Maria, Lisbon, Portugal
Multimodality Cardiac Imaging—When Is Echo Not Enough?

Anna E. Bortnick, MD, PhD
Cardiology Fellow, Cardiovascular Division, Department of Medicine, The Hospital of the University of Pennsylvania, Philadelphia, Pennsylvania
Intracardiac Echocardiography for Common Interventions on Structural Heart Disease

Nuno Cortez Dias, MD
Assistant Lecturer, Lisbon University Medical School; Department of Cardiology, University Hospital Santa Maria, Lisbon, Portugal
Multimodality Cardiac Imaging—When Is Echo Not Enough?

Veronica Lea J. Dimanno, MD
Senior Research Fellow, Division of Cardiology, Department of Medicine, Johns Hopkins University, Baltimore, Maryland
Echocardiographic Tools for Cardiac Resynchronization Therapy

Kristian Eskesen, MD
Senior Research Fellow, Department of Medicine, Johns Hopkins University, Baltimore, Maryland
Echocardiographic Tools for Cardiac Resynchronization Therapy

Linda D. Gillam, MD
Vice Chair of Cardiovascular Medicine, Morristown Medical Center, Atlantic Health System, Morristown, New Jersey; Professor of Clinical Medicine, Columbia University College of Physicians, New York, New York
Transthoracic and Transesophageal Echocardiography in the Catheterization Laboratory

Rebecca Hahn, MD
Assistant Professor of Clinical Medicine, Division of Cardiology, Weill Medical College of Cornell University, New York, New York
Transthoracic and Transesophageal Echocardiography in the Catheterization Laboratory

Judy Hung, MD
Associate Professor of Medicine, Associate Director, Echocardiology, Massachusetts General Hospital, Harvard Medical School, Boston, Massachusetts
Advanced Echocardiography Approaches: 3D Transesophageal Assessment of the Mitral Valve

Roberto M. Lang, MD
Professor of Medicine, Director of Cardiac Imaging Laboratories, Department of Medicine, Section of Cardiology, University of Chicago Medical Center, Chicago, Illinois
Transthoracic Three-Dimensional Echocardiography

Thomas H. Marwick, MD, PhD, FACC
Professor of Medicine, Cleveland Clinic, Cleveland, Ohio
Strain and Strain Rate Imaging

Victor Mor-Avi, PhD
Professor, Director of Cardiac Imaging Research, Department of Medicine, Section of Cardiology, University of Chicago Medical Center, Chicago, Illinois
Transthoracic Three-Dimensional Echocardiography

Sherif F. Nagueh, MD
Professor of Medicine, Department of Medicine, Weill Cornell Medical College; Director, Echocardiography Laboratory, Methodist DeBakey Heart and Vascular Center, Houston, Texas
Assessing Twist and Torsion

Joan J. Olson, RDCS
Lead Cardiac Sonographer, Nebraska Medical Center Echocardiography Lab, Nebraska Medical Center, Omaha, Nebraska
Contrast Perfusion Echocardiography

Catherine M. Otto, MD
J. Ward Kennedy-Hamilton Endowed Chair in Cardiology, Professor of Medicine, Director, Cardiology Fellowship Programs, University of Washington School of Medicine; Associate Director, Echocardiography Laboratory, University of Washington Medical Center, Seattle, Washington
Stress Testing for Structural Heart Disease

David S. Owens, MD
Assistant Professor, Department of Medicine, Division of Cardiology, University of Washington, Seattle, Washington
Stress Testing for Structural Heart Disease

Jonathan J. Passeri, MD
Instructor in Medicine, Harvard Medical School; Co-Director, Heart Valve Program, Department of Medicine, Cardiology Division, Massachusetts General Hospital, Boston, Massachusetts
Advanced Echocardiography Approaches: 3D Transesophageal Assessment of the Mitral Valve

Fausto J. Pinto, MD, PhD
Professor, Deparment of Medicine/Cardiology, Lisbon University Medical School; Senior Consultant, Cardiology, University Hospital Santa Maria, Lisbon, Portugal
Multimodality Cardiac Imaging—When Is Echo Not Enough?

Thomas Porter, MD
Thomas F. Hubbard Distinguished Chair of Cardiology and Professor of Medicine, University of Nebraska Medical Center, Omaha, Nebraska
Contrast Perfusion Echocardiography

Takahiro Shiota, MD
Clinical Professor, Department of Medicine, University of California, Los Angeles; Professor of Medicine, Department of Cardiology, Cedars-Sinai Medical Center, Los Angeles, California
Two-Dimensional and Three-Dimensional Echocardiographic Evaluation of the Right Ventricle

Frank E. Silvestry, MD
Associate Professor of Medicine, Cardiovascular Medicine, Department of Medicine, University of Pennsylvania School of Medicine, Philadelphia, Pennsylvania
Intracardiac Echocardiography for Common Interventions on Structural Heart Disease

Nozomi Watanabe, MD, PhD, FACC
Assistant Professor of Medicine, Department of Cardiology, Kawasaki Medical School, Kurashiki, Japan
Evaluation of Coronary Blood Flow by Echo Doppler

Feng Xie
Assistant Professor of Medicine, Division of Cardiology, University of Nebraska Medical Center, Omaha, Nebraska
Contrast Perfusion Echocardiography

Foreword

Echocardiography is a core component of every aspect of clinical cardiology and now plays an essential role in daily decision making. Both echocardiographers and clinicians face unique challenges in interpretation of imaging and Doppler data and in integration of these data with other clinical information. However, with the absorption of echocardiography into daily patient care, there are some voids in our collective knowledge base. First, clinicians caring for patients need to understand the value, strengths, and limitations of echocardiography relevant to their specific scope of practice. Second, echocardiographers need a more in-depth understanding of the clinical context of the imaging study. Finally, as new methods are developed, there often is a lag in transmission of the expertise needed for optimal application from the research to the clinical setting. The books in the Practical Echocardiography Series are aimed at filling these knowledge gaps, with each book focusing on a specific aspect of the clinical utility of echocardiography.

In addition to *Advanced Approaches in Echocardiography*, edited by Linda D. Gillam, MD, and myself, other books in the series are *Intraoperative Echocardiography*, edited by Donald C. Oxorn, MD; *Echocardiography in Congenital Heart Disease*, edited by Mark B. Lewin, MD, and Karen Stout, MD; and *Echocardiography in Heart Failure*, edited by Martin St. John Sutton, MD, and Susan E. Wiegers, MD. Information is presented as concise bulleted text accompanied by numerous illustrations and tables, providing a practical approach to data acquisition and analysis, including technical details, pitfalls, and clinical interpretation, supplemented by web-based video case examples. Each volume in this series expands on the basic principles presented in the *Textbook of Clinical Echocardiography, fourth edition*, and can be used as a supplement to that text or can be used by physicians interested in a focused introduction to echocardiography in their area of clinical practice.

Over the past decade a number of new echocardiographic modalities have been developed that have the potential to provide information not available with standard imaging and Doppler approaches. Some of these new methodologies have rapidly gained wide acceptance; others are still in development but are expected to become more feasible as instrumentation evolves. In this book, Linda Gillam and I sought out experts in each new echocardiographic modality, with the goal of providing the information you will need to apply these new approaches in your own clinical practice. We hope this information will both provide the context for optimal utilization of these new imaging modalities and allow further dissemination of these powerful new techniques in our clinical toolbox.

Catherine M. Otto, MD

Preface

Echocardiographic imaging and Doppler data are essential to the practice of clinical cardiology and are available to every medical center and cardiologist caring for patients with cardiovascular disease. In addition to these standard echocardiographic modalities, advances in imaging technology over the past few years also allow more sophisticated image analysis and display, including modalities such as three-dimensional (3D) and strain rate imaging. In addition, echocardiography has moved beyond the diagnostic imaging laboratory into the interventional cardiology arena, where it now is an integral component of transcatheter interventions for structural heart disease. Despite a wealth of research literature on these new applications of echocardiography, the knowledge needed for the clinician to start using and to optimize use of these new techniques has been lacking.

This book provides a practical approach to the integration of these new imaging modalities in your echocardiography laboratory. For each topic, a detailed step-by-step approach to clinical implementation is provided in a concise and easy-to-read bulleted format. Technical details and clinical pearls are highlighted in key points sections, and numerous illustrations show how to apply these new approaches in your daily practice. Authors for each chapter were selected on the basis of their clinical expertise in each of these modalities, as well as their research accomplishments in development and validation of these newer echocardiographic approaches.

The first section of the book focuses on 3D echocardiography, with separate chapters on transthoracic and transesophageal approaches, including assessment of the mitral valve and evaluation of the right ventricle. The next section details the use of transthoracic, transesophageal, and intracardiac echocardiography for monitoring cardiac interventions for structural heart disease. Several chapters address the utility of newer imaging modalities for evaluation of left ventricular function and coronary artery disease, including the applications of strain and strain rate imaging, approaches to measurement of ventricular twist and torsion, echocardiographic evaluation of cardiac resynchronization therapy, the use of contrast perfusion echocardiography, and direct Doppler assessment of coronary blood flow. The final section includes a chapter on stress echocardiography for structural heart disease and one on multimodality cardiac imaging. This last chapter provides the overall context for the use of newer echocardiographic approaches compared with other imaging modalities, such as cardiac computed tomography and cardiac magnetic resonance imaging.

We hope this book will allow wider application of these newer echocardiographic approaches. Given the ongoing rapid advances in this field, readers are encouraged to supplement the material in this book with publications from the current literature.

Linda D. Gillam, MD
Catherine M. Otto, MD

Contents

Glossary

2D two-dimensional
2DE two-dimensional echocardiography
3D three-dimensional
3DE three-dimensional echocardiography
a' late diastolic tissue velocity
A2C apical two-chamber view
A3C apical three-chamber view
A4C apical four-chamber view
AA ascending aorta
AC atrial contraction
AL amyloid light chain
AL-C anterolateral commissure
A_m late diastolic myocardial (tissue) velocity
AML anterior mitral valve leaflet
Ao aorta
A-P anterior-posterior
AR aortic regurgitation
AROA anatomic regurgitant orifice area
AS aortic stenosis
ASA alcohol septal ablation
ASD atrial septal defect
AV atrioventricular; aortic valve
AVA aortic valve area
AVC aortic valve closure
AVO aortic valve opening
BAV balloon aortic valvuloplasty
BP blood pressure
CAD coronary artery disease
CCT cardiac computed tomography
CFR coronary flow reserve
CHD congenital heart disease
CHF coronary heart failure
CI confidence interval
CMR cardiac magnetic resonance imaging
CPET cardiopulmonary exercise testing
CRT cardiac resynchronization therapy
CSA cross-sectional area
CT computed tomography
CTCA computed tomography coronary angiography
CW continuous wave
Cx circumflex coronary artery
ΔP transmitral gradient

DA descending aorta
DCM dilated cardiomyopathy
DE-CMR delayed contrast enhancement cardiac magnetic resonance
DHF diastolic heart failure
DICOM Digital Imaging and Communications in Medicine
DLC delayed longitudinal contraction
dP/dt rate of change in pressure over time
DSE dobutamine stress echocardiography
DSVR diastolic-to-systolic flow velocity ratio
DT deceleration time
E early diastolic velocity
e' early diastolic tissue velocity
ECG electrocardiogram, electrocardiographic, electrocardiography
EDV end-diastolic volume
EF ejection fraction
E_m tissue Doppler E wave at the basal septal mitral annulus
EMC electromechanical coupling
EROA effective regurgitant orifice area
ESS end-systolic strain
ESV end-systolic volume
ETT exercise treadmill
Ex exercise
FAC fractional area change
FAI functional aerobic impairment
fps frames per second
FR frame rate
GCS global circumferential strain
GLS global longitudinal strain
%GR percent grade
GS global strain
HCM hypertrophic cardiomyopathy
HR heart rate
HT hormone therapy
IAS interatrial septum
ICD intracardiac defibrillator; implantable cardioverter defibrillator
ICE intracardiac echocardiography
Is ischemia

IVA isovolumic acceleration
IVC inferior vena cava; isovolumic contraction
IVR isovolumetric relaxation
IVRT isovolumetric relaxation time
IVUS intravascular ultrasound
LA left atrial; left atrium
LAA left atrial appendage; left aortic arch
LAD left anterior descending (coronary artery)
LAP left atrial pressure
LAX long axis view
LBBB left bundle branch block
LCA left main coronary artery
LCO left coronary ostium
LCx left circumflex (artery)
LIMA left internal mammary artery
LIPV left inferior pulmonary vein
LM left main (coronary artery)
LMT left main trunk
LRV lower reference value
LSPV left superior pulmonary vein
LV left ventricular, left ventricle
LVESV left ventricular end-systolic volume
LVH left ventricular hypertrophy
LVOT left ventricular outflow tract
MCE myocardial contrast echocardiography
MET metabolic equivalent
MI mechanical index; myocardial infarction
M-L medial-lateral
MPH miles per hour
MPI myocardial perfusion imaging; myocardial performance index
MPR multiplanar reconstruction
MR mitral regurgitant, mitral regurgitation,
MRI magnetic resonance imaging
MS mitral stenosis
MSCT multislice spiral computed tomography
MV mitral valve
MVA mitral valve area
MVI myocardial videointensity
MVO mitral valve opening
MVP mitral valve prolapse
MVR mitral valve replacement
PA pulmonary artery
PAP pulmonary artery pressure
PBMV percutaneous balloon mitral valvuloplasty
PDA posterior descending coronary artery
PDE pulsed Doppler echocardiography
PEP pre-ejection period
PET positron emission tomography
PFO patent foramen ovale
PISA proximal isovelocity surface area
PLAX parsternal long axis view
PM papillary muscle
PM-C posteromedial commissure
PMVL posterior mitral valve leaflet
PR pulmonic regurgitation

PSI postsystolic index
PT pulmonary trunk
pulmV pulmonic valve
PV pulmonary vein
PW pulsed wave
R rest
RA right atrium
RAA right aortic arch
RCA right coronary artery
RCO right coronary ostium
RE rapid emptying
RF reservoir function
RIPV right inferior pulmonary vein
ROI region of interest
RPA right pulmonary artery
RSPV right superior pulmonary vein
RT3DE real-time three-dimensional echocardiography
RTPE real-time perfusion echocardiography
RV right ventricle; right ventricular
RVAC right ventricular arrhythmogenic cardiomyopathy
RVD right ventricle diameter
RVEF right ventricular ejection fraction
RVOT right ventricular outflow tract
s' systolic tissue velocity
SAM systolic anterior motion
SAX short axis view
SD standard deviation
SDI systolic dyssynchrony index
SHF systolic heart failure
S$_m$ myocardial systolic velocity
SPECT single-photon emission computed tomography
SPWMD septal-to-posterior wall motion delay
SR strain rate
SR$_a$ late diastolic strain rate
SR$_e$ early diastolic strain rate
SR$_s$ systolic strain rate
SRI strain rate imaging
SSFP steady state in free precession
STE speckle tracking echocardiography
STJ sinotubular junction
SV stroke volume
SVG saphenous vein graft
T trachea
TAPSE tricuspid annular plane systolic excursion
TAVI transcatheter aortic valve implantation
TAVR transcatheter aortic valve replacement
TDE tissue Doppler echocardiography
TDI tissue Doppler imaging
TEE transesophageal echocardiography
TGC time gain compensation
THV transcatheter heart valve
TIMI thrombolysis in myocardial infarction
TR tricuspid regurgitation, tricuspid regurgitant

Ts time-to-peak systolic velocity
TS transverse sinus
TSI tissue synchronization imaging
TTE transthoracic echocardiography
TV tricuspid valve
TVI tissue velocity imaging

UCA ultrasound contrast agent
VC vena contracta
VO² peak oxygen uptake
VTI velocity time integral
WMA wall motion abnormalities; wall motion analysis

Transthoracic Three-Dimensional Echocardiography

Victor Mor-Avi and Roberto M. Lang

Background

- Because the heart is three-dimensional (3D), it has been recognized that imaging the heart in three rather than two dimensions can be advantageous for the detailed evaluation of cardiac anatomy and function and better understanding of its pathophysiology.
- After a decade of research using time-consuming off-line 3D reconstruction from cumbersome acquisition of multiple two-dimensional (2D) planes, today's imaging technology has evolved to near real-time three-dimensional (RT3D) ultrasound imaging of the beating heart (Fig. 1-1).
- To overcome the technological challenges associated with the motion of the beating heart, two approaches have been implemented to create a dynamic 3D image throughout the cardiac cycle (Fig. 1-2) by (A) combining subvolumes that are scanned during consecutive cardiac cycles; (B) acquiring the entire heart in a single cardiac cycle by reducing the number of frames.
  - Currently, most manufacturers offer both approaches A and B in their imaging systems.
  - Approach A is better for visualization of rapidly moving structures, such as cardiac valves.
  - While approach B may be problematic in this regard because fast motion appears "choppy," it is advantageous over approach A in patients with irregular heart rhythms because it circumvents "stitch artifacts" and creates cohesive images at any phase of the cardiac cycle.
  - Approach A is difficult to use with stress testing because of rapid changes in the inotropic and chronotropic state of the heart, which frequently result in stitch artifacts.
  - Approach B is useful in the setting of stress testing because of its speed and ease of acquisition, but can be suboptimal because of the limited frame rates.

KEY POINTS

- There are two general approaches to RT3D echocardiography (RT3DE): combining subvolumes that are acquired from consecutive cycles (approach A) and acquiring the heart volume in single cardiac cycle (approach B).
- Approach A has better temporal resolution but is limited by linear artifacts where the subvolumes are joined (stitch artifacts), particularly when the heart rhythm is irregular or where cardiac function is changing quickly (stress echo).
- Approach B has poorer temporal resolution but is rapidly and easily acquired and is better suited in situations such as stress testing, where stitch artifacts are common.

Left Ventricular Volume

- The evaluation of left ventricular (LV) volumes is an integral part of clinical echocardiography, since accurate estimates of LV volumes provide important information for multiple clinical scenarios.
- The accuracy of the traditional 2D techniques for LV volume quantification is limited by their reliance on geometric modeling and by foreshortening of apical views of the left ventricle (LV).
- There are two approaches that are commonly used for LV quantification from RT3DE datasets (Fig. 1-3): (A) 3D-guided biplane technique—by selecting from a pyramidal dataset two anatomically correct non-foreshortened 2D views, from which LV volumes are calculated using a biplane approximation, and (B) direct volume quantification—based on semi-automated detection of LV endocardial surfaces followed by calculation of the volume contained within this surface.
- When compared with conventional 2D echocardiographic measurements, RT3DE-derived LV volumes and ejection fraction (EF) show higher levels of agreement with

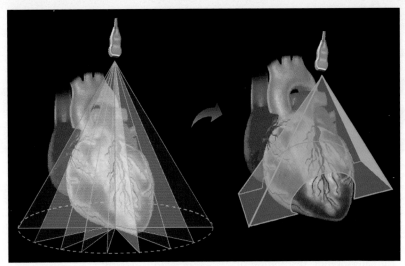

Figure 1-1. Originally, three-dimensional (3D) echocardiography was based on reconstruction from a sequential multiplane acquisition, gated to electrocardiography and respiration (*left*). This approach was tedious, time consuming, and prone to motion artifacts. This approach was later replaced by real-time volumetric imaging that allows acquisition of a pyramid of data (*right*) using matrix array transducers.

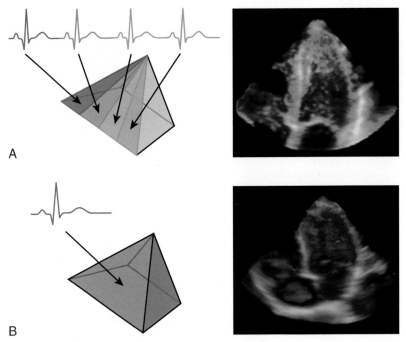

Figure 1-2. Two currently available approaches to create a dynamic 3D image of the beating heart: (**A**) by "stitching" dynamic subvolumes scanned during consecutive cardiac cycles, and (**B**) by decreasing the number of cardiac phases to allow imaging of the entire heart in a single cardiac cycle. Approach A allows imaging at higher frame rates (higher temporal resolution), with the potential disadvantage of having "stitch artifacts" as a result of changes in the position of the heart relative to the transducer. Approach B avoids motion artifacts but suffers from intrinsically lower frame rates (lower temporal resolution).

the respective reference technique, such as radionuclide ventriculography or cardiac magnetic resonance imaging (MRI).
- RT3DE-derived LV volumes and EF are more reproducible than 2D measurements.

- The improved accuracy and reproducibility of RT3DE-based LV volume and EF measurements is of vital importance because clinical decision making relies heavily on these measurements.

3D-GUIDED BIPLANE ANALYSIS

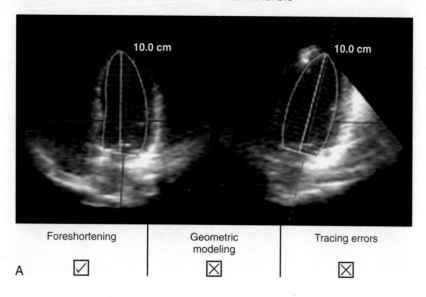

Foreshortening	Geometric modeling	Tracing errors
☑	☒	☒

A

VOLUMETRIC ANALYSIS

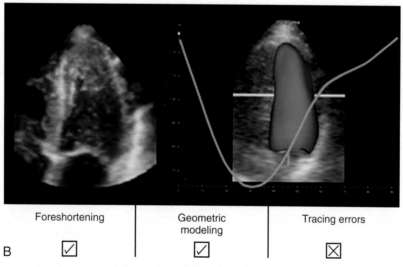

Foreshortening	Geometric modeling	Tracing errors
☑	☑	☒

B

Figure 1-3. Two approaches to measure left ventricular (LV) volume from real-time three-dimensional echocardiography (RT3DE) datasets: (**A**) 3D-guided biplane analysis based on selecting from the entire 3D dataset anatomically correct, nonforeshortened, apical two- and four-chamber views and then using the biplane calculation identical to that used with 2D imaging, and (**B**) direct phase-by-phase volumetric analysis based on counting pixels contained inside the 3D endocardial surface, which results in a volume over time curve (*green* curve). Key: √, resolved; ×, remains unresolved. *(Reproduced from Mor-Avi V, Lang RM. The use of real-time three-dimensional echocardiography for the quantification of left ventricular volumes and function. Curr Opin Cardiol. 2009;24:402-409, Figure 2.)*

- Despite the improved accuracy and reproducibility, recent studies have reported that RT3DE consistently underestimates LV volumes.
- Tracing errors were identified as the main cause of volume underestimation, since the spatial resolution of RT3DE images may not be sufficiently high to differentiate between the myocardium and endocardial trabeculae in all patients (Fig. 1-4).

Technical Considerations
- While the 3D-guided biplane technique (A) can minimize LV foreshortening, it still relies on geometric modeling to calculate volumes, and is thus likely to be inaccurate in distorted ventricles.
- Because direct volumetric quantification (B) is not affected by LV foreshortening and does not rely on geometric modeling, this approach is more accurate even in the presence of wall

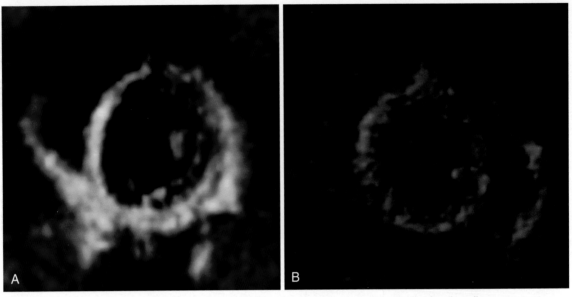

Figure 1-4. RT3DE images obtained in two patients: (**A**) with optimal endocardial visualization that allows accurate differentiation between the myocardium and the papillary muscle and endocardial trabeculae, and (**B**) with suboptimal endocardial visualization that is likely to result in inaccurate LV volume measurements. *(Reproduced from Mor-Avi V, Jenkins C, Kühl HP, et al. Real-time 3-dimensional echocardiographic quantification of left ventricular volumes: multicenter study for validation with magnetic resonance imaging and investigation of sources of error. J Am Coll Cardiol Imaging. 2008;1:413-423, Figure 4.)*

motion abnormalities and distorted ventricular shape.

- While volumetric quantification requires specialized software, the 3D-guided biplane technique is a reasonably accurate alternative for LV volume measurements.
- Tracing errors can be minimized by learning how to identify the true endocardial boundary beyond the blood-trabeculae interface and trace it as far out as possible, so as to include the papillary muscles and endocardial trabeculae in the LV cavity.

Left Ventricular Mass

- LV mass is an important predictor of morbidity and mortality, especially in patients with systemic hypertension.
- However, similar to the accuracy of 2D echocardiographic measurements of LV volume, measurements of LV mass are also limited by the frequent inability to obtain anatomically correct apical views and geometric modeling of asymmetrical ventricles.
- In addition to accurate detection of the endocardial boundaries, LV mass measurements rely on accurate detection of the epicardium (Fig. 1-5, left and middle),

which in most patients is extremely challenging.

- LV mass can also be measured using either one of the two approaches utilized to measure LV volumes from RT3DE datasets: the 3D-guided biplane technique or volumetric analysis (see Fig. 1-3).
- RT3DE-derived LV mass measurements avoid the use of foreshortened apical views (see Fig. 1-5, right).
- As a result, RT3DE-derived LV mass measurements are more accurate than the conventional biplane 2D techniques (Fig. 1-6, left).
- Also, RT3DE-derived LV mass measurements are more reproducible (see Fig. 1-6, right), because they are less view dependent.

Technical Considerations

- To obtain accurate LV mass measurements from RT3DE datasets, the same guidelines for endocardial tracing as for LV volume measurements (see above) should be strictly followed to avoid underestimation of LV mass.
- In addition, epicardial boundaries should be carefully initialized and adjusted when necessary in multiple views.
- While volumetric quantification requires specialized software, the 3D-guided biplane technique is a reasonably accurate alternative for LV mass measurements.

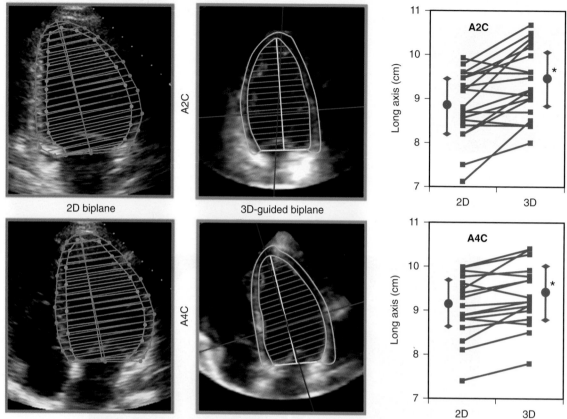

Figure 1-5. Comparison between 2D biplane (*left*) and 3D-guided biplane calculation of LV mass (*middle*). Because in the majority of patients LV apical views are foreshortened by 2D imaging (*right*), the calculated LV mass is underestimated when compared with magnetic resonance imaging (MRI) reference values. In contrast, RT3DE imaging allows avoiding foreshortened views and results in more accurate measurements. (*Reproduced from Mor-Avi V, Sugeng L, Weinert L, et al. Fast measurement of left ventricular mass with real-time three-dimensional echocardiography: comparison with magnetic resonance imaging. Circulation. 2004;110:1814-1818, Figures 1 and 5.*)

KEY POINTS

- There are two approaches to using 3D echocardiography to determine LV volumes and mass: the 3D-guided biplane or the volumetric technique.
- The volumetric approach should be used in patients with irregularly shaped ventricles.
- Both approaches provide measures of volume and mass that are more reproducible and correlate better with gold standard (MRI) values than those derived with 2D echocardiography, in part because they avoid foreshortening the apex.
- RT3DE approaches to determining LV volume underestimate gold standard values due to difficulty defining blood pool–trabecular interfaces.

Left Ventricular Wall Motion

- Echocardiography is the most widely clinically used imaging modality for the evaluation of regional LV function. This is usually achieved

by visual inspection of the beating ventricle in multiple cross-sectional planes that depict all 17 myocardial segments.

- The ability to capture the complete dynamic information of the LV in a single heartbeat lends itself to the analysis of regional wall motion.
- RT3DE allows visualization and evaluation of LV wall motion in different planes. Once the 3D dataset is acquired, image planes can be extracted in any desired orientation.
- Importantly, the ability to visualize the same LV segment in multiple planes can help in determining the extent and severity of the wall motion abnormality.
- Beyond visual interpretation, dynamic RT3DE datasets can be analyzed to obtain objective quantitative measurements of regional LV function. One such measure is segmental EF, which can be accurately calculated from segmental volumes (Fig. 1-7).

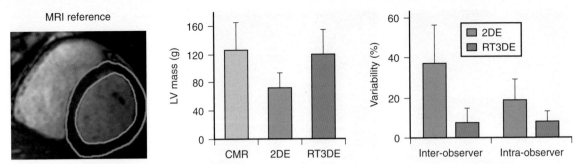

MRI reference

Figure 1-6. Side-by-side comparison between 2D biplane and 3D-guided biplane calculation of LV mass to MRI reference values in a group of patients (*left*), showing that the 2D technique underestimates LV mass, while the 3D technique results in more accurate measurements compared with a reference technique (*middle*). In addition, the 3D technique showed better reproducibility compared with the 2D methodology (*right*).

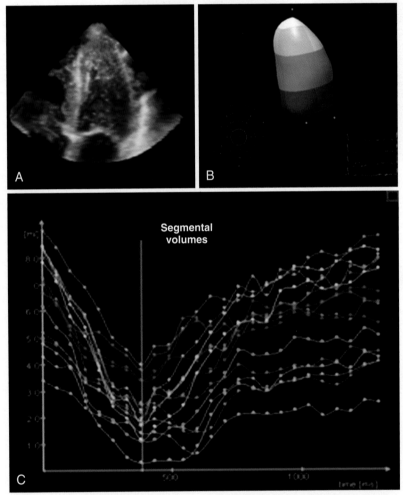

Figure 1-7. Endocardial surface extracted from an RT3DE dataset (**A**) can be divided into segments corresponding to specific LV walls (**B**). For each wall, segmental volume can be obtained over time throughout the cardiac cycle (**C**). From these curves, a variety of quantitative indices of regional LV systolic and diastolic function, including segmental ejection fraction, can be calculated.

- A decrease in segmental EF reflects reduced regional wall motion.
- All these features translate into improved accuracy of the echocardiographic diagnosis of ischemic heart disease.

Technical Consideration

- To allow accurate visual interpretation or quantitative analysis of regional wall motion from RT3DE datasets, it is important to ensure that the entire LV is included in the scan volume if possible and that drop-out artifacts are minimized.

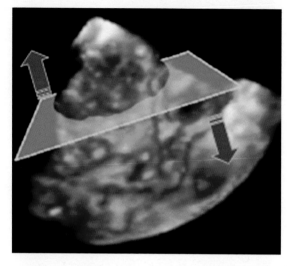

KEY POINTS
- RT3DE allows visualization of regional LV wall motion in any desired cross-sectional plane. - RT3DE datasets allow quantitative volumetric analysis of regional LV function.

Stress Testing

- Although stress echocardiography has become a widely used technique for the diagnosis and risk stratification of patients with suspected or known coronary artery disease, 2D stress echocardiography has methodologic limitations.
- 2D image acquisition during peak exercise may be impaired by: (1) probe positioning errors resulting in inadequate image planes; (2) reduced quality of transthoracic images with poor visualization of LV walls; (3) time-consuming acquisition of multiple imaging planes that need to be acquired within a narrow time window, while wall motion abnormalities are still present; and (4) subjectivity of image interpretation leading to poor interobserver agreement.
- Several of these limitations can be solved using RT3DE, which allows simultaneous visualization and evaluation of LV wall motion in different planes at different levels of the LV. Besides the conventional two-, three- and four-chamber views, multiple parallel short axis slices can be used for systematic assessment of regional wall motion, including side-by-side comparisons of rest and stress (Fig. 1-8).
- While acquisition of a complete pyramidal dataset greatly reduces the time required to capture a complete set of views during a stress test, serial acquisition of subvolumes during consecutive heartbeats is not ideal because of the rapid changes in heart rate.
- The alternative of simultaneous acquisition of multiple planes using either biplanar imaging (two orthogonal or nonorthogonal views) or

Rest   Stress

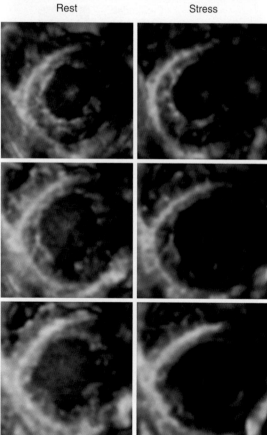

Figure 1-8. Off-line viewing of RT3DE data obtained during stress test allows extracting multiple short axis views at different levels of the left ventricle (LV) (*top*) simultaneously acquired at rest (*bottom left*) or during peak stress (*bottom right*). (*Reproduced from Lang RM, Mor-Avi V, Sugeng L, et al. Three-dimensional echocardiography: the benefits of the additional dimension. J Am Coll Cardiol. 2006;48:2053-2069, Figure 6.*)

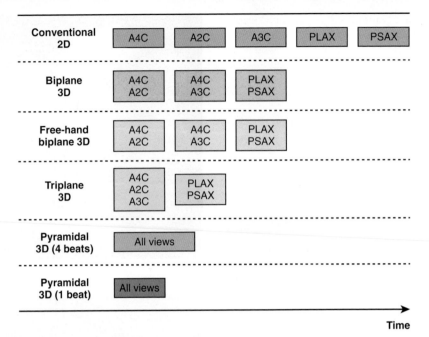

Figure 1-9. Gradual decrease in the time required for different acquisition modes currently used with stress testing, beyond the conventional 2D protocol that images one plane at a time and involves changes of transducer position from plane to plane. Time is saved by imaging more than one plane at a time and also by reducing the number of transducer positions.

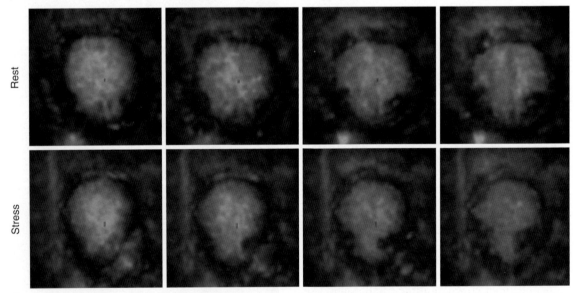

Figure 1-10. Example of LV short-axis slices extracted from a contrast-enhanced RT3DE pyramidal dataset at rest (*top*) and peak stress (*bottom*) from apex (*left*) to base (*right*). Contrast was used to improve the visualization of LV wall motion, which was achieved in all segments with a single injection.

triplanar imaging (three planes at 60-degree increments) also represents an improvement over 2D imaging (Fig. 1-9).

- Both exercise stress (either bicycle or treadmill) and pharmacological stress (mainly dobutamine plus atropine), which improves image quality and increases the available time for imaging during peak stress, have been used with RT3DE techniques.

- To improve endocardial delineation when necessary, left heart contrast agents have been used with stress RT3DE as well (Fig. 1-10).
- One advantage of contrast-enhanced biplane or triplane imaging for stress testing is that conventional 2D harmonic settings can be used, while acquisition of pyramidal volume datasets with contrast enhancement relies on settings that are not yet well defined and optimized.

- The biggest advantage of the RT3DE stress test with contrast is that the improvement in endocardial visualization is achieved with a single contrast injection.

Intraventricular Dyssynchrony

- Another evolving clinical application of RT3DE imaging is the use of segmental LV volume curves (see Fig. 1-7C) for the evaluation of intraventricular dyssynchrony and guidance of cardiac resynchronization therapy (CRT).
- To eliminate heart rate dependency and allow comparisons between patients or between serial measurements, these curves are frequently displayed with percent of the RR interval (from 0 to 100), rather than actual time in msec, in the time axis.
- LV dyssynchrony is reflected by the spread in the times at which segmental volume curves reach their minimal values.
- This temporal spread can be quantified by calculating the standard deviation of the times

to segmental end of ejection, frequently referred to as the systolic dyssynchrony index (SDI) (Fig. 1-11).
- Successful resynchronization therapy reduces LV dyssynchrony and consequently results in an increase in LV EF and a decrease in LV volumes (Fig. 1-12).
- The ease and speed of RT3DE analysis of LV synchrony lends itself to online guidance of CRT, as it can be used to aid the determination of the optimal location of the pacing leads.
- Limitations of this approach include (1) poor image quality leading to inadequate tracking and (2) poor quality of segmental volume curves in patients with severely reduced LV function, both resulting in inaccurate segmental end of ejection times.

3D Speckle Tracking Echocardiography

- Speckle tracking echocardiography is a relatively new technique that tracks the motion of distinct image features from frame to frame.
- Speckle tracking is an off-line technique that has been previously mostly applied to 2D echocardiographic images.
- Speckle tracking allows quantitative evaluation of LV deformation in terms of strain and strain rate. The main advantage of these indices over the traditional wall motion measures is that they are less affected by cardiac translation.
- Today, speckle tracking can be applied to RT3DE datasets, which allows measurements of deformation parameters in 3D space.
- The main advantage of 3D speckle tracking over 2D speckle tracking is that while the latter is "blinded" to out-of-plane motion, the 3D approach can track speckles in whichever direction they move, and thus allows an accurate evaluation of 3D myocardial deformation (Fig. 1-13).
- As a result, while 2D speckle tracking may erroneously depict out-of-plane motion as a wall motion abnormality, 3D speckle tracking avoids this problem (Fig. 1-14).

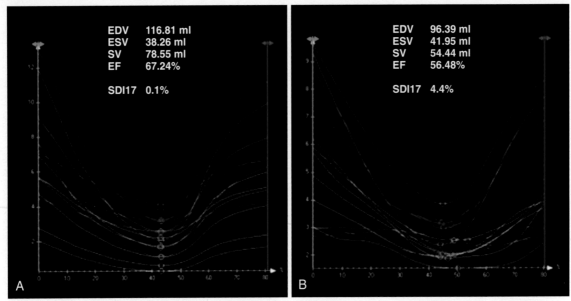

EDV 116.81 ml	EDV 96.39 ml
ESV 38.26 ml	ESV 41.95 ml
SV 78.55 ml	SV 54.44 ml
EF 67.24%	EF 56.48%
SDI17 0.1%	SDI17 4.4%

Figure 1-11. Segmental LV volume curves obtained from RT3DE datasets in a patient with normal conduction (**A**) and in a patient with left bundle branch block (**B**). Note the synchronized pattern of contraction with all segments reaching minimal values nearly simultaneously in the patient with normal conduction, and a dyssynchronous pattern where different segments reach their minima at different times in the patient with conduction abnormality. Hence the differences in the systolic dyssynchrony index calculated as a standard deviation of the time to end ejection measured in 17 segments (SDI17). *(Reproduced from Sonne C, Sugeng L, Takeuchi M, et al. Real-time 3-dimensional echocardiographic assessment of left ventricular dyssynchrony: pitfalls in patients with dilated cardiomyopathy. J Am Coll Cardiol Imaging. 2009;2:802-812, Figure 3.)*

- Currently, only selected manufacturers have commercial versions of 3D speckle tracking software.
- The relatively low spatial and temporal resolution of the RT3DE images may affect the accuracy and reproducibility of 3D speckle tracking.
- Despite these limitations, 3D speckle tracking is a promising new tool that allows more accurate measurements of myocardial deformation than 2D speckle tracking because of its intrinsic ability to detect all spatial components of the 3D motion of the heart.

KEY POINTS

- Speckle tracking can be applied to RT3DE datasets, which allows measurements of deformation parameters in 3D space.
- The major advantage over 2D speckle tracking is the ability to track out-of-plane motion.
- Major disadvantages are low spatial and temporal resolution.

Left Atrial Volume

- Left atrial (LA) enlargement is a marker of long-term LA pressure elevation. Enlargement of the left atrium (LA) is associated with an increased incidence of atrial fibrillation, ischemic stroke, and poor cardiovascular outcomes, including increased risk for overall mortality in patients post-myocardial infarction.
- LA volume is incompletely characterized by one- or two-dimensional approaches, which are based on geometric assumptions. LA volume measurements are preferred over linear dimensions because they allow more accurate assessment of the asymmetrical remodeling of the LA.
- Both the area-length and the biplane method of disks are dependent on the selection of the location and direction of the LA minor axis and the ability to clearly visualize the LA boundaries, as well as on geometric modeling. With its independence of geometric assumptions, RT3DE imaging is ideally suited for LA volume measurements.
- Similar to the LV, LA boundaries can be identified in the 3D space and LA endocardial surface can be reconstructed (Fig. 1-15).
- This reconstruction allows direct volumetric quantification of LA volume.
  - Although there is clear evidence of the prognostic value of LA enlargement as assessed by 2D echocardiography, currently no such data exist for RT3DE-derived LA volumes.

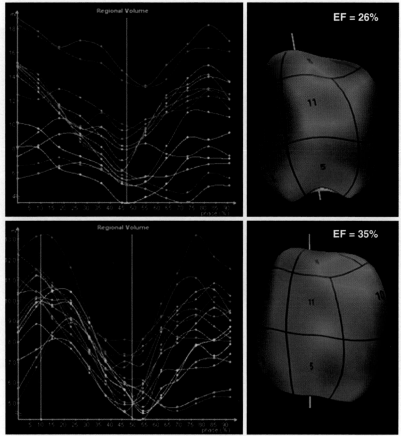

Figure 1-12. Assessment of the improvement in synchrony of LV contraction with pacing. Segmental volume time curves (*left*) obtained in a patient with LV dyssynchrony without (*top*) and with (*bottom*) biventricular pacing. Endocardial surfaces reconstructed from each dataset are shown with segmentation and color-coding according to regional time to end ejection (*right*). Note the change from a disorganized to a more organized pattern of segmental volume curves and the change in colors with pacing reflecting the effects of resynchronization therapy. *(Reproduced from Lang RM, Mor-Avi V, Sugeng L, et al. Three-dimensional echocardiography: the benefits of the additional dimension. J Am Coll Cardiol. 2006;48:2053-2069, Figure 7.)*

KEY POINTS

- Direct 3D quantification of LA volume is feasible and accurate.
- As opposed to 2D-derived LA volumes, the prognostic value of 3D volumes has not been established

Left Ventricular Shape

- Outcomes after myocardial infarction and heart failure are directly related to an adverse LV remodeling process. Patient survival has been shown to correlate with changes in LV volume and EF.
- New pharmacologic therapies, resynchronization devices, and remodeling surgery are all aimed at slowing down or reversing adverse remodeling.
- At a more basic level, remodeling is a complex process determined by the balance between distending LV dilatation forces and restraining forces resulting from the viscoelastic collagen composition of the extracellular matrix and intracellular myocyte sarcomeres.
- Clinically, LV remodeling is predominantly assessed using 2D echocardiographic evaluation of chamber size and volumes. These 2D techniques are limited by the use of foreshortened views and geometric assumptions, which limit their reproducibility and predictive power. Newer methods based on RT3DE imaging largely overcome these limitations.
- Until now, changes in LV shape have been assessed with a 2D-derived sphericity index, which fails to reflect regional changes in LV shape.
- It has been shown that RT3DE-based characterization of the LV endocardium better reflects both global and regional LV shape (Figs. 1-16 and 1-17).

2D STE   3D STE

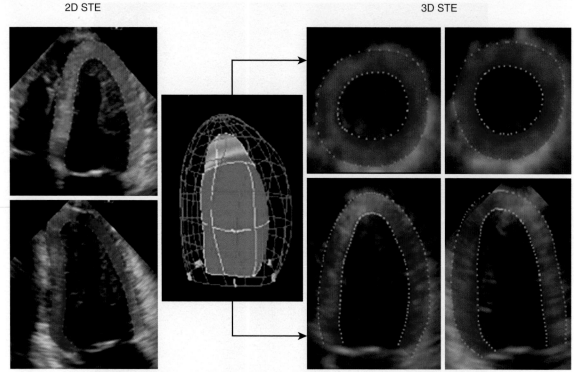

Figure 1-13. In this patient with normal LV wall motion, 2D speckle tracking (STE) showed uneven color distribution, indicating nonuniform deformation (*left panels*). In contrast, cut planes extracted from the 3D STE data (*center*) showed very even color distribution, indicating uniform contraction with a gradual decrease toward the apex (*right panels*). This can most likely be explained by the fact that 2D STE misinterprets changes detected in the imaging plane simply because it is "blinded" to the out-of-plane motion of the heart. *(Reproduced from Nesser HJ, Mor-Avi V, Gorissen W, et al. Quantification of left ventricular volumes using three-dimensional echocardiographic speckle tracking: comparison with MRI. Eur Heart J. 2009;30:1565-1573, Figure 1.)*

- Recently, a new 3DE-based sphericity index was shown in patients post-myocardial infarction to be a more accurate predictor of LV remodeling compared with other 2D echocardiographic parameters.

Mitral Stenosis

- Rheumatic mitral valve stenosis (MS) continues to be an important public health concern in developed countries due to the continuous immigration of patients from underdeveloped countries. In these latter countries, rheumatic valve disease continues to be extremely prevalent.
- To define the best therapeutic strategy, accurate measurements of the MV orifice area are required. Currently employed methods to obtain data on MV orifice area, such as 2D planimetry, pressure half-time, and flow convergence, have multiple limitations. The Doppler-based methods are heavily influenced by hemodynamic variables, LV hypertrophy, and associated valvular heart disease.
- Therefore, direct measurements of MV orifice area are more accurate. To date, this has been predominantly performed using planimetry of the MV orifice area on 2D images. However, this methodology is limited by the frequent use of incorrect image plane orientation relative to the cone-shaped mitral apparatus. This can result in overestimations of the MV orifice area.
- RT3DE allows visualization of the MV anatomy in any desired plane and orientation (Fig. 1-18). Among these, an anatomically correct *en face* view of the mitral valve apparatus at the tip of the leaflets improves

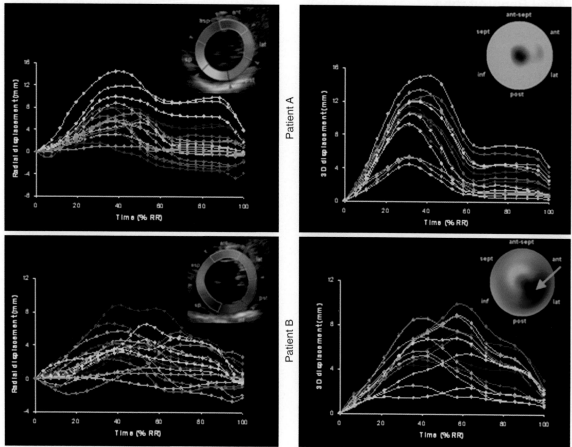

Figure 1-14. Segmental endocardial displacement curves obtained by 2D (*left*) and 3D (*right*) speckle tracking (STE) in two patients: patient A with normal wall motion and patient B with a hypokinetic apex and inferolateral wall due to ischemic heart disease. While 2D STE shows uneven color distribution and disorganized regional curves, potentially indicating wall motion abnormalities in both patients, 3D STE showed a normal pattern of contraction with synchronized curves in patient A, similar to that shown in Figure 1-11, but clearly depicted the area of hypokinesis and dyssynchronized curves in patient B (*green arrow*). *(Reproduced from Maffessanti F, Nesser HJ, Weinert L, et al. Quantitative evaluation of regional left ventricular function using three-dimensional speckle tracking echocardiography in patients with and without heart disease. Am J Cardiol. 2009;104:1755-1762, Figures 2 and 3.)*

the operator's ability to perform accurate MV area planimetry (Fig. 1-19).

- RT3DE improves the assessment of rheumatic MV stenosis, particularly in patients who have discordant results between different methods.
- Multiple studies have demonstrated discrepancies between MV orifice area measurements obtained with the pressure half-time and invasive methods immediately after percutaneous mitral valvuloplasty.
- RT3DE is a feasible and accurate technique for measuring MV area in patients undergoing balloon valvuloplasty. This methodology has the best agreement with the invasively determined MV area, particularly after percutaneous mitral valvuloplasty.

- RT3DE can also be used to estimate MV area in patients with MS secondary to severe calcification of the MV annulus.

KEY POINTS

- Transthoracic RT3DE is a feasible and accurate technique for measuring MV area in patients with rheumatic MS.
- In patients with rheumatic MS, the accuracy for measuring the MV area by 3D planimetry is superior to that of the invasive Gorlin method and other classic noninvasive methods, such as 2D planimetry, pressure half-time, and flow convergence methods. This modality should be considered as the preferred noninvasive method to measure MV area, particularly after mitral valvuloplasty.

3D Color Flow Assessment of Mitral Regurgitation

- Because of the complex geometry of the mitral apparatus, RT3DE is uniquely suited for the assessment of mitral regurgitation (MR) because it allows simultaneous data collection and 3D display of gray scale and color flow information (Fig. 1-20).

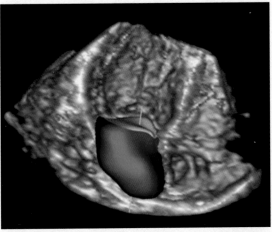

Figure 1-15. Left atrial endocardial surface reconstructed in 3D space (*green*) is shown superimposed on the original RT3DE dataset.

- Assessment of the effective regurgitant orifice area (EROA) and the vena contracta (VC) can be performed using RT3DE. 2D methods for EROA quantification require two major assumptions: (1) that the convergence zone is hemispherical and (2) that the regurgitant orifice is circular and centrally located.
- RT3DE-based measurements showed that these assumptions can be inaccurate; as a result, 2D EROA is frequently underestimated. The use of hemiellipsoidal flow convergence models reduces this underestimation. Today, direct tracing of radial planes of the proximal isovelocity surface area (PISA) zone and reconstruction of the total surface area from RT3DE datasets is possible, obviating the need for geometric assumptions.
- Transthoracic RT3DE has revealed that the VC is noncircular in most patients, especially in ischemic MR (Fig. 1-21). RT3DE-derived VC area was shown to correlate more closely with Doppler-derived EROA than with the 2D VC diameter.
- In most studies, the VC area has been measured using planimetry of 3D color flow jets using multiplanar views. However, the use of backscattered Doppler power from multiple beams in the flow convergence region to calculate VC area takes advantage of the concept that flow through the VC is laminar.

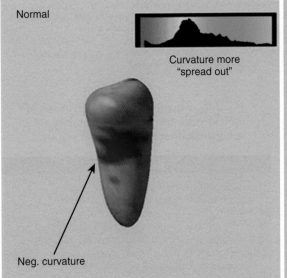
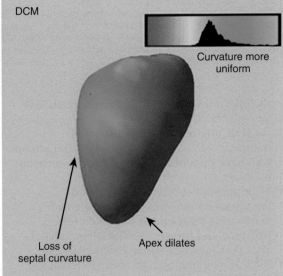

Normal — Curvature more "spread out" — Neg. curvature

DCM — Curvature more uniform — Loss of septal curvature — Apex dilates

Figure 1-16. 3D cast of the LV endocardium color encoded using regional 3D curvature information obtained at end systole in a normal subject (*left*) and in a patient with dilated cardiomyopathy (DCM, *right*). Note in the normal ventricle, the negative curvature in the area corresponding to the interventricular septum at the mid-ventricular level combined with the acutely conical apex. In contrast, in the patient with DCM, note the loss of negative curvature in the former area and the more rounded apex. *(Courtesy of Dr. Ivan S. Salgo.)*

Pre-operative   6 months

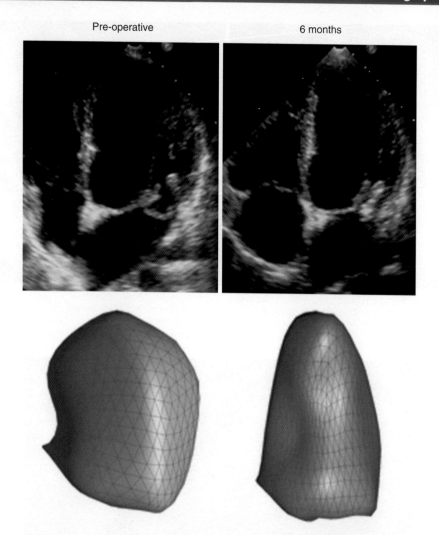

Figure 1-17. Apical four-chamber views obtained in a patient with normal LV ejection fraction undergoing mitral valve repair before and 6 months after surgery (*top*) and the corresponding RT3DE-derived endocardial surfaces. Note that preoperatively, the LV has a spherical shape that remodels into a more conical shape after surgery. (*Courtesy of Dr. Francesco Maffessanti.*)

- With RT3DE color flow imaging, it is possible to also quantify MR jet volumes. Comparison of 2D-derived jet areas and 3D-based jet volumes showed that the latter correlates better with the angiographic reference standard, particularly in patients with eccentric jets.
- An emerging method for MR quantification by RT3DE is delineation of the anatomic regurgitant orifice area (AROA) by direct volumetric *en face* visualization of the MV orifice (Fig. 1-22). The potential advantage of the AROA is that it directly measures the true anatomic orifice in 3D, taking into account the complex nonplanar geometry of this orifice.
  - In contrast, the 2D flow convergence (FC) method relies on the quantification of the narrowest flow emerging from the orifice, which is expected to be smaller by the coefficient of contraction and is also subject to orifice geometry and flow constraints.
- Drawbacks of 3DE color flow include (1) its limited availability and the fact that, as a new technology, it requires specific skills not yet widely available; and (2) image acquisition requires multiple cardiac cycles, which can be problematic in patients with arrhythmias, difficult acoustic windows, or uncooperative patients.
- As of now, online quantification of the flow convergence zone, VC, or AROA must be done manually. A semi-automated method of assessment is needed to make data analysis more efficient and user friendly.

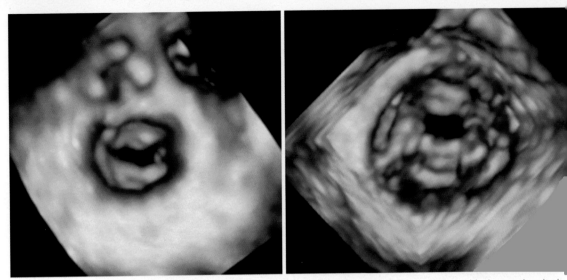

Figure 1-18. Transthoracic RT3DE narrow angle dataset of the mitral valve obtained in a patient with rheumatic mitral stenosis (MS), as viewed from the left atrial (*left*) and LV (*right*) perspectives. Note the increased leaflet thickness, as well as the fusion of the mediolateral commissures, typical of rheumatic MS.

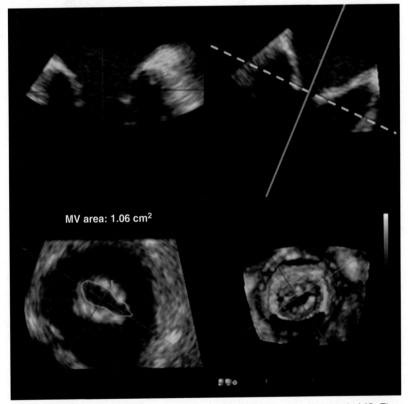

Figure 1-19. Multiplanar reconstruction views of the mitral valve in a patient with rheumatic MS. These views allow identification of an *en face* view of the mitral valve orifice in an anatomically correct plane at the tip of the leaflets (*dashed yellow line*), from which the mitral valve orifice area can be accurately measured using 3D planimetry (*bottom left panel*).

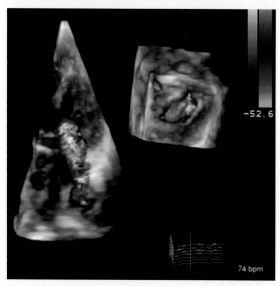

Figure 1-20. Example of RT3DE color flow information superimposed on the 3D rendered gray scale dataset obtained in a patient with moderate mitral regurgitation (MR).

• Furthermore, presently there are no professional society guidelines to assist in 3D quantification of MR, nor is there a validated reference standard for comparison of 2D or 3D findings.

• Despite these obstacles, 3DE can be a valuable tool in the assessment of MR, particularly when MR is felt to be underestimated by conventional 2D methods.

KEY POINTS

• EROA, VC, MR jet volumes, and AROA can be accurately assessed using RT3DE.

• 2D echocardiography tends to underestimate the EROA compared with RT3DE, particularly for eccentric jets.

• With its superior reproducibility, 3D volumetric analysis of the AROA is a useful alternative to quantify MR when 2D FC measurements are challenging.

• Drawbacks are the need for multibeat acquisitions and manual analysis.

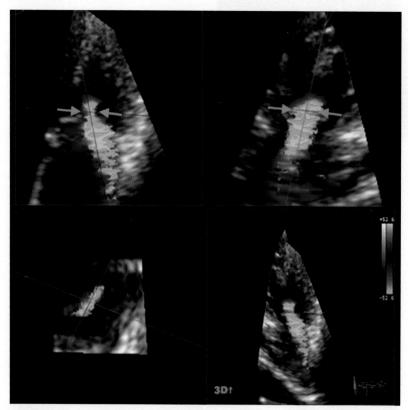

Figure 1-21. Multiplanar views of the 3D color flow obtained in a patient with MR. Note that in the apical four- (*top left*) and two-chamber (*top right*) views, the vena contracta has significantly different diameters (distance between green arrows). As a result, in the *en face* view of the mitral valve from the left atrial perspective (*bottom left*), the vena contracta has an elliptical rather than a circular shape, as frequently assumed with 2D echocardiography.

3D Evaluation of Myocardial Perfusion

- The ability of contrast echocardiography to image myocardial perfusion has been demonstrated by multiple investigators. However, the determination of the extent of perfusion defects is limited by the 2D nature of this methodology, which mandates repeated multiplane acquisition during repeated contrast maneuvers, such as boluses or transient microbubble destruction and replenishment.
- Because RT3DE technology allows volumetric imaging without reconstruction, it offers an opportunity for improved 3D perfusion imaging, without the need for repeated contrast maneuvers (Fig. 1-23).
- Perfusion defects may be visualized as dark areas in contrast-enhanced RT3DE datasets (Fig. 1-24).
- To allow quantitative analysis of regional myocardial contrast, 3D myocardial regions of interest can be defined by segmenting the 3D shell contained between the endo- and epicardial surfaces. Myocardial contrast enhancement curves can then be obtained from these 3D segments by measuring beat-by-beat contrast intensity during a transition from no contrast to fully enhanced myocardium (Fig. 1-25).
- Quantitative indices of myocardial perfusion, such as peak contrast inflow rate, obtained from myocardial contrast enhancement curves, were shown to reflect changes in coronary flow in experimental animals and in normal volunteers during vasodilator stress.
- The use of this methodology to detect myocardial ischemia induced by vasodilator stress in patients with coronary artery disease is currently limited to the research area and needs further testing and validation prior to clinical application.

Technical Considerations
- Interpretation of reduced videointensity as a perfusion abnormality can be hindered by drop-out artifacts that are commonly seen with contrast and are even more difficult to interpret with 3D imaging.
- Visualizing perfusion defects in different planes extracted from the 3D dataset helps identify such artifacts and also allows more complete evaluation of the extent of the defect.

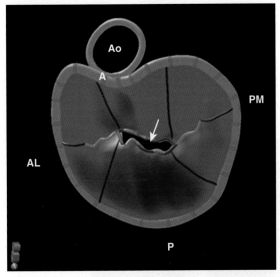

Figure 1-22. Color-coded 3D parametric display of the mitral valve leaflets in a patient with severe MS showing the anatomic regurgitant orifice area (AROA) (*arrow*). Note that the regurgitant orifice is irregular and nonplanar.

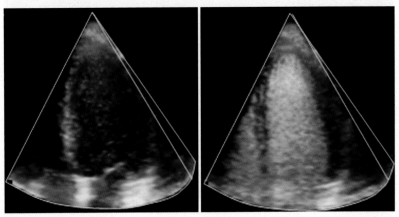

Figure 1-23. RT3DE datasets obtained in a normal volunteer before (*left*) and during peak contrast enhancement (*right*). (*Reproduced from Toledo E, Lang RM, Collins MS, et al. Imaging and quantification of myocardial perfusion using real-time three-dimensional echocardiography. J Am Coll Cardiol. 2006;47:146-154, Figure 7.)*

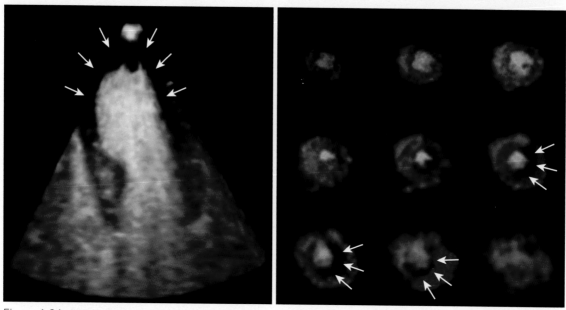

Figure 1-24. RT3DE dataset obtained in a patient with severe discrete left anterior descending (LAD) stenosis (*left*). The apex shows lack of contrast enhancement, indicating a perfusion defect. This defect was visible in multiple cross sections (*right*), allowing easy estimation of its extent.

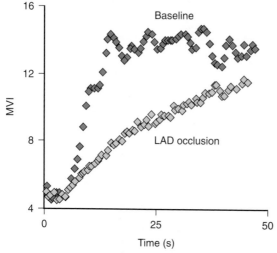

Figure 1-25. Myocardial videointensity (MVI) time curves measured in a 3D anteroseptal segment in an experimental animal during transition from no contrast enhancement to steady-state contrast enhancement at baseline and during LAD occlusion. Note the difference in the rate of contrast inflow between the two curves. (*Reproduced from Toledo E, Lang RM, Collins MS, et al. Imaging and quantification of myocardial perfusion using real-time three-dimensional echocardiography. J Am Coll Cardiol. 2006;47:146-154, Figure 5.*)

- Visualization of perfusion defects can be difficult to achieve with high mechanical index imaging. However, contrast-targeted modes such as power modulation help improve the visualization of perfusion defects.

KEY POINTS

- Contrast-enhanced RT3DE imaging provides the basis for volumetric imaging and quantification of myocardial perfusion.
- While 3D perfusion imaging can be performed in any laboratory with RT3DE equipment and experience with contrast echocardiography, quantitative analysis requires specialized software, and is not ready for clinical use.

Acknowledgment

We are thankful to Lissa Sugeng, MD, and Lynn Weinert, RDCS, for their expert contributions.

Suggested Reading

1. Lang RM, Mor-Avi V, Sugeng L, et al. Three-dimensional echocardiography: the benefits of the additional dimension. *J Am Coll Cardiol.* 2006;48:2053-2069.
   In this article, the authors review the published reports that have provided the scientific basis for the clinical use of 3D ultrasound imaging of the heart and discuss its potential future applications.
2. Mor-Avi V, Sugeng L, Lang RM. Real-time 3D echocardiography: an integral component of the routine echocardiographic examination in adult patients? *Circulation.* 2009;119:314-329.
   This is a review of the most recent RT3DE literature and provides readers with an update on the latest developments and the current status of this noninvasive imaging tool.
3. Jacobs LD, Salgo IS, Goonewardena S, et al. Rapid online quantification of left ventricular volume from real-time three-dimensional echocardiographic data. *Eur Heart J.* 2006;27:460-468.
   This paper validates online measurement of LV volumes from RT3DE data using cardiac magnetic resonance (CMR) as

the reference and demonstrates the superior accuracy and reproducibility of this approach relative to standard 2DE measurements.

4. Mor-Avi V, Sugeng L, Weinert L, et al. Fast measurement of left ventricular mass with real-time three-dimensional echocardiography: comparison with magnetic resonance imaging. *Circulation.* 2004;110:1814-1818.
This paper validates RT3DE as a method of calculating LV mass.

5. Corsi C, Lang RM, Veronesi F, et al. Volumetric quantification of global and regional left ventricular function from real-time three-dimensional echocardiographic images. *Circulation.* 2005;112:1161-1170.
This human study demonstrates that volumetric analysis of RT3DE data is clinically feasible and allows fast, semi-automated, dynamic measurement of LV volume and automated detection of regional wall motion abnormalities.

6. Nesser HJ, Sugeng L, Corsi C, et al. Volumetric analysis of regional left ventricular function with real-time three-dimensional echocardiography: validation by magnetic resonance and clinical utility testing. *Heart.* 2007;93:572-578.
This study, using prototype software to analyze RT3DE data, reports that quantification of regional LV function and semi-automated detection of regional wall motion abnormalities are as accurate as the same algorithm applied to CMR images.

7. Sawada SG, Thomaides A. Three-dimensional stress echocardiography: The promise and limitations of volumetric imaging. *Curr Opin Cardiol.* 2009;24:426-432.
This review focuses on the advantages and disadvantages of 3D volumetric imaging and the current and future role of the technique in stress echocardiography.

8. Matsumura Y, Hozumi T, Arai K, et al. Non-invasive assessment of myocardial ischaemia using new real-time three-dimensional dobutamine stress echocardiography: comparison with conventional two-dimensional methods. *Eur Heart J.* 2005;26:1625-1632.
This study validates real-time 3D dobutamine stress echocardiography for the diagnosis of ischemia using exercise 201Tl single-photon emission computed tomography as the reference standard.

9. Ahmad M, Xie T, McCulloch M, et al. Real-time three-dimensional dobutamine stress echocardiography in assessment of ischemia: comparison with two-dimensional dobutamine stress echocardiography. *J Am Coll Cardiol.* 2001;37:1303-1309.
This study reports the feasibility and efficacy of using RT3DE to detect ischemia during dobutamine-induced stress using conventional 2D stress echocardiography as the reference.

10. Sugeng L, Mor-Avi V, Weinert L, et al. Quantitative assessment of left ventricular size and function: side-by-side comparison of real-time three-dimensional echocardiography and computed tomography with magnetic resonance reference. *Circulation.* 2006;114:654-661.
This study compares cardiac computed tomography (CCT) and RT3DE measurements of left ventricular size and function to a CMR reference. It reports that CCT provides highly reproducible measurements of LV volumes, which are significantly larger than CMR values, and notes that RT3DE measurements compare more favorably with the CMR reference, albeit with higher variability.

11. Kapetanakis S, Kearney MT, Siva A, et al. Real-time three-dimensional echocardiography: a novel technique to quantify global left ventricular mechanical dyssynchrony. *Circulation.* 2005;112:992-1000.
This study validates a RT3DE method to assess global LV mechanical dyssynchrony based on the dispersion of the time to minimum regional volume for all 16 LV segments, the LV mechanical dyssynchrony index.

12. Sonne C, Sugeng L, Takeuchi M, et al. Real-time three-dimensional echocardiographic assessment of left ventricular dyssynchrony: pitfalls in patients with dilated cardiomyopathy. *J Am Coll Cardiol Imaging.* 2009;2:802-812.
This study reports normal values for the RT3DE-derived LV dyssynchrony index and notes the limitations of applying this index in patients with reduced LV function because of the inability to accurately detect end-ejection in low-amplitude regional volume curves in these patients.

13. Nesser HJ, Mor-Avi V, Gorissen W, et al. Quantification of left ventricular volumes using three-dimensional echocardiographic speckle tracking: comparison with MRI. *Eur Heart J.* 2009;30:1565-1573.
This is the first study to validate a 3D-speckle tracking echocardiographic technique for LV volume measurements using a magnetic resonance gold standard. It reports that this approach has superior accuracy and reproducibility over previously used 2D speckle tracking echocardiographic techniques.

14. Maffessanti F, Nesser HJ, Weinert L, et al. Quantitative evaluation of regional left ventricular function using three-dimensional speckle tracking echocardiography in patients with and without heart disease. *Am J Cardiol.* 2009;104:1755-1762.
This is the first study to evaluate a 3D speckle tracking echocardiographic technique for measurement of regional wall motion indexes (displacement and strain) in normal and abnormal LVs. It reports that this approach correlates well with a CMR gold standard and is superior to 2D speckle tracking echocardiography.

15. Jenkins C, Bricknell K, Marwick TH. Use of real-time three-dimensional echocardiography to measure left atrial volume: comparison with other echocardiographic techniques. *J Am Soc Echocardiogr.* 2005;18:991-997.
This study reports a good correlation between 2D and 3D echocardiographic LA volume determinations.

16. Chu JW, Levine RA, Chua S, et al. Assessing mitral valve area and orifice geometry in calcific mitral stenosis: a new solution by real-time three-dimensional echocardiography. *J Am Soc Echocardiogr.* 2008;21: 1006-1009.
This study uses RT3DE to measure mitral valve area (MVA) in calcific mitral stenosis, validating it against MVA determined by the continuity equation. The report notes that, in contrast with the doming valve shape present in rheumatic mitral stenosis, the limiting anatomic orifice area occurs at the annulus in calcific mitra mitral stenosis.

17. Little SH, Pirat B, Kumar R, et al. Three-dimensional color Doppler echocardiography for direct measurement of vena contracta area in mitral regurgitation: in vitro validation and clinical experience. *J Am Coll Cardiol Cardiovasc Imaging.* 2008;1:695-704.
This study evaluates a RT3DE method of measuring the mitral regurgitant vena contracta in both in vitro and human studies (gold standard = Doppler-derived effective regurgitant orifice area), proposing that this parameter would be particularly valuable clinically in eccentric jets and other situations where geometric assumptions may be incorrect.

18. Toledo E, Lang RM, Collins KA, et al. Imaging and quantification of myocardial perfusion using real-time three-dimensional echocardiography. *J Am Coll Cardiol.* 2006;47:146-154.
This study reports the feasibility of using RT3DE perfusion imaging and an algorithm for volumetric analysis of myocardial contrast inflow to assess myocardial perfusion in ex vivo and in vivo animal studies of variable global and regional flow as well as normal human volunteers subjected to adenosine-mediated hyperemia.

Advanced Echocardiography Approaches: 3D Transesophageal Assessment of the Mitral Valve

Jonathan J. Passeri and Judy Hung

2

Background

- Mitral valve (MV) function is important for filling and ejection of the left ventricle (LV).
- Proper MV function depends on a balance between closing forces generated by the LV and tethering forces generated by the chordal attachments to the papillary muscles, which prevent the leaflets from prolapsing into the left atrium (LA) (Fig. 2-1).
- The force created by the attachment of the chordae is termed tethering force.
- Each papillary muscle (PM) sends chordae to both leaflets. The posteromedial PM sends chordae to the posteromedial aspect of both leaflets, and the anterolateral PM sends chordae to the anterolateral aspect of both leaflets.
- During ventricular systole, the PMs contract to offset the loosening of the chordal forces that occurs with movement of the MV annulus toward the left ventricular (LV) apex in systole.
- The mitral annulus has a bimodal "saddle" shape, with high or superior points at the anterior and posterior parts of the annulus and the low or inferior points located at the medial and lateral parts of the annulus.
  - Finite element modeling of the annulus has demonstrated that a bimodal shape is optimal to minimize stress on the MV during opening and closing.
  - Three-dimensional (3D) echocardiography helped to define the bimodal shape and correlate the high and low points of the annulus to two-dimensional (2D) imaging planes.
- The broad anterior leaflet accounts for most of the closing surface area.
- Mitral leaflets have inherent redundancy in order to have overlap of the leaflets at the coaptation line.
  - This overlap region, often termed the "coaptation zone," is felt to be important for the leaflets to properly "seal" the mitral

orifice and prevent pathological mitral regurgitation (MR).
  - Although it is unclear what the optimal coaptation length is, a coaptation length of at least 1 cm is thought to be important for the mitral leaflets to form an appropriate seal.
- Transmitral gradients are determined by flow across the MV, which in turn is influenced by the left atrial (LA) to LV pressure gradient.
  - Clinical factors such as cardiac output, LA enlargement and pressure, LV compliance, and mitral stenosis (MS) influence transmitral gradients.

KEY POINTS

- MV function is based on a force balance relationship between closing and tethering forces.
- The mitral annulus has a bimodal "saddle" shape.
- A coaptation zone is important for mitral leaflet closure.
- Transmitral gradients are flow dependent.

Overview of the 3D Transesophageal Echocardiographic Approach

Historically, 3D imaging required gated reconstruction of multiple 2D imaging planes acquired by rotation around a fixed axis.

- Although accurate 3D reconstructions were obtained, this approach involved significant post-processing and careful respiratory and echocardiographic gating.
- In addition, this process did not allow for real-time imaging.
- The development of matrix array transducers allowed for real-time 3D imaging.
- 3D transthoracic echocardiography (TTE) provides standard and nonstandard imaging

planes. It can be used as the only imaging modality but more often is used in a complementary role to 2D imaging.

- Although real-time 3D imaging represents a significant advance in echocardiographic technique, image resolution remains a limitation of 3D TTE.
- However, the recent introduction of 3D transesophageal echocardiography (TEE) has improved image resolution and is ideally suited to assess MV anatomy and function.
- 3D TEE provides the same views as 2D TEE in addition to views that are unique to 3D imaging.
- The matrix array 3D TEE probe allows for several 3D imaging modes, each of which has advantages and limitations.
  - **Live 3D:** This mode displays a real-time fixed-volume, 50 × 30 degree, pyramidal dataset (Fig. 2-2A). Simplicity is the major advantage of the live 3D mode. A 3D image is displayed in real time without need for optimization of the image alignment in the display field. The major disadvantage is that the fixed volume size of the live 3D mode may not be of adequate size to capture the structure or area of interest.
  - **3D Zoom:** This mode displays a truncated pyramidal dataset of variable size (see Fig. 2-2B). The advantage of this mode is that the 3D volume can be adjusted by the operator to include the entire area of interest (e.g., the MV). However, as the volume is set larger, the frame rate and thus image resolution decrease.
  - **Full-volume:** This mode displays a 100 × 100 degree pyramidal dataset (Fig. 2-3). The MV should be aligned optimally in the middle of the image field using the biplane display, and, if possible, respiration should be suspended prior to full volume. Acquisition of a full volume dataset requires merging of smaller 3D pyramidal datasets obtained from 4–7 gated cardiac cycles (Fig. 2-4). The number of cycles can be

Normal

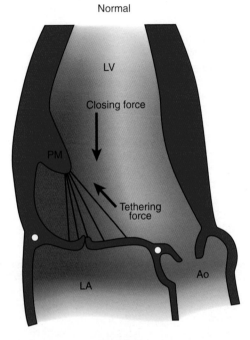

Figure 2-1. Mitral valve (MV) function results from a balance of closing forces and tethering forces.

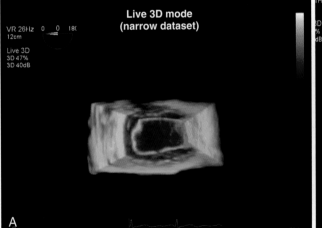
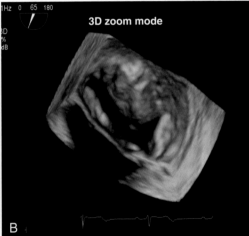

Figure 2-2. **A,** Narrow beam (live three-dimensional [3D] mode). **B,** 3D zoom mode.

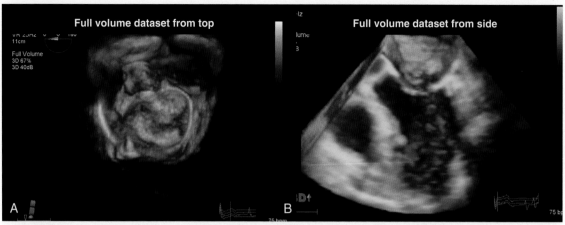

Figure 2-3. Full volume mode allows for large volume dataset. **A,** View of pyramidal dataset from top. **B,** View of 3D dataset from side.

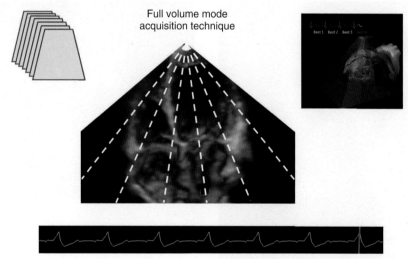

Figure 2-4. Full volume mode 3D dataset is acquired by merging of four to seven narrower pyramidal datasets (*dashed lines*).

preset. The greater the number of cycles, the higher the frame rate; however, the acquisition time is longer. The advantage of the full-volume mode is that it displays a large volume of data at a higher frame-rate than is possible with the 3D zoom mode. Because a full volume dataset is obtained by "stitching" together smaller pyramidal datasets, it is subject to "stitching artifacts" due to poor merging of the smaller pyramidal volumes caused by respiratory/transducer motion and/or arrhythmia (Fig. 2-5). Significant stitch artifacts will make the 3D datasets uninterpretable. Another disadvantage is that the dataset is not truly a "live" image.

- **3D Color Doppler**: This mode displays a pyramidal volume of color Doppler data superimposed upon a volume of gray scale data (Fig. 2-6). Due to the low frame rate, 3D color Doppler is acquired by volume rendering. This gated reconstruction requires 7 to 14 cardiac cycles. The greater the number of cardiac cycles, the better the frame rate. However, the increase in cardiac cycles comes with a greater risk of a stitching artifact. Additional disadvantages include a significantly smaller pyramidal color volume compared with full volume imaging mode, which limits a comprehensive display of the complete color Doppler signals.

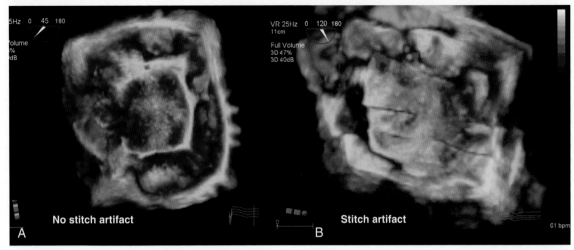

Figure 2-5. **A,** 3D dataset without stitch artifact. **B,** 3D dataset with significant stitch artifact.

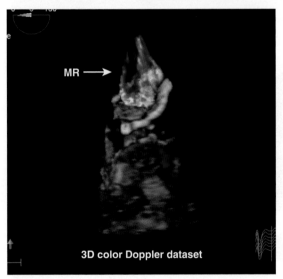

Figure 2-6. 3D transesophageal color Doppler dataset showing mitral regurgitation (MR) (*arrow*).

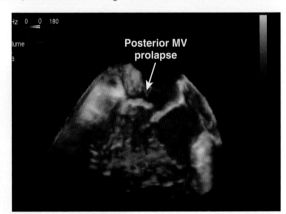

Figure 2-7. 3D dataset obtained in long axis plane (120 degree) showing posterior leaflet prolapse.

Suggested 3D TEE Protocol of the Mitral Valve

Image Acquisition

- Obtaining an optimal 3D TEE image of a given cardiac structure is best done by first optimizing the 2D image. First, depth and sector size should be optimized for frame rate. Adjustment of the focus, frequency, overall gain, and compression should be performed to optimize the image resolution. Time gain compensation should be reserved for additional fine tuning.
- Full-volume datasets of the MV in the horizontal (0 degree) plane (Fig. 2-7), commissural plane (generally between 40 and 60 degrees), and long axis plane (generally between 120 and 135 degrees).
  - Because the system acquires sector slices in a sweeping motion parallel to the reference image, 3D images viewed parallel to the

reference image will appear normal, whereas the artifacts will be most noticeable when viewed from a plane orthogonal to the reference image. Obtaining full-volume datasets using reference images viewed from multiple planes is one method to help avoid the pitfalls of interpreting datasets with this artifact.

- Narrow beam mode (3D zoom or live 3D) of the MV with the plane guided by MV pathology.
  - As with full-volume acquisition, multiple 3D zoom datasets should be obtained from multiple 2D reference planes.
  - A suggested basic format includes horizontal, commissural, and long axis imaging planes.
  - Additional views should be based on the particular mitral pathoanatomy of interest.
  - The volume should be set large enough to include the relevant MV pathology and pertinent adjacent structure(s), but small enough to maximize frame rate.
- 3D TEE color Doppler of MV regurgitant flow.
  - Depth and sector size should be adjusted to maximize frame rate.
  - The image should contain magnified views of the proximal jet and MV.
  - The Nyquist limit can be adjusted lower to capture the full range of MR flows.
  - Because the pyramidal dataset is narrower with 3D TEE color Doppler, more than one dataset may need to be acquired to obtain a complete assessment of the MV regurgitant data.

Cropping the Images

Once a 3D dataset has been obtained, the image should be cropped to display the MV structures

in standard orientations. Recommended orientations for viewing are:

- *En face* view of the MV: LA and LV aspects. The view from the LA aspect is oriented as a surgeon would view the MV from the open LA, with the aortic valve at midline and at the top of MV. The LA appendage is on the left of the field (surgeon's view, Figs. 2-8 and 2-9A). This view is best obtained by cropping in from the LA until the MV leaflets and annulus are seen without extraneous LA tissue. For the LV aspect, the view is oriented similarly to the 2D short axis plane of the MV. The aortic valve is midline and at the top of the MV. The medial portion of the MV is to the left and the lateral part is to the right (see Fig. 2-9B).

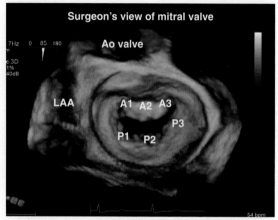

Figure 2-8. Surgeon's view of the MV as viewed from the left atrial aspect. The aorta is the midline at the top of the image (12 o'clock position) and the left atrial appendage (LAA) is on the left. Leaflet segments are categorized as 1, 2, and 3, with 1 denoting the lateral segments, 2 the middle segments, and 3 the medial segments.

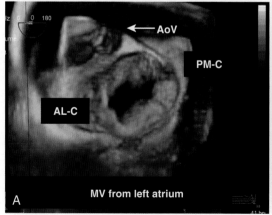
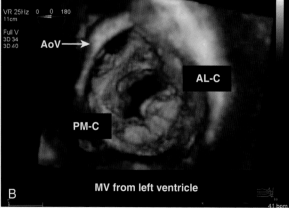

Figure 2-9. **A,** Orientation of the MV from the left atrial aspect. **B,** Orientation of the MV from the left ventricular aspect. AL-C, anterolateral commissure; PM-C, posteromedial commissure.

- Full volume datasets should be cropped along the anterior-posterior plane to display the long axis view. For a commissural view, datasets should be cropped along the medial to lateral plane (Fig. 2-10).

3D TEE is ideally suited to examine the complex pathoanatomy of the MV (see Suggested Reading 3). It allows direct visualization of the MV without the need for reconstruction of multiple planes as is necessary with 2D TEE imaging. This is especially helpful for identifying pathology at the commissures (areas in which it can be difficult to localize pathology by 2D TEE) and prominent clefts. *En face* views display the entire coaptation surface, making it ideal for localization of regurgitant leaks. 3D imaging of the LV aspect of the MV provides views of the subvalvular region not possible with 2D imaging. Figure 2-11 shows a 3D TEE view from the left atrial perspective of prolapse of the P2 segment.

KEY POINTS

- Images can be cropped to recreate 2D imaging planes or display views not obtainable with 2D echocardiography.
- *En face* views from both the atrial and ventricular perspective are particularly helpful.

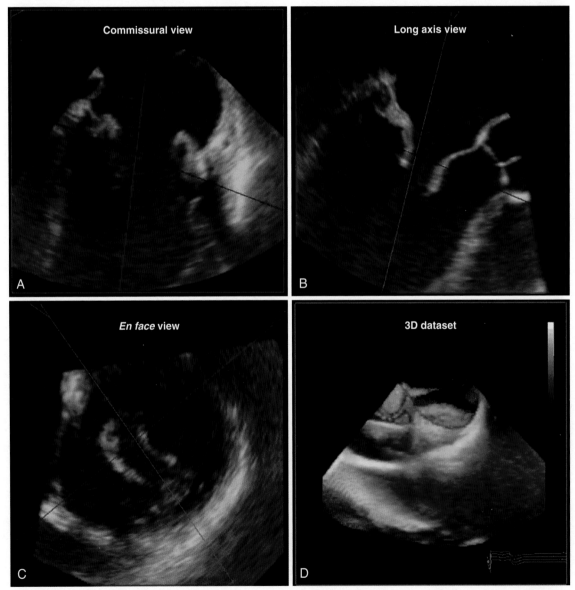

Figure 2-10. Multiplanar reconstruction (MPR) display. **A,** Commissural plane. **B,** Long axis plane. **C,** *En face* plane. **D,** 3D dataset.

Physiologic and Quantitative Data: Integrated Practical Approach to Data Acquisition and Analysis

Assessment of Mitral Regurgitation

- 3D TEE assessment of MR is complementary to 2D imaging.
- Cropping of 3D TEE color Doppler datasets should follow a similar protocol to that described above.
- The 3D TEE *en face* views from both the LA and LV perspectives are key views for localizing MR regurgitant jets.
- Matching the location of the regurgitant jets with the anatomic data can confirm the localization of the abnormal segments in complex cases. Nonstandard orientation displays may be needed for eccentric jets.
- For quantitation of the severity of MR, 3D-guided color Doppler measurement of the vena contracta area has been demonstrated to be feasible with good correlation to magnetic resonance imaging (MRI) quantitation of MR (see selected reading 4). Direct measurement of the vena contracta area (a measure of regurgitant orifice area) by 3D guidance obviates the need for geometric assumptions necessary with 2D calculation of the regurgitant orifice area.
- This is performed using multiplanar imaging to align the cropping plane at the level of the vena contracta for measurement using quantification software.
- Further validation data are necessary to determine clinical application.

Quantification of Mitral Stenosis

- 3D TEE offers the advantage of 3D-guided planimetry of the MV area. 3D echocardiography has demonstrated feasibility and decreased variability in mitral area measurement in MS due to the ability to align the imaging plane to the narrowest point of the leaflet orifice (see Suggested Reading 5) (Fig. 2-12).

In addition to 3D-guided planimetry of the MV area in MS, commercial software systems are available to perform more sophisticated, and in some cases semi-automated, quantitative measures of the MV that are best quantitated using

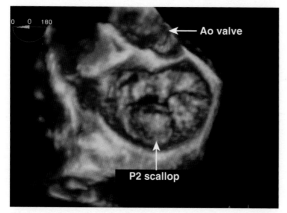

Figure 2-11. View of MV with posterior leaflet prolapse of P2 segment (*arrow*).

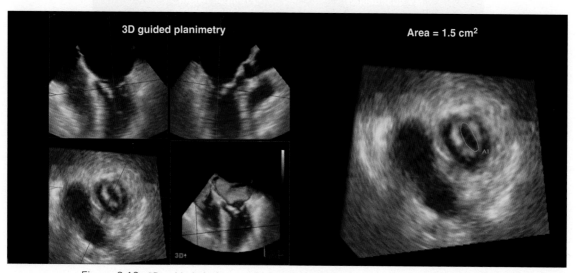

Figure 2-12. 3D guided planimetry of MV area at the narrowest orifice in rheumatic MS.

a 3D dataset. Examples include annular area, height, leaflet area and angles, and prolapse volume and height (Figs. 2-13 and 2-14). Validation and correlation of MV quantitative measures to clinical outcome measures are ongoing.

KEY POINTS

- For MR, 3D echocardiography provides a method for directly measuring the regurgitant orifice area.
- For MS, 3D echocardiography can directly measure the flow-limiting cross-sectional area.
- Commercially available software can provide sophisticated measures to better define mitral pathoanatomy.

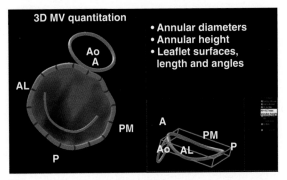

Figure 2-13. 3D quantitative MV measures using commercial software.

Alternate Approaches: Alternative Imaging Modalities for Assessing the Mitral Valve

Cardiac MRI and computed tomography (CT) offer alternative imaging modalities for assessing the MV. Both CT and MRI have superior spatial resolution compared with echocardiography. However, echocardiography has better temporal resolution than MRI and CT, which is an advantage when assessing highly mobile structures such as the MV apparatus. In patients where the echocardiography windows are poor, MRI and CT may provide a better assessment of the MV due to their superior spatial resolution despite a temporal resolution lower than that of echocardiography.

Both CT and MRI have demonstrated feasibility in assessing MV pathoanatomy. Recent studies have also validated MR quantification by cardiac MRI and CT using flow quantitation methods and direct measurement of the MR regurgitant orifice area.

KEY POINTS

- CT and MRI have superior spatial resolution relative to echocardiography.
- The greater temporal resolution of echocardiography provides an advantage when assessing mobile cardiac structures such as the MV and high-flow jets such as MR.
- The feasibility of using both CT and MRI to assess MV pathoanatomy and to quantitate MS and regurgitation has been demonstrated.

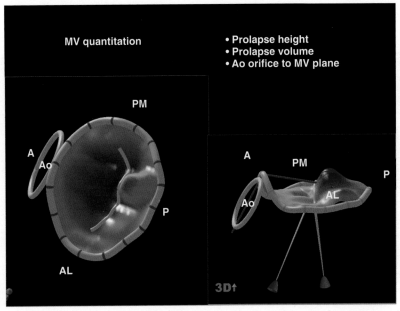

Figure 2-14. 3D quantitative MV measures using commercial software.

Suggested Reading

1. Levine R, Schwammenthal E. Ischemic mitral regurgitation on the threshold of a solution. *Circulation.* 2005;112:745-758.
   This review article provides a comprehensive discussion of the pathophysiology of ischemic mitral regurgitation and preliminary studies of innovative therapeutic strategies.

2. Sugeng L, Shernan SK, Salgo IS, et al. Live 3-dimensional transesophageal echocardiography initial experience using the fully-sampled matrix array probe. *J Am Coll Cardiol.* 2008;52:446-449.
   This paper reports the initial experience with the real-time 3D TEE probe, supporting its use for mitral surgical planning and guidance of percutaneous interventions.

3. Chandra S, Salgo IS, Sugeng L, et al. Characterization of degenerative mitral valve disease using morphologic analysis of real-time three-dimensional echocardiographic images: Objective insight into complexity and planning of mitral valve repair. *Circ Cardiovasc Imaging.* 2011;4:24-32.
   The study reports the utility of real time 3D TEE assessment of mitral leaflet billowing height and volume in distinguishing normal versus fibroelastic deficiency versus Barlow's disease valves. This information may be useful in planning surgical repair.

4. Shanks M, Siebelink HM, Delgado V, et al. Quantitative assessment of mitral regurgitation: Comparison between three-dimensional transesophageal echocardiography and magnetic resonance imaging. *Circ Cardiovasc Imaging.* 2010;3:694-700.
   Using an MRI gold standard, this study reports that quantification of mitral effective regurgitant orifice area and regurgitant volume with 3D TEE is feasible and accurate and results in less underestimation of the regurgitant volume as compared with 2D TEE.

5. Zamorano J, Perez de Isla L, Sugeng L, et al. Non-invasive assessment of mitral valve area during percutaneous balloon mitral valvuloplasty: Role of real-time 3D echocardiography. *Eur Heart J.* 2004;25(23):2086-2091.
   This study reports that real-time 3D transthoracic echocardiography is a feasible and accurate technique for measuring MVA in patients with rheumatic mitral stenosis. MVA calculated invasively using the Gorlin equation was the gold standard.

6. Veronesi F, Corsi C, Sugeng L, et al. A study of functional anatomy of aortic-mitral valve coupling using 3D matrix transesophageal echocardiography. *Circ Cardiovasc Imaging.* 2009;2:24-31.
   This is the first study to report quantitative 3D assessment of mitral-aortic valve dynamics from matrix array transesophageal images and to describe the mitral-aortic coupling in a beating human heart.

Two-Dimensional and Three-Dimensional Echocardiographic Evaluation of the Right Ventricle

3

Takahiro Shiota

Background

- The right ventricle (RV) originates embryologically from different progenitor cells and different sites than the left ventricle (LV).
- The inflow part of the RV is derived from the ventricular portion of the primitive cardiac tube, whereas the infundibulum is derived from the conus cordis.

Anatomy of the Right Ventricle

- The RV has a circumferential arrangement of myofibers in the subendocardium and longitudinal myofibers in the subendocardium (Fig. 3-1).
- The RV has three components (Fig. 3-2):
  - The inlet, which consists of the tricuspid valve (TV), chordae tendineae, and papillary muscle.
  - The trabecular apical myocardium.
  - The infundibulum or conus, which refers to the smooth myocardial outflow region.
- As shown by three-dimensional (3D) study, the infundibular part consists of 25% to 30% of the total right ventricular (RV) volume. The shape of the RV is complex (see Fig. 3-2). In the apical view the RV looks triangular, while in the cross-sectional view it appears crescentic in the normal condition.
- The three parts of the RV are not in the same plane as seen in a 3D echocardiogram from a normal subject (Fig. 3-3). A curved septum is seen in Figure 3-3 because the RV inflow contracts earlier than the infundibulum.

Coronary Artery

The coronary artery supply to the RV myocardium is shown in Figure 3-4, and the RV segments are shown in Figure 3-5.

Coronary flow to the RV is primarily from the right coronary artery (RCA) (dominant in 80% of the population) (Fig. 3-5):
- Conus branch of RCA (and left anterior descending [LAD] branches) to the outflow tract.
- Acute marginal branches to the anterior and lateral walls of the RV.
- Posterior descending coronary artery (PDA) to the posterior wall of the RV and posterior interventricular septum (the posterior interventricular septum will be supplied by the left circumflex when the left coronary artery is dominant).

As compared to the LV, the RV is more resistant to ischemic insult because of its lower oxygen consumption, more extensive collateral system, and ability to increase oxygen extraction.

Determinants of Right Heart Function

The function of the right heart is governed by the following four factors:
1. Preload (RV volume overload)
   - RV preload is the load present before RV contraction and is determined by venous return, shunt, tricuspid and pulmonic valve regurgitation and the distensibility of the RV's thin myocardial wall.
   - Tricuspid regurgitation (TR) can be categorized as:
     a. Primary TR due to organic TV disease such as prolapse, carcinoid, or trauma (i.e., a car accident).
     b. Functional TR caused by pulmonary hypertension and left-sided heart diseases such as mitral valve regurgitation and stenosis.

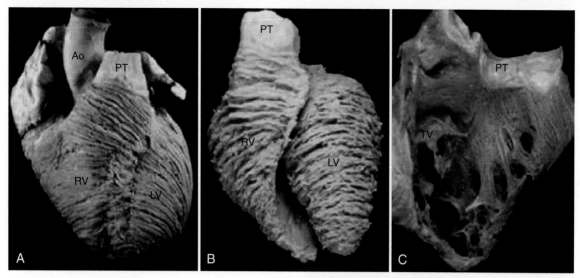

Figure 3-1. Myocardial fiber arrangement of the right ventricle (RV). Circumferential arrangement of subepicardial myofibril fibers (**A, B**) and longitudinal fibers (**C**) in the endocardium. *(From Ho SY, Nihoyannopoulos P. Anatomy, echocardiography, and normal right ventricular dimensions. Heart. 2006;92:i2-i13.)*

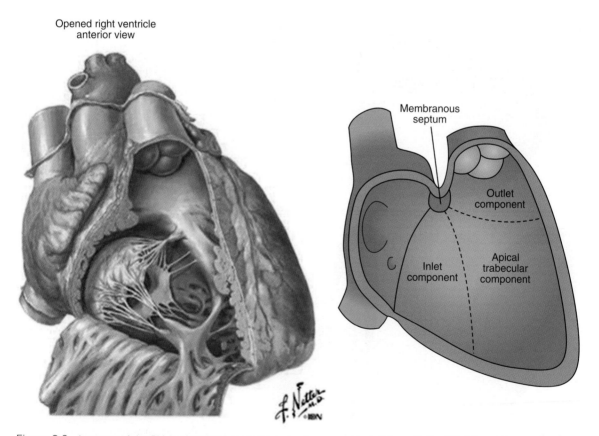

Figure 3-2. Anatomy of the RV, having three separate parts. *(Image on the left from Netter FH, Atlas of Human Anatomy, second edition. Philadelphia, Novartis, 1997; Plate 208.)*

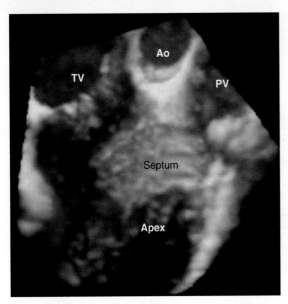

Figure 3-3. 3D echocardiographic presentation of the RV.

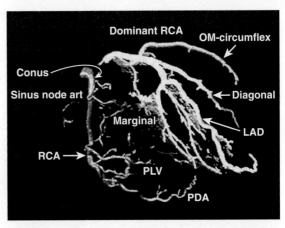

Figure 3-4. Coronary arteries to the RV. *(From Mangion JR. Right ventricular imaging by two-dimensional and three-dimensional echocardiography. Curr Opin Cardiol. 2010;22:423-429.)*

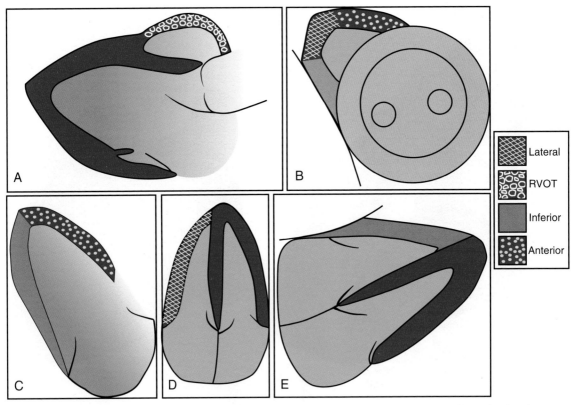

Figure 3-5. Segmentation of the RV wall. *(From Mangion JR. Right ventricular imaging by two-dimensional and three-dimensional echocardiography. Curr Opin Cardiol. 2010;22:423-429.)*

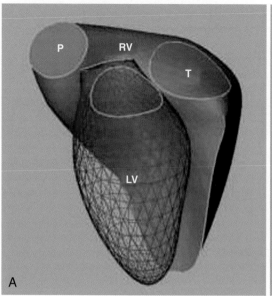
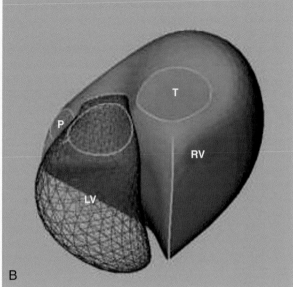

Figure 3-6. 3D reconstructions of the RV illustrating its complex shape in a normal subject (**A**). RV remodeling in diseased hearts can result in profound shape change, as in this patient (**B**) with a dilated RV due to severe PR following repair of tetralogy of Fallot. The mesh surface is the left ventricle. *(From Sheehan F, Redington A. The right ventricle: Anatomy, physiology and clinical imaging. Heart. 2008;94:1510-1515.)*

- Shunt. Atrial septal defect is the most common cause of RV volume overload in adult congenital heart disease. Other congenital diseases that cause RV volume overload are partial anomalous pulmonary venous return and Ebstein's anomaly.
- Pulmonic regurgitation (PR) is also seen in patients who have had repair of tetralogy of Fallot or who have carcinoid heart disease. In a patient with severe PR following repair of tetralogy of Fallot, 3D reconstruction with magnetic resonance imaging (MRI) showed a uniquely enlarged RV (Fig. 3-6). Septal flattening during diastole and right ventricular enlargement are markers of RV volume overload.

2. Afterload (RV pressure overload)
   - RV afterload represents the load that the RV has to overcome during ejection. Clinically speaking, RV afterload is considered to be pulmonary vascular resistance, which is affected by pulmonary flow and vasculature.
   - RV pressure overload can be determined with 2D echocardiography. RV and pulmonary systolic pressure are commonly estimated using continuous wave (CW) Doppler and the simplified Bernoulli equation as follows:

RV systolic pressure (mm Hg)
$$= 4V^2 \text{ (m/s)} + \text{right atrial (RA)}$$
$$\text{pressure (mm Hg)}.$$

where RA pressure is estimated using the American Society of Echocardiography (ASE) standard (Table 3-1).

- Acute pulmonary embolism is a common cause of acute RV pressure overload.
- The normal RV wall is thin and very compliant. Therefore, when pulmonary vascular resistance is increased acutely, such as in acute pulmonary embolism, the RV cavity will dilate before pulmonary pressure increases.
- Septal flattening only during systole is a sign of RV pressure overload.
- Septal flattening during diastole and systole is a sign of RV pressure/volume overload.
- A distinct echocardiographic pattern of regional RV dysfunction in which the apex is spared may occur in acute pulmonary embolism.
- Primary and secondary pulmonary hypertension, chronic obstructive pulmonary disease, Eisenmenger's syndrome, and pulmonary stenosis are causes of chronic RV pressure overload.
- Chronic RV pressure overload causes RV hypertrophy.

- A thick RV wall (>5 mm) is compatible with RV hypertrophy.
3. RV myocardial function
    - The RV inflow tract contracts earlier than the infundibulum, based on the study by Geva et al.[1] (Fig. 3-7).
    - The response of the three RV segments to medications, sympathetic stimulation, and volume and pressure overload may be different. For example, animal and human studies have suggested that the inotropic response of the infundibulum may be greater than that of the inflow tract.
    - Compliance is abnormal in RV hypertrophy and cardiomyopathy. RV diastolic abnormalities can be evaluated with echocardiography (Table 3-2).
    - RV ejection may depend on the degree to which the RV walls are stretched during diastole (preload).
    - Contractile abnormalities are caused by myocardial ischemia/infarction and cardiomyopathy.

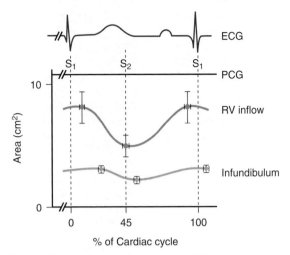

Figure 3-7. Timing of right ventricular (RV) contraction. RV inflow has earlier contraction than the infundibular RV. *(From Geva T, Powerll AJ, Crawford EC, et al. Evaluation of regional differences in right ventricular systolic function by acoustic quantification echocardiography and cine magnetic resonance imaging. Circulation. 1998;98: 339-345.)*

TABLE 3-1   ESTIMATION OF RA PRESSURE

Variable	Normal (0–5 [3] mm Hg)	Intermediate (5–10 [8] mm Hg)		High (15 mm Hg)
IVC diameter	≤2.1 cm	≤2.1 cm	>2.1 cm	>2.1 cm
Collapse with sniff	>50%	<50%	>50%	<50%
Secondary indices of elevated RA pressure		• Restrictive filling • Tricuspid E/E′ > 6 • Diastolic flow predominance in hepatic veins (systolic filling fraction < 55%)		

Ranges are provided for low and intermediate categories, but for simplicity, midrange values of 3 mm Hg for normal and 8 mm Hg for intermediate are suggested. Intermediate (8 mm Hg) RA pressures may be downgraded to normal (3 mm Hg) if no secondary indices of elevated RA pressure are present, upgraded to high if minimal collapse with sniff (<35%) and secondary indices of elevated RA pressure are present, or left at 8 mm Hg if uncertain.

From Rudski LG, Lai WW, Afilalo J, et al. Guidelines for the echocardiographic assessment of the right heart in adults: a report from the American Society of Echocardiography endorsed by the European Association of Echocardiography, a registered branch of the European Society of Cardiology, and the Canadian Society of Echocardiography. *J Am Soc Echocardiogr.* 2010;23:685-713.

TABLE 3-2   ECHOCARDIOGRAPHIC RV DIASTOLIC FUNCTION INDICES

RV Index	Normal Values	Age (years)	Clinical Meaning
RV E/A	1.50 ± 0.3	20–86 (57 ± 12)	>2 suggests restriction
RV DT	198 ± 23 ms	20–86 (57 ± 12)	<160 ms suggests restriction
Hepatic vein S/D	>1 in SR, <1 in AF	21–84	Reversal in diastolic dysfunction
Respiratory variation in E velocity	TV ≤ 15%insp.↑ MV ≤ 10%insp.↓	55 ± 15	Ventricular interdependence

RV, right ventricle; DT, deceleration time; S, systole; D, diastole; TV, tricuspid valve; MV, mitral valve; E, early diastolic filling velocity; A, velocity of diastolic filling after atrial contraction.

Modified from Vitarelli A, Terzano C. Do we have two hearts? New insights in right ventricular function supported by myocardial imaging echocardiography. *Heart Fail Rev.* 2010;15:39-61.

- Cardiomyopathy includes right ventricular arrhythmogenic cardiomyopathy (RVAC) and Uhl's anomaly.
- RVAC is a cardiomyopathy characterized pathologically by fibrofatty replacement primarily of the RV and clinically by life-threatening ventricular arrhythmias in young people. Echocardiographic findings include dilation of the RV and localized aneurysms of the free wall during diastole. 3D echocardiographic findings are compared with pathology in Figure 3-8.
- Uhl's anomaly is cardiomyopathy specific to the RV and may be an extreme manifestation of RVAC.
4. Pericardium or extracardiac force (constriction and pericardial effusion).
   - Pericardial abnormalities typically directly impact ventricular filling though indirectly affect ejection due to altered preload. There is enhanced ventricular interdependence and respiratory changes in chamber sizes and Doppler indices of filling and ejection (RV parameters increase with inspiration while LV parameters decrease with inspiration).

KEY POINTS

RV function is governed by:
- Preload (volume overload, due to shunt and tricuspid/pulmonic regurgitation)
- Afterload (pressure overload, due to pulmonary hypertension)
- Myocardial factors (myocardial infarction, cardiomyopathy, RVAC)
- Pericardial factors (pericardial effusion, constriction)

- Echocardiographic indices of RV diastolic function are shown in Table 3-2.

Importance of Assessing RV Function

RV size and function are important prognostic factors in many cardiopulmonary conditions as follows:
- RV dysfunction noted at the time of diagnosis of pulmonary embolism is associated with a high mortality rate.
- RV dysfunction defined as a tricuspid annular plane systolic excursion (TAPSE) of less than 14 mm is an independent predictor for long-term mortality in patients with ST elevation myocardial infarction.
- In patients with idiopathic dilated cardiomyopathy, a dilated hypocontractile RV is a poor prognostic sign.
- In patients with inferior myocardial infarction, RV infarction is an independent predictor of major complications and in-hospital mortality.
- In patients undergoing mitral valve surgery, preoperative right ventricular ejection fraction (RVEF) of less than 20% predicts late postoperative death.
- RV dysfunction is associated with decreased cardiac output and a greater requirement for inotropic agents after surgery in patients with aortic stenosis.

Echocardiographic Assessment of RV Size and Function

- 2D echocardiography is widely used to evaluate RV size and function in daily cardiac practice.

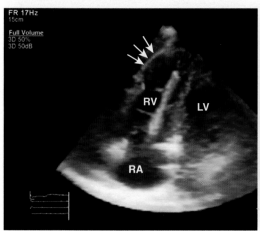
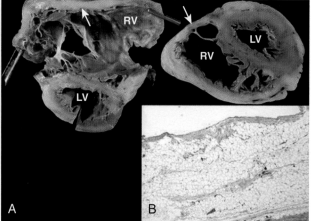

Figure 3-8. 3D echocardiography showing RV aneurysm in a patient with arrhythmogenic right ventricular dysplasia. Findings include RV apical dilation on 3D echocardiography (*left*), anatomic findings of RV dilation and wall thinning (**A**) and histologic evidence of fibrofatty replacement of the myocardium (**B**). *(From Goland S, Czer LS, Luthringer D, Siegel RJ. A case of arrhythmogenic right ventricular cardiomyopathy. Can J Cardiol. 2008;24:61-62.)*

- For the assessment of RV size and function, 2D echocardiography uses multiple views, including parasternal long axis and short axis views, TV inflow view, and apical four-chamber view (Fig. 3-9).
- The size of the RV is evaluated in multiple 2D views, including parasternal long and short axis, and apical four-chamber views.
- Normal values for RV size and function are shown in Table 3-3.

- In the apical four-chamber and parasternal long axis view, the normal RV area is approximately two-thirds that of the LV. When the RV appears larger than the LV and/or shares the apex, RV dilation may be present.
- Systolic function is determined by the following 2D echocardiography methods (Box 3-1).
  1. TAPSE, movement of the tricuspid annulus (Fig. 3-10)

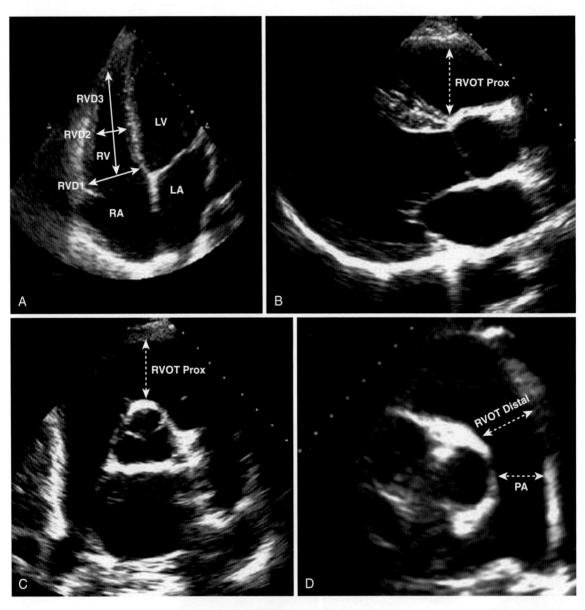

RV Dilation

Figure 3-9. RV standard views for estimation of RV size, showing (**A**) measurement of RV length and diameter (RVD) in the apical 4-chamber view, (**B**) the proximal (Prox) RV outflow tract (RVOT) in the parasternal long axis view, and (**C**) the short axis and (**D**) pulmonary artery bifucation views. *(From Rudski LG, Lai WW, Afilalo J, et al. Guidelines for the echocardiographic assessment of the right heart in adults: a report from the American Society of Echocardiography endorsed by the European Association of Echocardiography, a registered branch of the European Society of Cardiology, and the Canadian Society of Echocardiography. J Am Soc Echocardiogr. 2010;23:685-713.)*

TABLE 3-3   2D ECHOCARDIOGRAPHY PARAMETERS FOR THE NORMAL RV SIZE

Dimension	Studies	n	LRV (95%)	Mean (95% CI)	URV (95% CI)
RV mid-cavity diameter (mm) (Fig. 3-9, RVD2)	12	400	20 (15–25)	28 (23–33)	35 (30–41)
RV basal diameter (mm) (Fig. 3-9, RVD1)	10	376	24 (21–27)	33 (31–35)	42 (39–45)
RV longitudinal diameter (mm) (Fig. 3-9, RVD3)	12	359	56 (50–61)	71 (67–75)	86 (80–91)
RV end-diastolic area (cm²) (Fig. 3-13)	20	623	10 (8–12)	18 (16–19)	25 (24–27)
RV end-systolic area (cm²) (Fig. 3-13)	16	508	4 (2–5)	9 (8–10)	14 (13–15)
RV end-diastolic volume indexed (mL/m²)	3	152	44 (32–55)	62 (50–73)	80 (68–91)
RV end-systolic volume indexed (mL/m²)	1	91	19 (17–21)	33 (31–34)	46 (44–49)
3D RV end-diastolic volume indexed (mL/m²)	5	426	40 (28–52)	65 (54–76)	39 (77–101)
3D RV end-systolic volume indexed (mL/m²)	4	394	12 (1–23)	28 (18–38)	45 (34–56)
RV subcostal wall thickness (mm)	4	180	4 (3–4)	5 (4–5)	5 (5–6)
RVOT PLAX wall thickness (mm)	9	302	2 (1–2)	3 (3–4)	5 (4–6)
RVOT PLAX diameter (mm) (Fig. 3-9)	12	405	18 (15–20)	25 (23–27)	33 (30–35)
RVOT proximal diameter (mm) (Fig. 3-9, RVOT-Prox)	5	193	21 (18–25)	28 (27–30)	35 (31–39)
RVOT distal diameter (mm) (Fig. 3-9, RVOT-Distal)	4	159	17 (12–22)	22 (17–26)	27 (22–32)
RA major dimension (mm)	8	267	34 (32–36)	44 (43–45)	53 (51–55)
RA minor dimension (mm)	16	715	26 (24–29)	35 (33–37)	44 (41–46)
RA end-systolic area (cm²)	8	293	10 (8–12)	14 (14–15)	18 (17–20)

CI, confidence interval; LRV, lower reference value; PLAX, parasternal long axis view; RA, right atrium; RV, right ventricle; RVD, right ventricular diameter; RVOT, right ventricular outflow tract; 3D, three dimensional; URV, upper reference value.
From Rudski LG, Lai WW, Afilalo J, et al. Guidelines for the echocardiographic assessment of the right heart in adults: a report from the American Society of Echocardiography endorsed by the European Association of Echocardiography, a registered branch of the European Society of Cardiology, and the Canadian Society of Echocardiography. *J Am Soc Echocardiogr.* 2010;23:685-713.

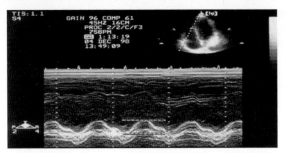

Figure 3-10. M-mode recording, showing how to measure tricuspid annular plane systolic excursion as shown by the two dashed lines on the M-mode recording of the annulus from an apical transducer position. *(From Kaul S, Tei C, Hopkins JM, Shah PM. Assessment of right ventricular function using two-dimensional echocardiography.* Am Heart J. *1984;107:526-531.)*

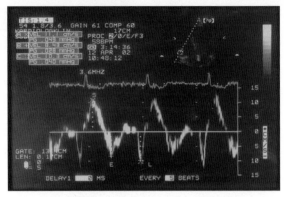

Figure 3-11. A pulsed Doppler tissue imaging of tricuspid annulus. *(From Kukulski T, Voigt JU, Wilkenshoff UM, et al. A comparison of regional myocardial velocity information derived by pulsed and color Doppler techniques: an in vitro and in vivo study.* Echocardiography. *2000;17:639-651.)*

BOX 3-1   2D Echocardiographic Signs of RV Dilation

- RV basal diameter in apical 4-chamber view > 42 mm (see Fig. 3-9)
- RV mid cavity diameter in apical 4-chamber view > 35 mm
- RV longitudinal diameter in apical 4-chamber view > 86 mm
- RVOT diameter in parasternal long axis view > 33 mm (see Fig. 3-9)
- RVOT proximal diameter in parasternal long and short axis view > 35 mm
- RVOT distal parasternal short axis pulmonary bifurcation view > 27 mm
- RV end-diastolic area in apical 4-chamber view > 25 cm^2
- RV end-systolic area in apical 4-chamber view > 14 cm^2
- Septal flattening in diastole is a sign of RV volume overload
- Dilatation along the free wall to septal minor axis as compared to RV long axis

---

- TAPSE is determined as the apical systolic motion of the TV annulus on M-mode recording. The movement of the tricuspid annulus in a standard apical four-chamber view is easy to recognize. This method is often used clinically for visual evaluation of RV systolic function without actual measurement.
- Normal TAPSE is greater than 15 mm.
- RV systolic dysfunction is suspected when TAPSE is less than 16 mm.
- However, this method assumes that the TV annular movement is representative of overall RV function, which may not hold true when regional RV dysfunction exists.

2. Peak systolic tricuspid annular velocity by pulsed and tissue Doppler (Fig. 3-11)
   - The evaluation of peak systolic tricuspid annular velocity using Doppler tissue imaging provides a simple, rapid, and noninvasive tool for assessing RV systolic function in patients with heart failure.
   - According to the ASE recommendation, RV systolic dysfunction (RVEF < 45%) is suspected when the peak systolic tricuspid annular velocity is less than 10 cm/s.
   - However, like TAPSE, this method assumes that the TV annular velocity represents the overall RV function, which may not hold true when regional RV dysfunction exists.
3. Myocardial performance index or Tei index (Fig. 3-12)
   - Myocardial performance index or Tei index is considered an index of global RV function.
   - The value is determined as the ratio of the total isovolumic time (isovolumic relaxation time and isovolumic contraction time) to RV ejection time (see Fig. 3-12).
   - The measurement can be performed with the pulsed Doppler and/or tissue Doppler method.
   - This method is relatively simple and does not require optimal RV imaging.
   - RV systolic dysfunction is suspected when:

   MPI > 0.40 by pulsed Doppler
   MPI > 0.55 by tissue Doppler

- However, this method may be inaccurate in patients with irregular heartbeats and also when RA pressure is increased.
4. RV area change (RAC) (Fig. 3-13)
   - The fractional area change (FAC) is defined as

$$(EDV - ESV)/EDV \times 100\%$$

where EDV and ESV are end-diastolic and end-systolic RV volumes. This value is determined by RV endocardial tracing in the apical four-chamber view.
   - Mean normal value is 49% (47–51%, 95% confidence interval, see Table 3-4).
   - RV systolic dysfunction is suspected with a FAC less than 35%.
   - However, this method does not reflect the right ventricular outflow tract (RVOT), which may react differently from the RV inflow to medications and pressure and volume overload as discussed earlier.
5. RV dP/dt (Fig. 3-14)
   - The rate of pressure rise can be estimated by CW Doppler recording of TR velocity.
   - RV dP/dt is determined by the ratio of the increase in pressure (12 mm Hg from 1 m/s to 2 m/s of TR velocity) to the time (from 1 m/s to 2 m/s).

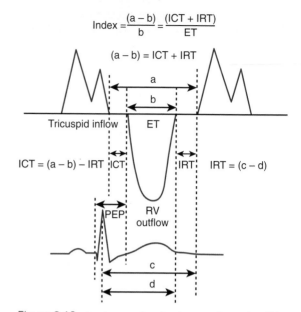

Figure 3-12. A schema, showing how to determine RV function using the Tei index. *(From Tei C, Dujardin KS, Hodge DO, et al. Doppler echocardiographic index for assessment of global right ventricular function. J Am Soc Echocardiogr. 1996;9:838-847.)*

- RV dP/dt less than 400 mm Hg/s may be considered to be abnormal (if other findings are consistent).
- However, this method is dependent on preload and less accurate in severe TR. Thus, no 2D echo method is reliably able to determine RV systolic function.

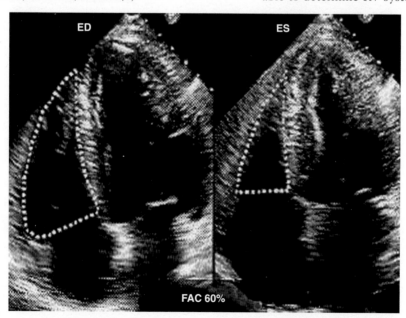

Figure 3-13. An example of how to measure fractional area change (FAC). *(From Rudski LG, Lai WW, Afilalo J, et al. Guidelines for the echocardiographic assessment of the right heart in adults: A report from the American Society of Echocardiography endorsed by the European Association of Echocardiography, a registered branch of the European Society of Cardiology, and the Canadian Society of Echocardiography. J Am Soc Echocardiogr. 2010;23:696.)*

TABLE 3-4   NORMAL VALUES OF 2D RV SYSTOLIC FUNCTION PARAMETERS

Variable	Studies	n	LRV (95% CI)	Mean (95% CI)	URV (95% CI)
TAPSE (mm) (Fig. 3-10)	46	2320	16 (15–18)	23 (22–24)	30 (29–31)
Pulsed Doppler velocity at the annulus (cm/s)	43	2139	10 (9–11)	15 (14–15)	19 (18–20)
Color Doppler velocities at the annulus (cm/s)	5	281	6 (5–7)	10 (9–10)	14 (12–15)
Pulsed Doppler MPI (Fig. 3-12)	17	686	0.15 (0.10–0.20)	0.28 (0.24–0.32)	0.40 (0.35–0.45)
Tissue Doppler MPI (Fig. 3-11)	8	590	0.24 (0.16–0.32)	0.39 (0.34–0.45)	0.55 (0.47–0.63)
FAC (%) (Fig. 3-13)	36	1276	35 (32–38)	49 (47–51)	63 (60–65)

CI, Confidence interval; EF, ejection fraction; FAC, fractional area change; IVA, isovolumic acceleration; LRV, lower reference value; MPI, myocardial performance index; RV, right ventricular; TAPSE, tricuspid annular plane systolic excursion; 3D, three-dimensional; URV, upper reference value.

From Rudski LG, Lai WW, Afilalo J, et al. Guidelines for the echocardiographic assessment of the right heart in adults: a report from the American Society of Echocardiography endorsed by the European Association of Echocardiography, a registered branch of the European Society of Cardiology, and the Canadian Society of Echocardiography. *J Am Soc Echocardiogr.* 2010;23:685-713.

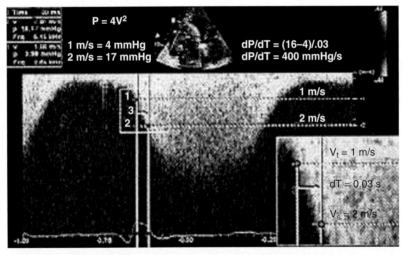

Figure 3-14. Continuous wave (CW) Doppler recording of tricuspid regurgitation and measurement of RV *dP/dt*. *(From Rudski LG, Lai WW, Afilalo J, et al. Guidelines for the echocardiographic assessment of the right heart in adults: A report from the American Society of Echocardiography endorsed by the European Association of Echocardiography, a registered branch of the European Society of Cardiology, and the Canadian Society of Echocardiography. J Am Soc Echocardiogr. 2010;23:685-713.)*

KEY POINTS

- TAPSE
  - RV systolic dysfunction is suspected when TAPSE is less than 16 mm
- Peak systolic tricuspid annular velocity by pulsed and tissue Doppler
  - RV dysfunction is present when S' velocity is less than 10 cm/s.
- Myocardial function index or Tei index; RV dysfunction when

- MPI is greater than 0.40 by pulsed Doppler
- MPI is greater than 0.55 by tissue Doppler
- RV area change
  - RV systolic dysfunction is suspected when FAC is less than 35%.
- RV *dP/dt*
  - RV *dP/dt* less than 400 mm Hg/s indicates RV systolic dysfunction.

2D and 3D Echocardiography for Determining RV Volume and Ejection Fraction

- Considering the complex geometry of the RV cavity (see Fig. 3-3), no 2D echocardiographic methods can provide true RV volumes.
- 2D echocardiography with the area length method and Simpson method was proposed to determine RV volume and EF (Fig. 3-15). As compared with MRI, however, this type of 2D approach to RV volume determination has been proven inaccurate.
- Therefore, 2D echocardiography-derived RV volume is not clinically used.
- 3D echocardiography has been proposed as a better method than 2D for determining RV volumes.

Step I: Anatomic Imaging with 3D Echocardiography

Acquisition
- 3D transthoracic echocardiography (TTE) uses apical (and subcostal) views to determine RV volume and function (Fig. 3-16).

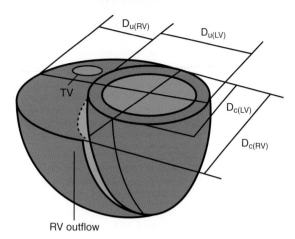

1. RV volume = 2/3 x area (apical view) x D (SAX)
2. RV volume by the Simpson method (4 and 2 AP)

Figure 3-15. *Area length method for estimating RV volume with 2D echocardiography. (From Panidis IP, Ren JF, Kotler MN, et al. Two-dimensional echocardiographic estimation of right ventricular ejection fraction in patients with coronary artery disease. J Am Coll Cardiol. 1983;911-918.)*

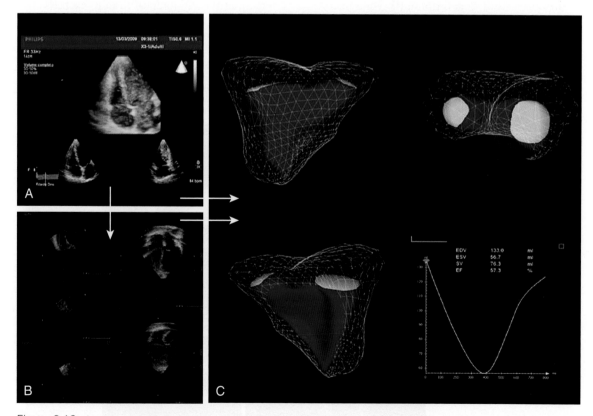

Figure 3-16. An example of how to measure RV volume with RV software. *(From Tamborini G, Marsan NA, Gripari P, et al. Reference values for right ventricular volumes and ejection fraction with real-time three-dimensional echocardiography: Evaluation in a large series of normal subjects. J Am Soc Echocardiogr. 2010;23:109-115.)*

- To include the entire RV, ECG-gated consecutive four-beat images are necessary, although a new echo system may include the entire RV in a single beat at the expense of temporal and spatial resolution.
- Discontinuity of these four volumes is a source of error. Careful acquisition is essential.
- When the study aims to determine the LV volume as well as that of the RV, the conventional apical four-chamber view is used to obtain 3D LV and RV imaging.
- However, only 30% of such 3D imaging may include the entire RV. Therefore, for the sole purpose of RV volume determination, slightly right-sided movement of the probe from the LV apex would be highly recommended to include the entire RV.
- With 3D transesophageal echocardiography (TEE), the apical four-chamber view, aortic short axis view (Fig. 3-17), and transgastric view would be used to include the entire RV to determine absolute RV volumes.
- Full volume acquisition with four consecutive ECG-gated cardiac cycles is necessary.

Analysis after Acquisition

- After the image acquisition, RV analysis software is used to determine RV volumes. Multiple software applications have been developed to this end. The most recent software has used multiple steps in common (Figs. 3-16 and 3-18).

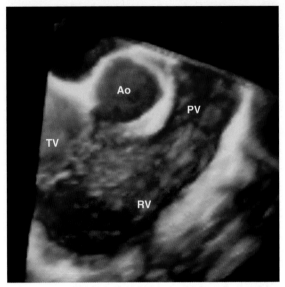

Figure 3-17. 3D transesophageal echocardiography (TEE) image acquisition of the RV for RV volume determination.

- First, three orthogonal RV planes (such as coronal, sagittal, and frontal planes) are generated from the original 3D dataset.
- Second, in end systole and end diastole, tracing of the RV endocardium in each RV plane is performed.
- Third, the software automatically detects RV endocardium throughout the cardiac cycle, providing RV volumes and EF.

NORMAL

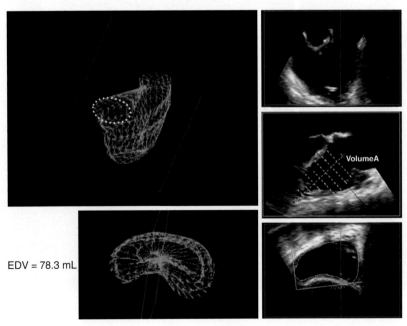

Figure 3-18. One type of software to determine absolute RV volume from 3D TEE volume.

- Manual correction to adjust the RV endocardial contours may be necessary when the automatic tracing is not reasonable.

Normal Values of RV Volumes by 3D Echocardiography

Normal values of RV volumes are reported in Tables 3-5 and 3-6.

- There were significant differences in RV end-diastolic volume (EDV) between men and women (129 ± 25 vs. 102 ± 33 mL, $P < .01$).
- However, adjusting to lean body mass (but not the body surface area or height) eliminated this difference (2.1 ± 0.5 vs. 2.2 ± 0.4 mL/kg, P = not significant).
- 3D RV volume determination with MRI has been well validated.

TABLE 3-5   NORMAL RV VOLUMES BY 3D ECHOCARDIOGRAPHY

Age Decile (y)	RV EDV (mL)			RV ESV (mL)			RV EF (%)		
	All	Men	Women	All	Men	Women	All	Men	Women
<30	92 ± 23	107 ± 22	78 ± 12	33 ± 13	41 ± 12	$24 \pm 8\,8$	66 ± 8	62 ± 6	69 ± 9
30–39	88 ± 20	99 ± 22	79 ± 11	30 ± 10	35 ± 10	25 ± 7	66 ± 8	64 ± 8	69 ± 7
40–49	88 ± 19	96 ± 20	76 ± 13	28 ± 10	34 ± 10	22 ± 7	68 ± 8	64 ± 8	71 ± 7
50–59	87 ± 20	99 ± 21	74 ± 8	30 ± 11	36 ± 11	24 ± 6	66 ± 7	65 ± 6	67 ± 8
60–69	82 ± 22	96 ± 13	68 ± 19	27 ± 10	31 ± 10	23 ± 10	67 ± 9	68 ± 9	67 ± 10
>70	80 ± 22	94 ± 23	70 ± 15	26 ± 11	33 ± 12	21 ± 7	68 ± 7	65 ± 6	71 ± 7
All	86 ± 21	99 ± 14	74 ± 14	29 ± 11	35 ± 7	23 ± 7	67 ± 8	64 ± 8	69 ± 8

RV EDV, right ventricular end-diastolic volume; RV ESV, right ventricular end-systolic volume; RV EF, right ventricular ejection fraction.

Data are expressed as mean ± SD.

From Tamborini G, Marsan NA, Gripari P, et al. Reference values for right ventricular volumes and ejection fraction with real-time three-dimensional echocardiography: evaluation in a large series of normal subjects. *J Am Soc Echocardiogr*. 2010;23:109-115.

TABLE 3-6   NORMAL RV VOLUMES BY 3D ECHOCARDIOGRAPHY

Volume	n	CMR (mL/m²)			RT 3D ECHO-DS (mL/m²)		
		Mean	SD	Reference Range, mean ± 2SD	Mean	SD	Reference Range, mean ± 2SD
EDV							
All	71	71.3	12.9	45.5–97.1	70.0	13.9	42.2–97.8
Female	36	67.1	12.1	42.9–90.2	65.4	13.4	38.6–92,2
Male	35	75.6	12.4	50.8–100.4	74.7	13.0	48.7–100
ESV							
All	71	33.5	9.9	13.7–55.3	33.4	10.3	12.8–54.0
Female	36	28.6	8.1	12.4–44.8	29.2	10.7	7.8–50.6
Male	35	38.4	9.1	20.2–56.6	37.8	7.4	23–52.6
SV							
All	71	37.8	8.7	20.4–46.5	36.6	9.3	18–45.9
Female	38	36.2	6.8	22.6–43.0	36.1	6.8	22.5–42.9
Male	34	37.2	9.9	17.4–47.1	37.0	11.4	14.2–48.4
EF							
All	71	53.3	8.7	35.9–62	52.6	9.9	32.8–62.5
Female	38	57.5	7.0	43.5–64.5	56.2	9.1	38–65.3
Male	34	49.0	8.8	31.4–57.8	48.9	9.5	29.9–58.4

CMR, cardiac magnetic resonance imaging; EDV, end-diastolic volume; EF, ejection fraction; ESV, end-systolic volume; RT 3D ECHO, real-time 3-dimensional echocardiography using disk summation method; SV, stroke volume.

From Gopal AS, Chukwu EO, Iwuchukwu CJ, et al. Normal values of right ventricular size and function by real-time 3-dimensional echocardiography: comparison with cardiac magnetic resonance imaging. *J Am Soc Echocardiogr*. 2007;20:445-455.

- In clinical studies there have been consistent underestimation of MRI-derived RV volumes by 3D echocardiography.[2]
- Meta-analysis shows that RV volumes are slightly underestimated by 3D echocardiography as compared with MRI (Fig. 3-19).[2]

Normal values of RVEF are reported by multiple authors (Tables 3-6 and 3-7).

- Gopal et al. reported normal RVEF of 56.6 ± 9.9% by 3D echocardiography and 53.3 ± 8.7% by MRI.[3]
- Tamborini et al. reported normal RVEF of 67 ± 8% by 3D echocardiography.[4]
- Our meta-analysis showed that EF was slightly underestimated (0.9%) by 3D echocardiography as compared with MRI (Fig. 3-20).

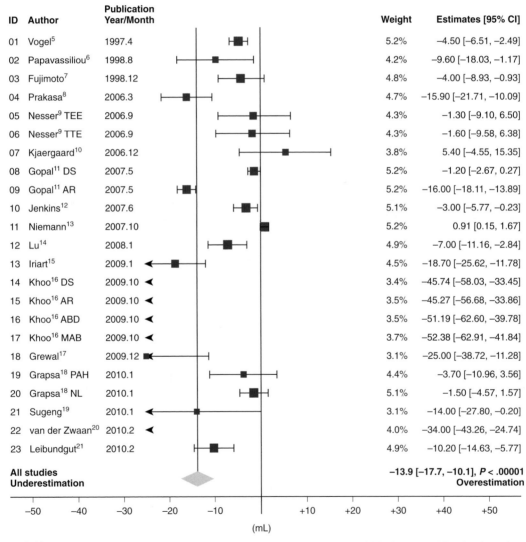

Figure 3-19. Meta-analysis of RV end-diastolic volume by 3D echocardiography. ABD, Automated border detection; AR, apical rotation; CI, confidence interval; DS, disk summation; MAB, manual adjustments of the detected borders; PAH, pulmonary artery hypertension; TEE, transesophageal echocardiography; TTE, transthoracic echocardiography. *(From Shimada YJ, Shiota M, Siegel RJ, et al. Accuracy of right ventricular volumes and function determined by three-dimensional echocardiography in comparison with magnetic resonance imaging: a meta-analysis study. J Am Soc Echocardiogr. 2010;23:943-953.)*

TABLE 3-7   COMPARISON BETWEEN 2D AND 3D ECHOCARDIOGRAPHY AND CMR

	2D Echocardiography		3D Echocardiography	CMR
RV size	Relatively simple measurement in multiple views and visual assessment	Easy to apply but not quantitative Moderate accuracy	Better estimate than 2D echocardiography Need more time to measure May underestimate RV volumes	Gold standard, but not for daily practice
RV volume	Area length or Simpson method	Not accurate	Need more time	Accurate
RV function	TAPSE TV annulus velocity (pulsed and tissue Doppler) MPI or Tei index Fractional area change CW *dP/dt*	All indices are limited due to localized information	Better estimate than 2D echocardiography May underestimate RVEF	Accurate RVEF, not used in daily practice

RV, right ventricle; TV, tricuspid valve; MPI, myocardial performance index; RVEF, RV ejection fraction; TAPSE, tricuspid annular plane systolic excursion.

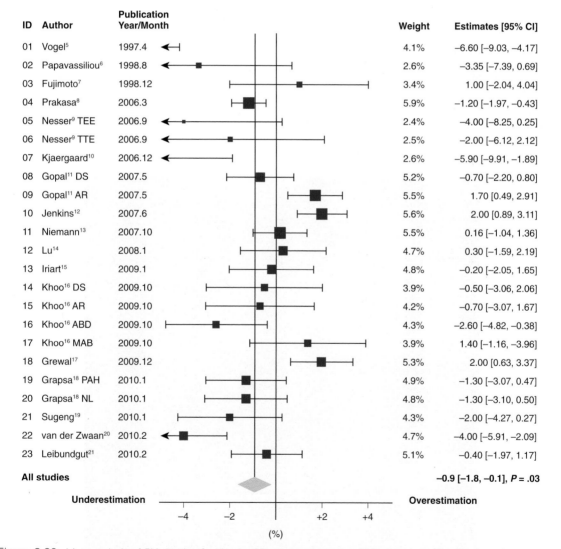

DIFFERENCE IN RVEF BETWEEN 3DE AND MRI

ID	Author	Publication Year/Month	Weight	Estimates [95% CI]
01	Vogel[5]	1997.4	4.1%	−6.60 [−9.03, −4.17]
02	Papavassiliou[6]	1998.8	2.6%	−3.35 [−7.39, 0.69]
03	Fujimoto[7]	1998.12	3.4%	1.00 [−2.04, 4.04]
04	Prakasa[8]	2006.3	5.9%	−1.20 [−1.97, −0.43]
05	Nesser[9] TEE	2006.9	2.4%	−4.00 [−8.25, 0.25]
06	Nesser[9] TTE	2006.9	2.5%	−2.00 [−6.12, 2.12]
07	Kjaergaard[10]	2006.12	2.6%	−5.90 [−9.91, −1.89]
08	Gopal[11] DS	2007.5	5.2%	−0.70 [−2.20, 0.80]
09	Gopal[11] AR	2007.5	5.5%	1.70 [0.49, 2.91]
10	Jenkins[12]	2007.6	5.6%	2.00 [0.89, 3.11]
11	Niemann[13]	2007.10	5.5%	0.16 [−1.04, 1.36]
12	Lu[14]	2008.1	4.7%	0.30 [−1.59, 2.19]
13	Iriart[15]	2009.1	4.8%	−0.20 [−2.05, 1.65]
14	Khoo[16] DS	2009.10	3.9%	−0.50 [−3.06, 2.06]
15	Khoo[16] AR	2009.10	4.2%	−0.70 [−3.07, 1.67]
16	Khoo[16] ABD	2009.10	4.3%	−2.60 [−4.82, −0.38]
17	Khoo[16] MAB	2009.10	3.9%	1.40 [−1.16, −3.96]
18	Grewal[17]	2009.12	5.3%	2.00 [0.63, 3.37]
19	Grapsa[18] PAH	2010.1	4.9%	−1.30 [−3.07, 0.47]
20	Grapsa[18] NL	2010.1	4.8%	−1.30 [−3.10, 0.50]
21	Sugeng[19]	2010.1	4.3%	−2.00 [−4.27, 0.27]
22	van der Zwaan[20]	2010.2	4.7%	−4.00 [−5.91, −2.09]
23	Leibundgut[21]	2010.2	5.1%	−0.40 [−1.97, 1.17]

All studies — **−0.9 [−1.8, −0.1], *P* = .03**

Underestimation   Overestimation

−4   −2   +2   +4

(%)

Figure 3-20. Meta-analysis of RV ejection fraction by 3D echocardiography. ABD, Automated border detection; AR, apical rotation; CI, confidence interval; DS, disk summation; MAB, manual adjustments of the detected borders; PAH, pulmonary artery hypertension; TEE, transesophageal echocardiography; TTE, transthoracic echocardiography. *(From Shimada YJ, Shiota M, Siegel RJ, et al. Accuracy of right ventricular volumes and function determined by three-dimensional echocardiography in comparison with magnetic resonance imaging: a meta-analysis study. J Am Soc Echocardiogr. 2010;23:943-953.)*

- RV systolic dysfunction is suspected when 3D EF is less than 44%.

Pitfalls of 3D Echo Measurement

- Inclusion of the entire RV is not automatic. In 40 patients planned for routine 2D TTE, parasternal, apical, and subcostal views were used for 3D echocardiography. In this study, the RV was adequately visualized in only 12 (30%) patients by 3D echocardiography.
- Tracing of the RV endocardium may be erroneous, although the typical views such as the apical four-chamber view show an optimal RV image for tracing (Fig. 3-21).
- Inclusion and exclusion of the moderator band may create confusion.

Additional Testing Based on Limitations of Echocardiographic Data

- MRI is the gold standard for determining RV volume and function (Table 3-7). This method should be considered when the image quality

of 3D echocardiography is not good enough for evaluation.

Clinical Evaluation of RV Volume and Function by 3D Echocardiography

- 3D echocardiography-derived RVEF correlated negatively with 2D-derived pulmonary arterial systolic pressure and positively with TAPSE, peak systolic velocity, and fractional shortening area (Box 3-2).
- TAPSE (15.5 ± 3, 16.5 ± 3, and 18.5 ± 4 mm at 3, 6, and 12 months, respectively) and peak systolic velocity of the tricuspid annulus (11.9 ± 2, 12 ± 2, and 12.8 ± 3 cm/s at 3, 6, and 12 months, respectively) were significantly ($P < .001$) lower after mitral valve surgery for prolapse in comparison with presurgical values. However, preoperative 3D-derived RVEF ($58.4 \pm 4\%$) did not change after surgery (56.9 ± 5, 59.5 ± 5, and $58.5 \pm 5\%$ at each step).
- 3D echocardiography showed that patients with pulmonary hypertension had the largest RV volumes and the lowest RVEF, and that

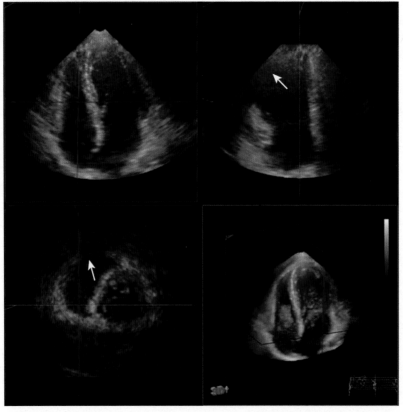

Figure 3-21. A pitfall of RV volume determination with 3D echocardiography. Unclear endocardial borders (*arrows*) is a cause of erroneous estimation of RV volume.

those with idiopathic dilated cardiomyopathy were characterized by lower RVEF than patients with valvular disease.
- In a clinical feasibility study, at least one good 3D acquisition of the RV was achieved in all subjects in a mean time of 3 ± 1 min, and the RV image quality was good in most subjects (85%).
- Transthoracic real-time 3D echocardiography revealed that patients with arrhythmogenic RV cardiomyopathy had a decreased RVEF (0.47 ± 0.08 vs. 0.53 ± 0.05, $P < .01$) as compared with controls.
- In 60 patients with tetralogy repair at 14.3 ± 7.2 years after surgery and in 29 healthy controls, multivariate analysis identified 3D echocardiography-derived RV EDV as a significant correlate of the LV systolic dyssynchrony index.

Various Clinical Applications of 3D Echocardiography Related to the Right Ventricle

- 3D echocardiography reportedly proved to be a reliable noninvasive modality to properly direct the bioptome to the desired site of biopsy within the RV.
- By real-time 3D echocardiography, the pulmonary valve was visualized sufficiently in 68% and the RVOT excellently in 40%.
- Real-time 3D echocardiography was a promising tool to offer insights into the morphology and to evaluate the efficacy of surgical valve repair in patients with Ebstein's malformation.
- 3D echocardiographic images revealed evidence of a free stent trapped in the tricuspid valvular apparatus causing severe tricuspid regurgitation.
- Real-time 3D TTE was useful to characterize the morphology and extent of masses in the right atrium and RV.

- In a case of traumatic TR, 3D echocardiography was useful not only for its diagnosis but also in providing important information for surgical decision making.
- These clinical studies are quite interesting and demonstrate unique images of the RV and RV-related cardiac abnormalities only possible with 3D echocardiography.

References

1. Geva T, Powell AJ, Crawford EC, et al. Evaluation of regional differences in right ventricular systolic function by acoustic quantification echocardiography and cine magnetic resonance imaging. *Circulation*. 1998;98:339-345.
2. Shimada YJ, Shiota M, Siegel RJ, et al. Accuracy of right ventricular volumes and function determined by 3-dimensional echocardiography in comparison with magnetic resonance imaging: a meta-analysis study. *J Am Soc Echocardiogr*. 2010;23:943-953.
3. Gopal AS, Chukwu EO, Iwuchukwu CJ, et al. Normal values of right ventricular size and function by real-time 3-dimensional echocardiography: Comparison with cardiac magnetic resonance imaging. *J Am Soc Echocardiogr*. 2007;20:445-455.
4. Tamborini G, Marsan NA, Gripari P, et al. Reference values for right ventricular volumes and ejection fraction with real-time three-dimensional echocardiography: Evaluation in a large series of normal subjects. *J Am Soc Echocardiogr*. 2010;23:109-115.
5. Vogel M, Gutberlet M, Dittrich S, et al. Comparison of transthoracic three dimensional echocardiography with magnetic resonance imaging in the assessment of right ventricular volume and mass. *Heart*. 1997;78:127-130.
6. Papavassiliou DP, Parks WJ, Hopkins KL, et al. Three-dimensional echocardiographic measurement of right ventricular volume in children with congenital heart disease validated by magnetic resonance imaging. *J Am Soc Echocardiogr*. 1998;11:770-777.
7. Fujimoto S, Mizuno R, Nakagawa Y, et al. Estimation of the right ventricular volume and ejection fraction by transthoracic three-dimensional echocardiography. A validation study using magnetic resonance imaging. *Int J Card Imaging*. 1998;14:385-390.
8. Prakasa KR, Dalal D, Wang J, et al. Feasibility and variability of three dimensional echocardiography in arrhythmogenic right ventricular dysplasia/cardiomyopathy. *Am J Cardiol*. 2006;97:703-709.
9. Nesser HJ, Tkalec W, Patel AR, et al. Quantitation of right ventricular volumes and ejection fraction by three-dimensional echocardiography in patients: comparison with magnetic resonance imaging and radionuclide ventriculography. *Echocardiography*. 2006;23:666-680.
10. Kjaergaard J, Petersen CL, Kjaer A, et al. Evaluation of right ventricular volume and function by 2D and 3D echocardiography compared to MRI. *Eur J Echocardiogr*. 2006;7:430-438.
11. Gopal AS, Chukwu EO, Iwuchukwu CJ, et al. Normal values of right ventricular size and function by real-time 3-dimensional echocardiography: comparison with cardiac magnetic resonance imaging. *J Am Soc Echocardiogr*. 2007;20:445-455.
12. Jenkins C, Chan J, Bricknell K, et al. Reproducibility of right ventricular volumes and ejection fraction using real-time three-dimensional echocardiography: comparison with cardiac MRI. *Chest*. 2007;131:1844-1851.

13. Niemann PS, Pinho L, Balbach T, et al. Anatomically oriented right ventricular volume measurements with dynamic three-dimensional echocardiography validated by 3-Tesla magnetic resonance imaging. *J Am Coll Cardiol.* 2007;50:1668-1676.

14. Lu X, Nadvoretskiy V, Bu L, et al. Accuracy and reproducibility of real-time three-dimensional echocardiography for assessment of right ventricular volumes and ejection fraction in children. *J Am Soc Echocardiogr.* 2008;21:84-89.

15. Iriart X, Montaudon M, Lafitte S, et al. Right ventricle three-dimensional echography in corrected tetralogy of Fallot: accuracy and variability. *Eur J Echocardiogr.* 2009;10:784-792.

16. Khoo NS, Young A, Occleshaw C, et al. Assessments of right ventricular volume and function using three-dimensional echocardiography in older children and adults with congenital heart disease: comparison with cardiac magnetic resonance imaging. *J Am Soc Echocardiogr.* 2009;22:1279-1288.

17. Grewal J, Majdalany D, Syed I, et al. Three-dimensional echocardiographic assessment of right ventricular volume and function in adult patients with congenital heart disease: comparison with magnetic resonance imaging. *J Am Soc Echocardiogr.* 2010;23:127-133.

18. Grapsa J, O'Regan DP, Pavlopoulos H, et al. Right ventricular remodelling in pulmonary arterial hypertension with three-dimensional echocardiography: comparison with cardiac magnetic resonance imaging. *Eur J Echocardiogr.* 2010;11:64-73.

19. Sugeng L, Mor-Avi V, Weinert L, et al. Multimodality comparison of quantitative volumetric analysis of the right ventricle. *JACC Cardiovasc Imaging.* 2010;3:10-18.

20. van der Zwaan HB, Helbing WA, McGhie JS, et al. Clinical value of real-time three-dimensional echocardiography for right ventricular quantification in congenital heart disease: validation with cardiac magnetic resonance imaging. *J Am Soc Echocardiogr.* 2010;23:134-140.

21. Leibundgut G, Rohner A, Grize L, et al. Dynamic assessment of right ventricular volumes and function by real-time three-dimensional echocardiography: a comparison study with magnetic resonance imaging in 100 adult patients. *J Am Soc Echocardiogr.* 2010;23: 116-126.

Suggested Reading

1. Ho SY, Nihoyannopoulos P. Anatomy, echocardiography, and normal right ventricular dimensions. *Heart.* 2006;92(Suppl 1):i2-i13.

2. Haddad F, Hunt SA, Rosenthal DN, Murphy DJ. Right ventricular function in cardiovascular disease, part I: Anatomy, physiology, aging, and functional assessment of the right ventricle. *Circulation.* 2008;117:1436-1448.

3. Mangion JR. Right ventricular imaging by two-dimensional and three-dimensional echocardiography. *Curr Opin Cardiol.* 2010;22:423-429.

4. Sheehan F, Redington A. The right ventricle: Anatomy, physiology and clinical imaging. *Heart.* 2008;94: 1510-1515.

5. Rudski LG, Lai WW, Afilalo J, et al. Guidelines for the echocardiographic assessment of the right heart in adults: A report from the American Society of Echocardiography endorsed by the European Association of Echocardiography, a registered branch of the European Society of Cardiology, and the Canadian Society of Echocardiography. *J Am Soc Echocardiogr.* 2010;23:685-713.

6. Vitarelli A, Terzano C. Do we have two hearts? New insights in right ventricular function supported by myocardial imaging echocardiography. *Heart Fail Rev.* 2010;15:39-61.

Transthoracic and Transesophageal Echocardiography in the Catheterization Laboratory

4

Rebecca Hahn and Linda D. Gillam

ALCOHOL SEPTAL ABLATION

Background

- In the setting of hypertrophic obstructive cardiomyopathy (HOCM), transcoronary alcohol septal ablation by injection of ethanol into the septal perforator supplying the muscle mass adjacent to the point of mitral leaflet-septal contact widens the outflow tract and relieves the obstruction.
- Echocardiography has become an essential tool, contributing to procedural success and reduction in complications.

Preprocedural Anatomic and Physiologic Imaging

- Confirm left ventricular (LV) anatomy and function:
  - Perform routine transthoracic imaging to exclude atypical forms of hypertrophic cardiomyopathy as well as fixed left ventricular outflow tract (LVOT) obstruction.
    - Patients with apical or mid-cavity hypertrophy with intracavitary (not subaortic) gradients are not candidates for alcohol septal ablation (ASA).
  - Measure the septal thickness at the site of obstruction from parasternal and apical views (Fig. 4-1).
    - Avoid measuring right ventricular (RV) trabeculations and papillary muscle tissue, which may merge with the RV side of the septum.
- Confirm mitral valve (MV) anatomy and function:
  - Document systolic anterior motion (SAM) of the mitral leaflet with proximal MV-septal contact (Fig. 4-2).
  - Document the direction and severity of mitral regurgitation (MR).

- Typical MR jet secondary to SAM is directed laterally and posteriorly (Fig. 4-3).
- Severity of MR is usually proportional to the severity of septal contact during SAM and thus to the severity of the LVOT obstruction.
- If atypical MR is seen, intrinsic valvular disease may be present.
- Determine the subaortic gradient:
  - Appropriate patients for ASA should have a gradient of 50 mm Hg or more measured with Doppler echocardiography either at rest and/or with physiologic provocative maneuvers and/or during exercise.
    - Avoid using dobutamine as a stressor since it can provoke significant subaortic gradients in normal hearts and may result in catastrophic adverse consequences in patients with significant obstructive disease.

Pitfalls

- RV trabeculations merging with the septum should not be included in measurements of the interventricular septum. Low parasternal views are particularly prone to this type of error. If in doubt, angulation of the imaging plane will help demonstrate the plane separating such trabeculations from the septum.
- When endocardial borders are not well imaged, consider using intravenous contrast agents for LV opacification to confirm ventricular anatomy. The apex may be particularly difficult to image.
- Discrete subaortic stenosis and valvular aortic stenosis must be excluded.
- Congenital abnormalities of the mitral apparatus (anomalous papillary muscle insertion or malpositioned enlarged papillary muscles) produce more distal muscular

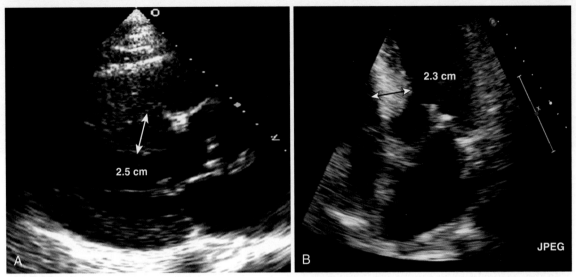

Figure 4-1. Septal thickness at the site of obstruction should be measured from parasternal (**A**) and apical (**B**) views (*arrows*).

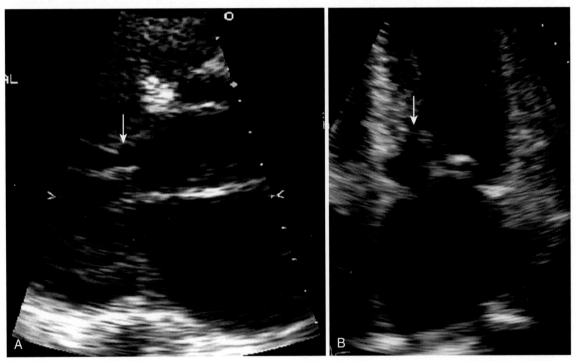

Figure 4-2. Document systolic anterior motion (SAM) of the mitral leaflet with proximal mitral valve (MV)-septal contact (*arrows*) from parasternal (**A**) and apical (**B**) views.

obstruction in the mid-cavity. These lesions are not candidates for ablation.

- Avoid contamination of the subaortic spectral Doppler with MR.
  - MR peak velocities are always higher than LVOT velocities.
  - Both MR and LVOT velocities may appear to peak late given the anatomy; however,

the duration of MR is typically greater than the duration of systolic ejection (Fig. 4-4).

- Use color Doppler to determine the direction of flow: MR and LVOT flows are typically in opposite directions unless intrinsic MV disease is present.

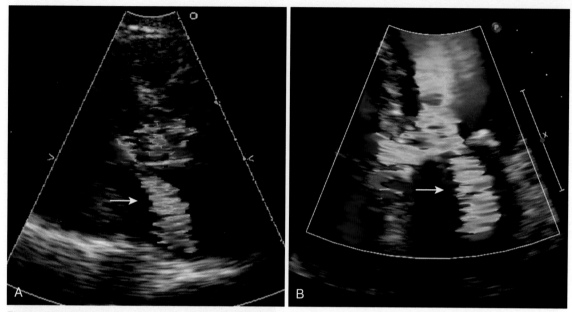

Figure 4-3. Typical mitral regurgitation (MR) jet secondary to SAM is directed posteriorly (**A,** parasternal view) and laterally (**B,** apical view).

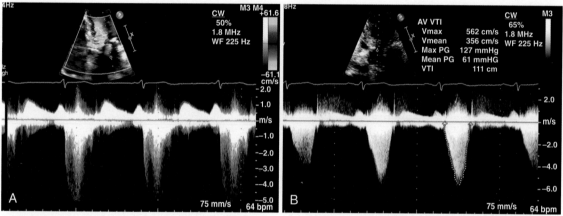

Figure 4-4. Both MR and left ventricular outflow tract (LVOT) velocities may appear to peak late given the close relationship between abnormal MV motion and outflow obstruction; however, the duration of MR (**A**) is typically longer and the velocity higher than transaortic (**B**) flow.

Intraprocedural Anatomic and Physiologic Imaging

- Identification of the appropriate septal perforator:
  - Balloon occlusion followed by myocardial contrast injection directly into the septal perforator by the angiographer should be performed during continuous transthoracic echocardiographic (TTE) or transesophageal echocardiographic (TEE) imaging.
    - Apical four- or five-chamber views are easiest to obtain during the procedure.

- The resulting hyperechoic region of the myocardium is identified (Fig. 4-5).
- Continuous wave (CW) Doppler is performed (again from the apical views).
  - An immediate fall in outflow gradient following balloon occlusion and/or contrast injection should be seen and aids in the decision to proceed with alcohol injection.
  - If no change in gradient is seen and/or the hyperechoic region of the septum does not correlate with the region of subvalvular

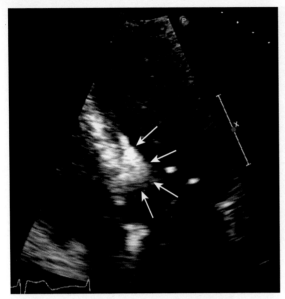

Figure 4-5. Following direct intracoronary contrast injection, the resulting hyperechoic region of the myocardium is identified.

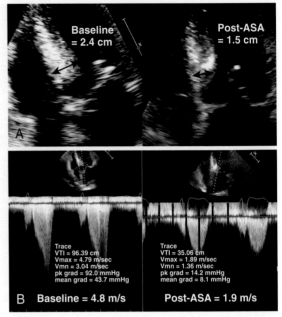

Figure 4-6. Following injection of alcohol, the area of infarction is identified by myocardial thinning (**A**) and hypokinesis with an immediate reduction in transaortic gradient (**B**).

obstruction, another target septal perforator should be chosen.

- Injection of alcohol with limited myocardial infarction:
  - Apical four- or five-chamber views are continuously imaged during and following injection of alcohol.
    - The area of infarction is identified by myocardial thinning and hypokinesis (Fig. 4-6).
  - CW Doppler is performed and an immediate fall in outflow gradient following septal ablation is frequently seen.

Pitfalls

- The selected septal perforator must perfuse the region of the septum in contact with the MV during SAM but should not perfuse other distant regions of the LV or RV myocardium or papillary muscles.
- Approximately 15% to 20% of patients will not have a successful procedure due to lack of suitable septal arteries in the region of obstruction.
- If a larger than expected region of anteroseptal hypokinesis is seen, the possibility of backward extravasation of alcohol producing occlusion or abrupt coronary no-flow should be considered.

Postprocedural Imaging

- Confirm LV anatomy and function:
  - Image basal septum from parasternal and apical views concentrating on septal anatomy following controlled infarction.
    - Measure the septal thickness in the region of infarction and, if different, in the region of mitral-to-septal contact.
    - Color Doppler imaging to exclude perforation (ventricular septal defect) should include the RV side of the septum.
    - Color Doppler imaging of the LVOT should show reduced turbulence.
- Confirm MV anatomy and function:
  - Document absence of SAM of the mitral leaflet.
  - Color Doppler to assess the severity of residual MR.
- Determine the subaortic gradient:
  - Following successful ASA, peak gradients should be <50 mm Hg.
  - Acute reduction in transaortic gradient in the catheterization laboratory may be followed by an increase in gradient within 24 hr, but typically is followed by significant reduction in the gradient over the ensuing 6 to 12 months due to further remodeling and thinning of the affected septum.

TABLE 4-1 THE MV SCORE HELPS PREDICT PERCUTANEOUS BALLOON MITRAL VALVULOPLASTY SUCCESS BY GRADING FOUR CHARACTERISTICS OF THE MV APPARATUS

Grade	Mobility	Subvalvular Thickening	Leaflet Thickening	Calcification
1	Highly mobile valve with only leaflet tips restricted	Minimal thickening just below the mitral leaflets	Leaflets near normal in thickness (4–5 mm)	A single area of echo brightness
2	Leaflet mid and base portions have normal mobility	Thickening of chordal structures extending up to $\frac{1}{3}$ of the chordal length	Mid-leaflets normal, considerable thickening of margins (5–8 mm)	Scattered areas of brightness confined to leaflet margins
3	Valve continues to move forward in diastole, mainly from the base	Thickening extending to the distal $\frac{1}{3}$ of the chords	Thickening extending the entire length of the leaflet (5–8 mm)	Brightness extending into the midportion of the leaflets
4	No or minimal forward movement of the leaflets in diastole	Extensive thickening and shortening of all chordal structures extending down the papillary muscles	Considerable thickening of all leaflet tissue (>8–10 mm)	Extensive brightness throughout much of the leaflet tissue

Adapted from Wilkins GT, Weyman AE, Abascal VM, Block PC, Palacios IF. Percutaneous balloon dilatation of the mitral valve: an analysis of echocardiographic variables related to outcome and the mechanism of dilatation. *Br Heart J*. 1988;60:299–308.

KEY POINTS

- Confirm LV anatomy (increased basal septal wall thickness) and MV anatomy (SAM) with documentation of a resting or provoked gradient of >50 mm Hg arising from septal-MV contact.
- Identify appropriate septal perforator supplying the region of septal-MV contact using direct injection of myocardial contrast and imaging the hyperechoic region of the septum.
- Image the area of infarction and document myocardial thinning and hypokinesis, as well as residual outflow gradient.

PERCUTANEOUS BALLOON MITRAL VALVULOPLASTY

Background

- Since the advent of percutaneous balloon mitral valvuloplasty (PBMV) in 1984, the technique has become the treatment of choice for mitral stenosis (MS); it is as effective as open valvotomy and more effective than closed valvotomy. Echocardiographic assessment is essential in patient selection, intraprocedural monitoring, and postprocedural follow-up.
- Echocardiographic characterization and quantitation of MV structure and function are key determinants of patient suitability for PBMV.

Preprocedural Imaging

- Assess severity and level of MV obstruction.
  - Both the pre-PBMV area and severity of MR are independent predictors of immediate post-PBMV success and should be assessed.
    - Planimeter MV area from parasternal short axis views.
    - Color Doppler MV to assess MR.
    - CW Doppler across MV to record peak and mean gradients and pressure halftime.
    - Record heart rate.
- Apply the Wilkins Echo Score to predict outcome of valvuloplasty (Table 4-1).
  - In Wilkins' original report,[1] patients with a score of less than or equal to 8 were more likely to have optimal results following valvuloplasty (post mitral valve area [MVA] >1.5 cm^2, left atrial pressure [LAP] <18 mm Hg). Patients with a score of greater than 8 had suboptimal outcomes, and a score of greater than 10 increased the chance of suboptimal results with complications.
- Apply MR score (Table 4-2) to predict development of significant MR.
- Assess presence of intracardiac thrombus.
  - Preprocedure TEE is performed to exclude left atrial thrombus (Fig. 4-7).
    - If a thrombus is found, PBMV is relatively contraindicated. The patient can be anticoagulated or surgical intervention considered.
  - Confirmation of MV anatomy is also performed; three-dimensional (3D) TEE may be useful for optimizing planimetry of the valve orifice (Fig. 4-8).

TABLE 4-2   FURTHER SCORING OF THE MV HELPS PREDICT THE OCCURRENCE OF THE PRIMARY COMPLICATION OF PBMV, MITRAL REGURGITATION

Grade	Subvalvular Thickening	Leaflet Thickening (Score Each Leaflet Separately)	Calcification
1	Minimal thickening just below the mitral leaflets	Leaflets near normal in thickness (4–5 mm)	Fibrosis and/or calcium in only one commissure
2	Thickening of chordal structures extending up to ⅓ of the chordal length	Leaflet fibrotic and/or calcified evenly; no thin areas	Both commissures mildly affected
3	Thickening extending to the distal ⅓ of the chords	Leaflets fibrotic and/or calcified with uneven distribution; thinner segments are mildly thickened (5–8 mm)	Calcium in both commissures, one markedly affected
4	Extensive thickening and shortening of all chordal structures extending down the papillary muscles	Leaflets fibrotic and/or calcified with uneven distribution; thinner segments are near normal (4–5 mm)	Calcium in both commissures, both markedly affected

Adapted from Padial LR, Freitas N, Sagie A, et al. Echocardiography can predict which patients will develop severe mitral regurgitation after percutaneous mitral valvulotomy. *J Am Coll Cardiol.* 1996;27:1225-1231.

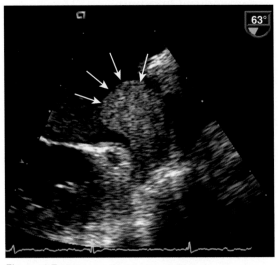

Figure 4-7. Preprocedural transesophageal echocardiography (TEE) must be performed to exclude left atrial thrombus (*arrows*).

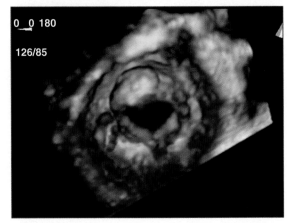

Figure 4-8. Three-dimensional (3D) TEE imaging may be utilized to assess the MV area.

Pitfalls

- Pressure half-time calculation of valve area has numerous limitations and should be used with caution in older patients, in atrial fibrillation, and in patients with prior MV interventions. An integrative approach to calculating valve area is always recommended.
- Peak and mean gradients are closely related to the amount of diastolic flow across the valve and the diastolic filling period and should be interpreted in relation to heart rate.

- Patients with degenerative MS (calcification of the annulus or body of the leaflets with little or no commissural fusion) should not undergo PBMV.
- Scores greater than 8 are not absolute contraindications to attempted PBMV.

Intraprocedural Imaging

- Transseptal puncture: although typically interventionalists can perform the transseptal puncture under fluoroscopy, occasionally TEE can help interventionalists position the puncture to avoid puncture of the aorta or atrial wall.

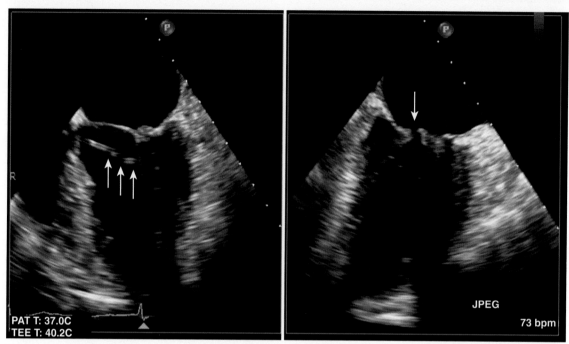

Figure 4-9. This biplane image following percutaneous balloon mitral valvuloplasty shows a noncommissural tear (*right panel, arrow*), which is the most common etiology of significant MR. In the *left panel* the *arrows* point to the intraventricular catheter.

- Assessing postvalvuloplasty results by TTE:
  - After each balloon inflation, imaging should be performed to assess MR severity, peak and mean transmitral gradients, and MV area by planimetry.
    - A suboptimal valvuloplasty result is defined as a final valve area of less than 1.0 cm², a final transmitral mean pressure gradient greater than 10 mm Hg, or a less than 25% increase in valve area.
    - Creation of more than mild MR is a relative contraindication to further balloon inflations.
    - In some cases, intracardiac echocardiography or TEE imaging (see Fig. 4-8) may be utilized to assess MV area.
  - Assess for complications of the procedure:
    - Hemopericardium (0.5–12%), embolism (0.5–5%), severe MR (2–10%, although 25% of patients increase severity by one grade) most often due to non-commissural tear, any of which might create a need for urgent surgery (<1%) (Fig. 4-9).
    - Transient atrial septal defects are common after transseptal access, but substantial shunting occurs in less than 5% of patients.

Pitfalls

- Pressure half-time calculation cannot be used immediately post-PBMV to assess area due to acute changes in compliance of the left atrium.

KEY POINTS
• Apply various echocardiography scores to predict procedural success and anticipate procedural complications. • Assess peak/mean gradient and presence/severity of MR following each balloon inflation and planimeter the final valve area. • Assess for complications.

PERCUTANEOUS VALVES: TRANSCATHETER AORTIC VALVE IMPLANTATION

Background

- Transcatheter aortic valve implantation (TAVI) has been shown to be superior to medical therapy in a population of patients with severe, symptomatic aortic stenosis at prohibitive risk for surgery.[2]

- Because echocardiography has largely replaced the invasive assessment of aortic stenosis, it is a necessary tool in the preprocedural, intraprocedural, and postprocedural evaluation of patients undergoing transcatheter valve procedures.
- Because the experience in the United States has to date been limited to the balloon expandable valve, the current review will outline the approach to preprocedural, intraprocedural, and postprocedural echocardiographic assessment of candidates for TAVI with the balloon expandable valve. Both the balloon expandable and a self-expanding valve are commercially available in Europe.

Preimplantation Echocardiographic Imaging for TAVI (Box 4-1)

- Measure the LVOT diameter in systole:
  - The LVOT diameter should be measured from parasternal long axis views in systole
    - The diameter is measured in parasternal long axis view typically between the annulus and 0.5 cm apical to the aortic

annulus in systole. The long axis view is used to measure the diameter of the LVOT since the septum and anterior leaflet of the MV are most parallel in this view; apical views should not be used.

- The largest measured diameter of the LVOT should be used in calculating the aortic valve area.
- In the setting of acoustic shadowing of the distal annulus, a lower or higher window can be used to better image the entire plane of the annulus.
- If the LVOT diameter cannot be accurately measured, the dimensionless index (cut-off of <0.25 for LVOT diameters of 2.4 cm and <0.2 for LVOT diameters of >2.4 cm) can be a more accurate indicator of aortic stenosis severity.
- Measure the aortic annulus diameter in systole:
  - The annulus should be measured from the long axis view in systole.
    - Measure the hinge point of the cusps.
    - Short axis views may be helpful in characterizing the appearance of the valve and aligning the long axis view perpendicular to the largest annular diameter (Fig. 4-10).

BOX 4-1 Preprocedural Echocardiographic Imaging Protocol for TAVI

AV and root
  Bicuspid vs trileaflet
    Bicuspid AV current contraindication to TAVR
  AV
    AV gradients and area
    Annular dimensions
      2 sizes for balloon-expandable transcatheter heart valve (THV)
      2 sizes for self-expanding THV
  Aortic calcification
    Extent and distribution
    Valve opening symmetric vs asymmetric
  Aortic root dimensions and calcification
    Location of coronary ostia
MV
  Severity of MR
  Severity of ectopic calcification
    Anterior leaflet calcification may affect placement of valve
LV size and function
  Wall motion
  Ejection fraction
  Wall thickness
    Upper septal hypertrophy
    LVOT morphology

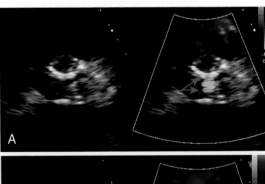

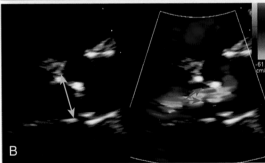

Figure 4-10. Short-axis views may be helpful in characterizing the appearance of the valve. Short axis images of the aortic valve (**A**) reveal aortic regurgitation in the commissure between the left and right coronary cups (*red arrows*). This same jet is imaged in the long axis view (**B**), which then helps identify the largest annular diameter (*yellow arrow*).

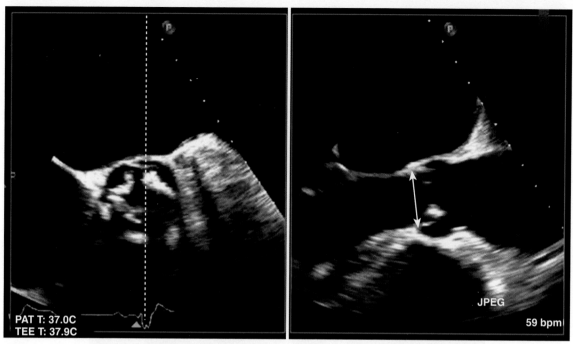

Figure 4-11. Using the biplane function of a real-time three-dimensional (RT3D) TEE probe allows simultaneous imaging of both long and short axis views and thus more accurate positioning of the longitudinal plane at the largest annular diameter.

- When TTE imaging does not allow a confident annular measurement to be made, TEE should be performed.
  - Using the biplane function of a real-time three-dimensional (RT3D) TEE probe allows more accurate positioning of the longitudinal plane at the largest annular diameter. The orthogonal short axis plane should be centered at its largest diameter (Fig. 4-11).
- Measure the aortic root in diastole:
  - Measure the length of the root (from annulus to sinotubular junction) and diameter of the sinotubular junction (STJ)
    - For the Edwards Sapien balloon expandable valve (Edwards Lifesciences, Irvine, CA), the height of the 23-mm valve is 14.5 mm and the height of the 26-mm valve is 16 mm.
- Measure the left main coronary artery ostium height:
  - Use RT3D volumes (TEE) to image the left main coronary ostium in the coronal plane.
    - Obtain a full volume or zoom volume of the entire aortic valve and aortic root (including the left main coronary artery).
    - In the multiplanar reconstruction mode, align any of the planes in the coronal view to include the ostium of the left main coronary artery.
  - Measure the distance between the annulus and the proximal ostium of the left main coronary artery in systole.
  - Attempt to measure the length of the left coronary cusp in systole (note: this may be difficult in the setting of severe calcification and significantly reduced mobility) (Fig. 4-12).
  - A distance of greater than 10 mm is desirable for the 23-mm balloon expandable valve, and a distance of greater than 11 mm is desirable for the 26-mm valve.
- Assess LV and RV size and function:
  - Although either no change or improvement in function is typically observed, an acute reduction in LV or RV function may be a clue to coronary artery compromise by the THV stent.
- Assess mitral and tricuspid regurgitation:
  - Although either no change or improvement in function is typically observed, an acute change in valvular function may be the first clue to an acute hemodynamic change. A full preimplantation assessment is always performed.
- Assess aortic valve function by Doppler.

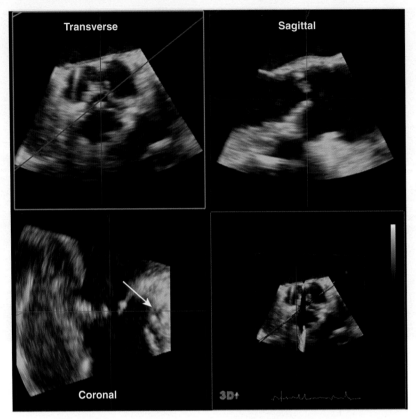

Figure 4-12. Multiplanar reconstruction images showing generation of a coronal plane view of the aortic root. This view, which cannot be obtained with two-dimensional (2D) imaging, provides a means for measuring the distance from the annulus to the left main coronary ostium.

Pitfalls

- Calcification of the anterior mitral leaflet should be excluded from LVOT diameter measurement (Fig. 4-13).
- The annulus measurement is the most critical for deciding the size of the valve to be used, and incorrect measurement is the most common reason for TAVI adverse outcome and residual aortic regurgitation (AR) following valve deployment.
  - There are currently two balloon expandable valve sizes available in the United States.
  - The 23-mm valve is typically placed for an annular measurement of 18 to 22 mm. The 26-mm valve is typically placed for an annular measurement of 22 to 25 mm.
  - Annular measurement of greater than 25 mm is an exclusion criterion for the balloon expandable valve
- Irregular calcification of the STJ may be best characterized by 3D imaging.
- The minimum and maximum dimensions of the STJ should be measured and may influence the size of the THV chosen.

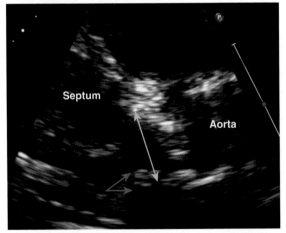

Figure 4-13. Calcification of the anterior mitral leaflet (*red arrows*) should be excluded from LVOT diameter measurement (*yellow arrow*).

- 3D echocardiography may be used in the future to planimeter the area of the LVOT or annulus; however, poor resolution compared with two-dimensional (2D) imaging limits the routine use of 3D imaging for this purpose.

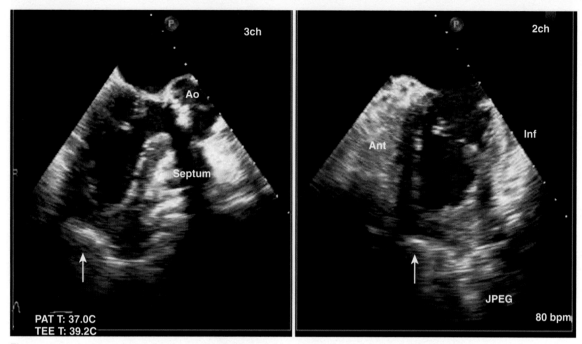

Figure 4-14. Imaging during transapical catheter insertion may be used to help confirm the location of apical cannulation: the surgeon may digitally identify the apex (*arrow*) prior to insertion of the apical cannula. *Left panel*: Three-chamber view; *right panel*: two-chamber view.

Intraprocedural Transesophageal Echocardiographic Imaging

- Intraprocedural imaging can be performed in single plane mode; however, biplane mode is highly recommended for rapid on-axis assessment of structures from simultaneous orthogonal views.
- There are two approaches to TAVI: transfemoral and transapical. Although imaging of catheter advancement is typically not required for the transfemoral approach, additional imaging is typically required for transapical TAVI.
  - Image the MV apparatus during transapical catheter insertion.
  - Confirm the location of apical cannulation (Fig. 4-14): (1) a mid-esophageal apical three-chamber view is typically used; (2) the apical cannulation site is typically anterolateral to the true apex.
  - Continuously image during needle insertion and advancement of the guidewire.
  - Use color Doppler to assess MV function, particularly following insertion of the stiff wire.
- Imaging the aortic valve apparatus during balloon aortic valvuloplasty (BAV):
  - Immediately following balloon deflation, increased mobility of the aortic cusps and assessment of aortic regurgitation severity are made from both long and short axis views of the aortic valve.
  - If using a RT3D TEE probe, biplane mode may be utilized for simultaneous imaging of mid-esophageal long and short axis views of the aortic valve.
- Balloon inflation may be imaged with color Doppler to confirm annular size and balloon inflation volume (Fig. 4-15).
  - Characterization of the regurgitant jets around the balloon may help focus post-TAVI imaging for AR.
- Imaging the aortic valve apparatus during positioning of the TAVI stent:
  - Long axis view of the aortic valve is used to confirm TAVI stent positioning prior to deployment.
  - The valve stent crimped on the balloon should typically be centered on the aortic annulus (50% above and below the annulus) (Fig. 4-16).
    - Typically, the LV edge of the THV should align with the hinge point of the anterior mitral leaflet.
    - Some operators may prefer to position the valve more than 50% below the annulus.
    - Optimal positioning of the valve should always be individualized based on the anatomy of the LVOT, annulus, and aortic root, and position of the coronary ostia.

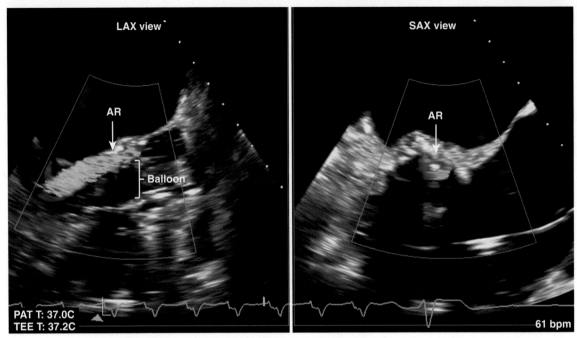

Figure 4-15. Balloon inflation may be imaged with color Doppler to confirm annular size and balloon inflation volume.

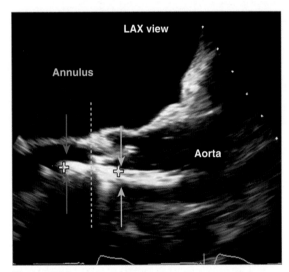

Figure 4-16. The valve stent crimped on the balloon (*between yellow and red arrows*) should typically be centered on the aortic annulus (*blue dashed line*).

Pitfalls

- Because of the significant acoustic density of the stent, reducing the overall gain may reduce the acoustic noise of the balloon, which enhances the borders of the stent.
- If using single plane imaging, the long axis of the aortic valve apparatus is recommended. In biplane mode either the short or long axis view may be the primary view; however, the long axis view is preferred to minimize probe manipulation for post-TAVI imaging.
- Use of 3D narrow sector or thin slice imaging may be helpful if the stent cannot be identified on 2D images.

Postprocedural Transesophageal Echocardiographic Imaging

- Although the position of the valve prior to deployment can be assessed using fluoroscopy alone, the immediate and precise assessment of both valve position and integrity, as well as coronary patency and LV function, is best accomplished by echocardiography.
- The biplane mode may be most useful for post-TAVI imaging; both long and short axis views of the THV must be rapidly assessed.
- Imaging the THV:
  - Immediately after valve deployment, image TAVI stent position and leaflet motion from long and short axis views (Fig. 4-17).
  - Color Doppler of the aortic valve from long and short axis views to assess:

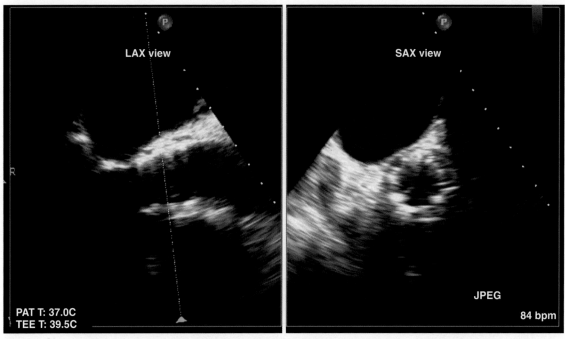

Figure 4-17. Immediately after valve deployment, TAVI stent position and leaflet motion from long and short axis views.

- Presence/severity of paravalvular regurgitation; short axis plane imaged should be just below the TAVI stent.
- Patency of the left main coronary artery; short axis plane imaged should be in the aortic root.
- Biplane mode, imaging the long axis aorta as the primary view allows rapid acquisition of both the above short axis views without moving or rotating the probe.
- If significant aortic regurgitation is seen, a repeat balloon dilatation of the stent may be performed.
- Confirmation of the severity of aortic regurgitation should always be performed from the deep gastric views (Fig. 4-18).
  - Acoustic shadowing of the anterior TAVI annulus in mid-esophageal views can underestimate the presence/severity of aortic regurgitation.
  - Imaging the entire annulus is mandatory and requires rotating 180 degrees while centered on the valve.
  - Alternatively, use biplane imaging, rotating 90 degrees.
- Assess THV by Doppler:
  - Pulsed wave Doppler of the LVOT and CW Doppler across the TAVI are obtained to calculate THV area.

- Quantitative Doppler is performed to determine the regurgitant volume using the RV outflow tract stroke volume as the forward stroke volume. Full-volume 3D color Doppler acquisition can be performed for planimetry of the regurgitant jet orifices using multiplanar reconstruction (Fig. 4-19).
- Reimaging of the MV, left ventricle, right ventricle, tricuspid valve, and aorta are performed.
  - The order of imaging of these structures may be dictated by the interventionalists, surgeon, or anesthesiologist, depending on the clinical status of the patient.
  - Abnormalities pre-TAVI should be imaged post-TAVI (i.e., mobile atheroma, significant MR, or tricuspid regurgitation).

Pitfalls

- If using a single plane mode, the short axis view is preferred. If using biplane mode, the primary image should be the long axis view with the second (biplane) image the short axis view. This allows the imager to rapidly steer the short-axis plane along the aortic valve and root.
- The right coronary artery is infrequently imaged because of acoustic shadowing.

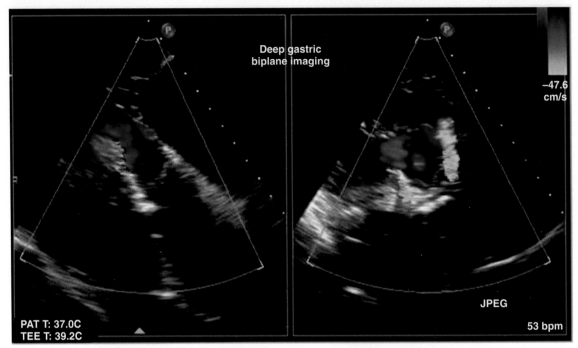

Figure 4-18. Confirmation of the severity of aortic regurgitation should always be performed from the deep gastric views.

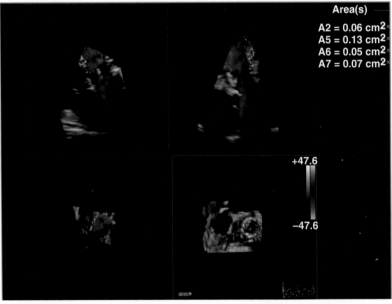

Figure 4-19. Full-volume 3D color Doppler acquisition can be performed for planimetry of the regurgitant jet orifices using multiplanar reconstruction.

<table>
<tr><td colspan="2">KEY POINTS</td></tr>
</table>

KEY POINTS

- Accurate measurement of the aortic annulus, aorta dimensions, and coronary locations is key to choosing the appropriate size transcatheter heart valve and plan for the appropriate positioning of the THV.
- Intraprocedural imaging using multiplane TEE or RT3D TEE is used primarily for confirming the

position of the THV prior to deployment, as well as to monitor for possible complications (including paravalvular aortic regurgitation) during the immediate postprocedural period.
- Multiple planes (including nonstandard views) are needed to confirm THV position and function.

ENDOVASCULAR MITRAL VALVE REPAIR

Background

- Although all parts of the mitral apparatus are potential targets for transcatheter repair in the setting of severe MR, the procedure that has the largest number of implantations and the greatest worldwide experience is percutaneous mitral leaflet repair with the MitraClip (Abbott Vascular, Abbott Park, IL).
- Reports of percutaneous MV repair with the MitraClip system show low rates of morbidity and mortality, as well as acute MR reduction to less than 2+ in the majority of patients and sustained freedom from death, surgery, or recurrent MR in a substantial proportion.[3]
- Echocardiography is the primary imaging tool for preprocedural patient selection and intraprocedural device positioning and implantation.

Preimplantation Echocardiographic Imaging for the Mitral Valve Clip

- Preprocedural TTE and TEE are performed to assess the MV leaflet anatomy and the severity of MR:
  - The optimal patient has MR originating from A2-P2 mal-coaptation, best seen in the parasternal long axis or apical three-chamber view.
  - Any MV imaging plane with the aorta in view images portions of the A2 and P2 scallops.
- Two TEE intraprocedural imaging techniques may be used for the standard imaging protocol:
  - Multiplane TEE:
    - Five key echocardiographic views are used to help position the endovascular device (Fig. 4-20): (1) Mid-esophageal long axis view (100–160 degrees): to position the device in the anterior-posterior (A-P) direction (note: both anterior and posterior MitraClip arms should be visible and of equal length in this view). (2) Mid-esophageal intercommissural view (55–75 degrees): this view guides positioning of the device in the medial-lateral (M-L) direction. (3) Mid-esophageal four-chamber view (0–20 degrees): this view allows determination of the transseptal height (above the annular plane). (4) Bicaval view (80–110 degrees): this view is used for transseptal A-P positioning and to determine the relation of the device to lateral structures. (5) Transgastric short axis views at the levels of the MV and LV (0–20 degrees): this view is used to align the MitraClip arms perpendicular to the leaflet line of coaptation.
  - RT3D TEE:
    - RT3D has significantly changed the imaging protocol for percutaneous mitral repair (Fig. 4-21).
    - RT3D TEE allows 3D visualization of the entire mitral leaflet line of coaptation from the surgical view of the left atrium (*en face*) and reduces the need to move between the multiple views to confirm catheter and clip position.
    - This same *en face* view allows for accurate alignment of the clip arms to the line of coaptation.
  - All imaging protocols require:
    - Measurement of the "tethering" height and coaptation length for functional MR (Fig. 4-22A).
    - Measurement of the flail width and flail gap for degenerative, flail MR (see Fig. 4-22B).
    - Note: patients with MR due to rheumatic disease, endocarditis, or congenital abnormalities are not candidates for the MitraClip.

Intraprocedural Standing Imaging Protocol

- Transseptal puncture and introduction of catheters:
  - Locate the position and direction of transseptal catheter puncture (Fig. 4-23).
    - 3.5 to 4 cm above the annular plane
    - Mid-posterior fossa
    - Posterior and superior direction of the catheter
  - Position the MitraClip guiding catheter so that the tip (double-echodensity) is across the interatrial septum (Fig. 4-24).
- Advancing the clip delivery system:
  - Continuously image the guide catheter as the delivery catheter system (with clip) is introduced into the left atrium.
    - The catheter should avoid contact with lateral structures in the left atrium.
  - Guide the manipulation of the steering mechanisms to position the clip above the A2-P2 scallops (Fig. 4-25).

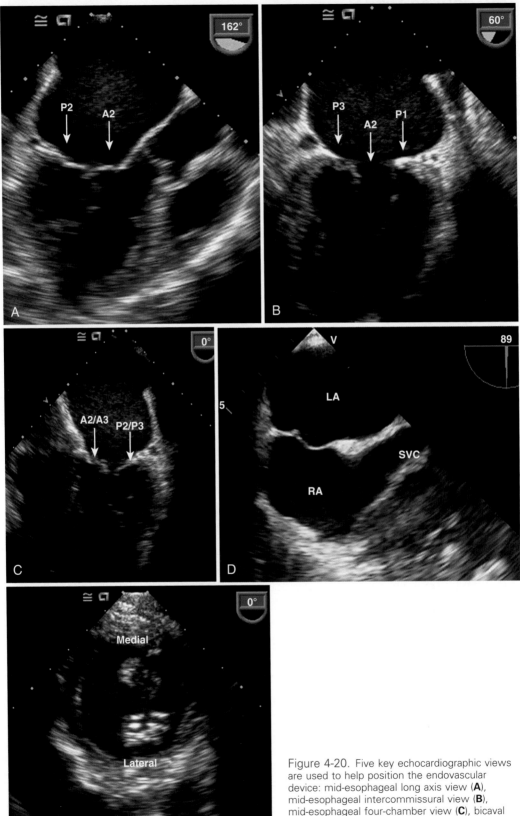

Figure 4-20. Five key echocardiographic views are used to help position the endovascular device: mid-esophageal long axis view (**A**), mid-esophageal intercommissural view (**B**), mid-esophageal four-chamber view (**C**), bicaval view (**D**), and transgastric short axis view at the MV and in the left ventricle (**E**).

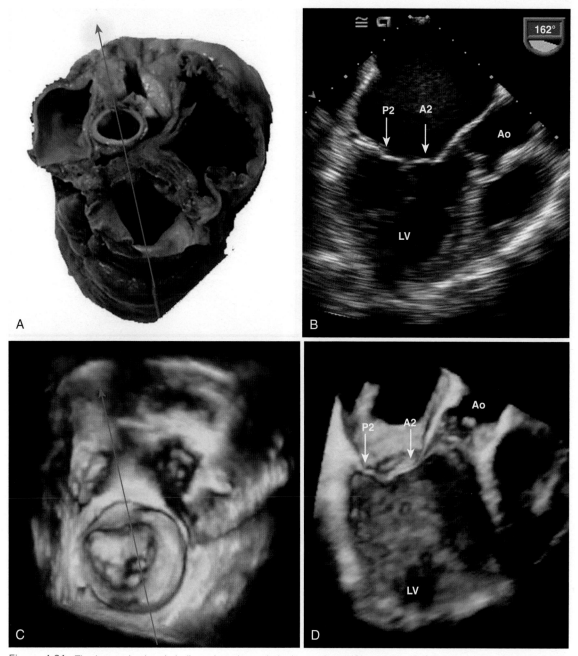

Figure 4-21. The long axis view is indicated on the pathologic specimen (**A**), and the 3D full-volume view (**C**) by the *red arrow*. The corresponding 2D (**B**) and 3D (**D**) views are shown. For MV procedures, imaging the *en face* view of the entire MV by RT3D has significantly changed the imaging protocol eliminating the need for mental reconstruction of the valve using 2D images.

- Position the clip and orient the clip arms:
  - Based on the preprocedural anatomic imaging (TEE) of the MV, the clip is positioned over the regurgitant orifice.
  - The clip arms are partially opened to determine orientation.
    - Echocardiographic imaging guides the orientation/rotation of the clip arms to be perpendicular to the leaflets at the site of the regurgitant orifice. (Note: although typically the clip is perpendicular to the commissures, maximum reduction in regurgitant volume may require an off-axis orientation of the clip.)
  - Use color Doppler to confirm positioning above the regurgitant jet (Fig. 4-26).

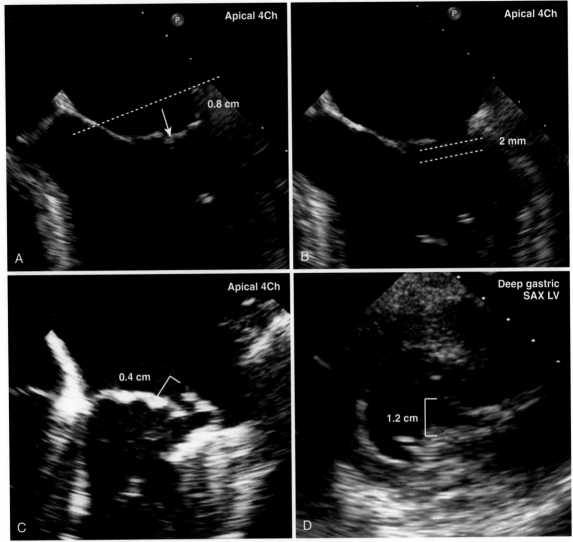

Figure 4-22. Anatomic measurements must be performed to assess the appropriateness of the MitraClip. For functional MR, measurements include the "tethering" height and coaptation length for (**A, B**). For degenerative MV disease, measurements include flail gap and flail width (**C, D**).

- Grasping the leaflets:
  - Follow the closed clip across the mitral orifice into the LV.
  - Once opened within the LV, document the orientation of the clip following these maneuvers and guide repositioning if needed.
  - Continuously image the two clip arms as the interventionalists withdraw the clip (toward the leaflets) and grasp both anterior and posterior leaflets with the device grippers.
  - Verify capture of both leaflets prior to full closure of the clip.
    - Multi-plane 2D imaging (Fig. 4-27A,B) or RT3D imaging (Fig. 4-28).
  - Recapture may be necessary if confirmation of capture cannot be made.
- With incremental closure of the clip:
  - Verify MR reduction (see Fig. 4-27C,D).
  - Planimetry of the double MV orifice area (Fig. 4-29).
- Deploy clip.
- Postdeployment assessment:
  - Verify MR reduction by multiple methods:
    - CW Doppler for peak and mean transmitral gradients
    - Color Doppler for mitral regurgitant jet area and vena contracta
    - Pulse-wave Doppler for reversal of pulmonary vein flow

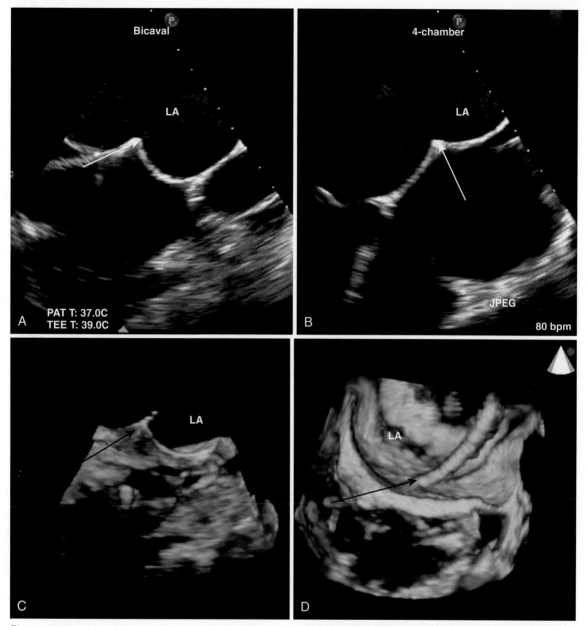

Figure 4-23. Locating the position and direction of the transseptal catheter puncture (*white arrows*) can be performed using alternating bicaval and four-channel views; however, the biplane mode (**A, B**) allows imaging of both views simultaneously. The height of the puncture above the annulus is measured. 3D imaging (**C, D**) is helpful in showing the direction of the transseptal catheter (*black arrows*).

- Planimetry of the regurgitant orifice using *en face* views of 3D color Doppler.
- Planimetry of the double MV orifice area:
  - 3D reconstruction and planimetry may be useful in the setting of non-planar orifices.
- Decide whether a second clip is required.
- Image the delivery catheter to ensure safe withdrawal (avoidance of lateral left atrial structures).
- Document the resulting interatrial defect.

Pitfalls

- Near-field imaging artifacts and other limitations may prevent adequate imaging of the transseptal puncture or guide catheter.
- Following clip deployment, acoustic shadowing from deep gastric views may limit the utility of this view for assessing both residual MR and the mitral diastolic area.

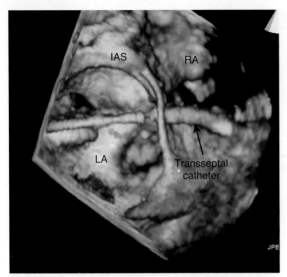

Figure 4-24. The MitraClip guiding catheter can be identified by the double echodensity at the tip. In this RT3D image, the catheter is well positioned across the interatrial septum.

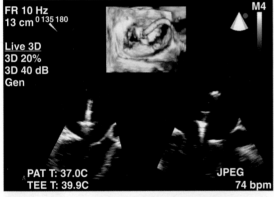

Figure 4-25. In this triplane imaging view, the RT3D image (*top*) shows the partially opened clip above the mitral orifice but not orthogonal to the commissures. The lower left panel shows the corresponding long axis view.

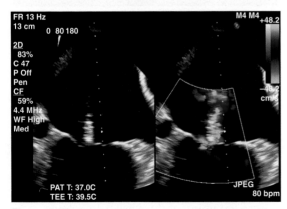

Figure 4-26. In this 2D and corresponding color Doppler image of the commissural view, color Doppler is used to confirm positioning of the clip above the regurgitant jet.

- Quantification of MR by 3D color Doppler in the setting of a mitral clip has not been validated.
- Continued discussion between the interventionalists and imager is required throughout the procedure.
- The interventionalists must understand and interpret the echocardiographic images obtained in order to accurately place the clip.

KEY POINTS

- Define MV anatomy and confirm severity and location of MR.
- Determine if the mitral anatomy is appropriate for MitraClip placement.
- Guide each step of clip placement: transseptal puncture, advancement of clip delivery system, positioning/orienting the clip arms, grasping the leaflets and deploying the clip.
- Measure the resulting double orifice MV area.
- Estimate the residual MR.

PERCUTANEOUS TRANSCATHETER REPAIR OF PARAVALVULAR REGURGITATION

Background

- Numerous reports of percutaneous transcatheter repair of paravalvular regurgitation have drawn attention to this nonsurgical option for high-risk patients. However, it must be noted that there are relatively few patients in whom this procedure has been performed and even fewer in whom the procedure has had long-term success.
- Multiple devices have been used in this procedure:
  - New devices to make this procedure more successful (crescent-shaped devices) are in development.
- Multiple procedural approaches are currently being used:
  - Retrograde (through the aortic valve)
  - Antegrade (through the interatrial septum)
  - Transapical (through the LV apex)
- Although theoretically paravalvular aortic regurgitation could be closed with percutaneous devices, in reality the constraint of the aorta will prevent placement of currently used devices in the majority of cases.
- The current section will be limited to a discussion of transcatheter treatment of paravalvular MR in the setting of mitral valve

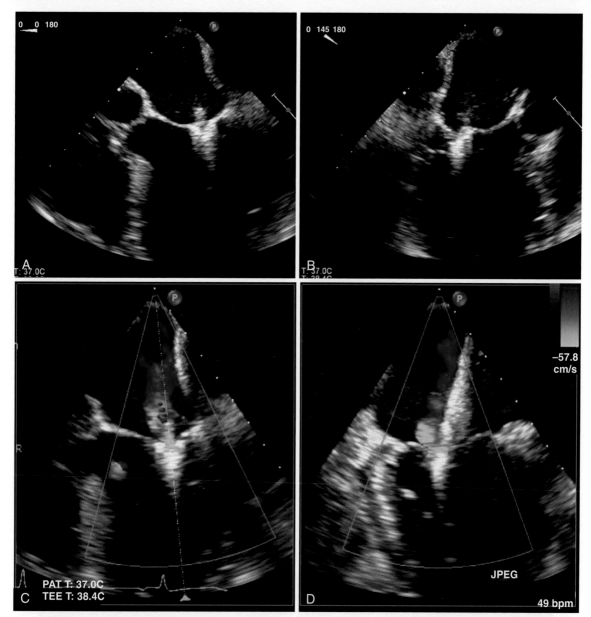

Figure 4-27. Prior to release, clip capture must be imaged from multiple views. The four-chamber (**A,** at 0 degrees) and long axis (**B,** at 145 degrees) views show clip capture of both anterior and posterior leaflets. Color Doppler of these same views (**C, D**) show minimal residual regurgitation around the clip, with incremental closure of the clip.

replacement (MVR). Imaging relies heavily on 3D reconstruction, and the basic approach to imaging (irrespective of the catheter approach) will be described.

Preprocedural Imaging

- RT3D imaging of the MV is preferred to reduce the number of multiplane images required to precisely define MVR anatomy.

- When using RT3D imaging, any modality (live/narrow volume, live/zoom volume, or full volume) may be used to image the MVR.
- Identify the location, number, and size of the paravalvular defect(s) (Fig. 4-30).
  - Determine type, size, and number of devices needed. The dimensions of the defect will determine the size of the devices used, realizing that the largest devices may interfere with prosthetic valve function.

- Determine optimal approach. Markedly anterior defects may be best approached by the transapical approach (Fig. 4-31).
- Image the regurgitant jets (Fig. 4-32).

Intraprocedural Imaging

- Image transseptal puncture (for antegrade approach).
  - TEE can help the interventionalists position the puncture to avoid puncture of the aorta or atrial wall.

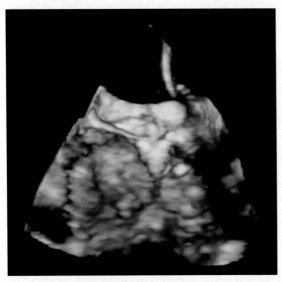

Figure 4-28. RT3D imaging can confirm clip capture with a single acquisition in any plane.

- Guide placement of guidewires across the paravalvular defect.
- Guide placement of devices within the paravalvular defect.
- Imaging of the MVR and device prior to and after deployment should include the following steps:
  - Determine device seating and stability.
  - Determine residual regurgitation and need for second device.
  - Determine function of the prosthetic valve.
    - Normal opening/closure of prosthetic valve leaflets/disks must be imaged prior to deployment (Fig. 4-33).

Pitfalls

- Mental reconstruction of the multiple 2D images may be inaccurate if the imaging plane is not aligned parallel to the apex. In addition, procedural guidance is more difficult using 2D imaging only.
- Echo dropout due to acoustic shadowing occurs in both 2D and 3D imaging and may appear as a defect but does not represent a true paravalvular dehiscence. It is imperative that the targeted defect be confirmed by color Doppler imaging.
- RT3D color Doppler is not currently available, and the narrow-angle volume that is generated by splicing subvolumes is rarely large enough to encompass the entire sewing ring; thus, reconstruction of portions of the annulus must be performed to image the entire sewing ring.

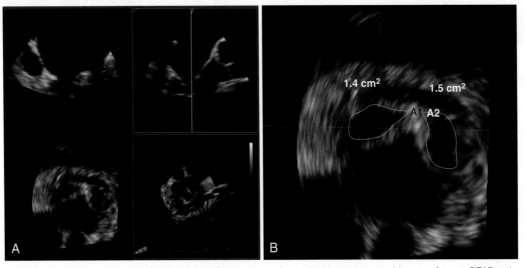

Figure 4-29. Planimetry of the double MV orifice (**B**) can be performed on reconstructed images from a RT3D volume set (**A**).

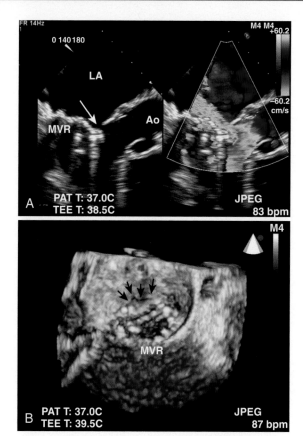

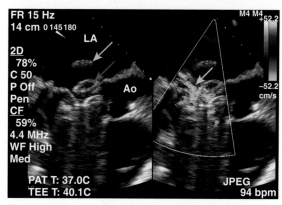

Figure 4-32. This 2D and corresponding color Doppler long axis view shows the first closure device (*red arrow*) in place with color Doppler continuing to show significant MR (*blue arrow*). A second device (*yellow arrow*) can be seen prior to positioning.

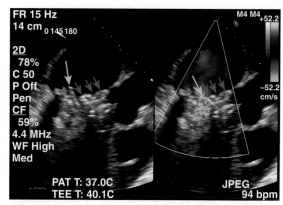

Figure 4-30. A 2D and corresponding color Doppler long axis view (**A**) with bileaflet mechanical MV replacement and an anterior paravalvular defect (*white arrow*). The RT3D image (**B**) better defines the location and size of the defect (*black arrows*).

Figure 4-33. This 2D and corresponding color Doppler long axis view shows the closure devices in place (*red arrows*); however, one disk fails to close (*blue arrow*), with corresponding turbulent diastolic color Doppler flow (*yellow arrow*).

KEY POINTS

- Define paravalvular anatomy and confirm paravalvular regurgitant orifice.
- Determine the appropriate approach to device placement based on paravalvular anatomy.
- Image device positioning with reduction of regurgitation prior to deployment.
- Confirm prosthetic valve function and any compromise to adjacent structures prior to device deployment.

References

1. Wilkins GT, Weyman AE, Abascal VM, et al. Percutaneous balloon dilatation of the mitral valve: an analysis of echocardiographic variables related to outcome and the mechanism of dilatation. *Br Heart J.* 1988;60:299-308.
   This is the original description and validation of the echo-based scoring system that remains the cornerstone of assessing the

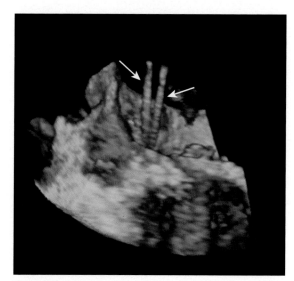

Figure 4-31. The defect imaged in Figure 4-30 is approached transapically with two wires crossing the defect (*arrows*).

probability of being able to successfully balloon dilate stenotic mitral valves.

2. Leon MB, Smith CR, Mack M, et al. Transcatheter aortic-valve implantation for aortic stenosis in patients who cannot undergo surgery. *N Engl J Med.* 2010;363: 1597-1607.
   This paper reports 1-year results from Cohort B (surgery vs. medical management in inoperable patients with severe symptomatic aortic stenosis) of the pivotal randomized trial of the Sapien balloon expandable transcatheter valve. Key findings were that transcatheter aortic valve implantation, as compared with standard therapy, significantly reduced the rates of death from any cause, the composite end point of death from any cause or repeat hospitalization, and cardiac symptoms, despite the higher incidence of major strokes and major vascular events.

3. Feldman T, Kar S, Rinaldi M, et al. Percutaneous mitral repair with the MitraClip system: safety and midterm durability in the initial EVEREST (Endovascular Valve Edge-to-Edge REpair Study) cohort. *J Am Coll Cardiol.* 2009;54:686-694.
   This study reports the mid-term results of Everest, the initial prospective multicenter single-arm study of the MitraClip device. Feasibility, safety and efficacy data are provided.

Suggested Reading

1. Sigwart U. Non-surgical myocardial reduction for hypertrophic obstructive cardiomyopathy. *Lancet.* 1995;346:211-214.
   This is the original report (12 patients) of alcohol septal ablation for the treatment of hypertrophic obstructive cardiomyopathy (HOCM).

2. Maron BJ. Role of alcohol septal ablation in treatment of obstructive hypertrophic cardiomyopathy. *Lancet.* 2000; 355:425-426.
   This commentary discusses treatment options for patients with HOCM, with an emphasis on the role for alcohol septal ablation.

3. Maron BJ, McKenna WJ, Danielson GK, et al. American College of Cardiology/European Society of Cardiology Clinical Expert Consensus Document on Hypertrophic Cardiomyopathy. A report of the American College of Cardiology Foundation Task Force on Clinical Expert Consensus Documents and the European Society of Cardiology Committee for Practice Guidelines. *Eur Heart J.* 2003;24:1965-1991.
   This document provides a consensus-driven overview of clinical aspects of hypertrophic cardiomyopathy. It includes a discussion of alcohol septal ablation and the role of echocardiography during this procedure. It may be downloaded from the website of the American College of Cardiology (www.cardiosource.org).

4. Padial LR, Freitas N, Sagie A, et al. Echocardiography can predict which patients will develop severe MR after percutaneous mitral valvulotomy. *J Am Coll Cardiol.* 1996;27:1225-1231.
   This is the original description and validation of an echocardiography-based score that can be used to predict the development of severe MR after percutaneous mitral valvulotomy.

5. Bonow RO, Carabello BA, Chatterjee K, et al. 2008 focused update incorporated into the ACC/AHA 2006 guidelines for the management of patients with valvular heart disease: a report of the American College of Cardiology/American Heart Association Task Force on Practice Guidelines (Writing Committee to revise the 1998 guidelines for the management of patients with valvular heart disease). Endorsed by the Society of Cardiovascular Anesthesiologists, Society for Cardiovascular Angiography and Interventions, and Society of Thoracic Surgeons. *J Am Coll Cardiol.* 2008;52:e1-e142.
   This is the latest version of the American College of Cardiology/American Heart Association guidelines for the management of patients with valvular heart disease and is available through the websites of the American College of Cardiology (www.cardiosource.org) and American Heart Association (www.myamericanheart.org)

6. Silvestry FE, Rodriguez LL, Herrmann HC, et al. Echocardiographic guidance and assessment of percutaneous repair for mitral regurgitation with the Evalve MitraClip: lessons learned from EVEREST I. *J Am Soc Echocardiogr.* 2007;20:1131-1140.
   This paper reports the importance of transesophageal echocardiography (TEE) guidance during placement of the MitraClip and emphasizes the use of predetermined standardized views.

7. Altiok E, Becker M, Hamada S, et al. Real-time 3D TEE allows optimized guidance of percutaneous edge-to-edge repair of the mitral valve. *JACC Cardiovasc Imaging.* 2010;3:1196-1198.
   This imaging vignette derived from 26 patients demonstrates the superior guidance of percutaneous edge-to-edge mitral valve repair using real-time 3D TEE versus 2D TEE.

8. Kim MS, Casserly IP, Garcia JA, et al. Percutaneous transcatheter closure of prosthetic mitral paravalvular leaks: are we there yet? *JACC Cardiovasc Interv.* 2009;2:81-90.
   This state-of-the-art paper examines the current state of transcatheter prosthetic mitral paravalvular leak closure, and describes the authors' experience using advanced imaging modalities for procedural guidance. It also illustrates some of the limitations associated with using existing devices for this procedure.

Intracardiac Echocardiography for Common Interventions on Structural Heart Disease

Anna E. Bortnick and Frank E. Silvestry

5

Introduction

- Intracardiac echocardiography (ICE) may be performed as a collaborative effort between the echocardiographer and interventionalist, or performed solo by a skilled interventionalist or electrophysiologist during a procedure.
- It is used as an alternative to transesophageal echocardiography (TEE) in guiding complex percutaneous noncoronary interventions (Box 5-1).
- Risks of ICE are listed in Box 5-2.
- Advantages of ICE include:
  - ICE may be used in a lightly sedated or nonsedated patient.
  - There is no risk of esophageal trauma or perforation.
  - There is no risk of overheating of the probe, as is possible with lengthy TEE procedures.
  - Many structures may be better visualized with ICE than on TEE, including the interatrial septum and its surrounding structures.
  - ICE may reveal abnormalities not appreciated on preprocedure transthoracic echocardiography (TTE), TEE, or other radiologic studies. For example, multiple fenestrations of an atrial septal defect (ASD), deficient rim, or anomalous pulmonary veins may all be better visualized with ICE than TEE.
  - ICE probes may be resterilized one to two times for multiple use, with the caveat that image quality may decline with successive resterilization.
- Certainly, real-time three-dimensional (3D) TEE images may be better in specific circumstances, such as percutaneous mitral valve (MV) repair with the MitraClip system, but most common interventional procedures do not need this degree of imaging precision.
- 3D ICE is currently being actively developed for clinical use (Biosense Webster SoundStar 3D ICE, Diamond Bar, CA).

- This chapter reviews how to obtain images with the Biosense Webster–distributed, Siemens-manufactured popular AcuNav catheter (Siemens Medical, Mountain View, CA), a commonly used phased array transducer, for ICE guidance of interventions on the interatrial septum, including ASD and patent foramen ovale (PFO) closure, transseptal puncture, and for guiding percutaneous balloon mitral valvuloplasty.
- A nearly identical approach can be used with the St. Jude Medical ViewFlex PLUS ICE catheter (St. Jude Medical, St. Paul, MN), with the exception that this catheter only offers two directions of steering (anterior and posterior), whereas the Biosense Webster catheter offers four directions of steering (anterior, posterior, rightward, and leftward). See the later discussion on the use of these steering directions.
- This chapter will not address the use of radial ICE with the Boston Scientific Ultra ICE catheter (Boston Scientific, Natick, MA). This system more closely resembles an intravascular ultrasound catheter as it provides radial ICE imaging and not phased array imaging. It is not steerable, nor does it offer full Doppler capabilities. Although it is used worldwide to guide procedures, it is exclusively used by interventionalists, electrophysiologists, and surgeons, and therefore not accessible to cardiac imagers per se.
- Table 5-1 lists the currently available ICE systems in greater detail.

Standard Views

- The Biosense Webster AcuNav catheter creates a standard, wedge-shaped display of imaging that is identical to that seen with the phased array catheters used for standard TTE and TEE.
  - It is a four-way steerable catheter, able to perform linear and Doppler measurements,

BOX 5-1 Procedures Guided by Intracardiac Echocardiography

Interventional cardiology
- Transseptal catheterization
- Percutaneous balloon valvuloplasty
- Percutaneous transcatheter closure of atrial and ventricular septal defect
- Alcohol septal ablation in hypertrophic obstructive cardiomyopathy
- Placement of percutaneous left ventricular support device
- Balloon or blade atrial septostomy
- Placement of left atrial appendage occlusion device
- Placement of stented valve prosthesis
- Echocardiographically guided right and left ventricular biopsy
- Congenital heart disease applications such as completion of Fontan and coarctation repair
- Placement of aortic endovascular graft
- Percutaneous mitral valve repair

Electrophysiology
- Pulmonary vein isolation for atrial fibrillation (including transseptal catheterization)
- Sinoatrial node modification for inappropriate sinus tachycardia
- Ablation of ventricular tachycardia originating from the left ventricular endocardium
- Ablation of ventricular tachycardia originating from the left ventricular epicardium
- Ablation of ventricular tachycardia originating from the aortic cusp
- Ablation of ventricular tachycardia originating from the right ventricular outflow tract

Diagnostic
- Alternative to transesophageal echocardiography in those with contraindication
- Aortic evaluation
- Tricuspid and pulmonic valve prosthetic valve evaluation
- Congenital heart disease

BOX 5-2 Potential Risks of Intracardiac Echocardiography

Vascular
- Vascular trauma at groin site
- Vascular bleeding and groin hematoma
- Retroperitoneal bleeding or hematoma
- Perforation of venous structures

Cardiac perforation
- Pericardial effusion
- Cardiac tamponade

Arrhythmia
- Atrial premature beats and atrial tachycardia
- Atrial fibrillation
- Ventricular ectopy
- Ventricular tachycardia
- Heart block

Thromboembolism
- Venous thromboembolism
- Arterial thromboembolism

Superficial cutaneous nerve palsy

and has full color Doppler flow imaging capability.
- The catheter is typically introduced into the right or left femoral vein in a neutral position and advanced into the right atrium (RA) using fluoroscopic guidance.
- The catheter may be placed in the aorta or other vascular structures that can accommodate its size.
- The catheter is then rotated clockwise in small 10- to 15-degree increments to image initially more posterior structures and flexed rightward or leftward as needed.

- The catheter also includes anterior and posterior flexion steering, allowing the catheter to move closer or away from structures, as well as "look up" (posterior deflection, which points the imaging array more cephalad or superiorly) or "look down" (anterior deflection, which points more caudad or inferiorly) at structures of interest.

Key Views

- Axially rotating the catheter to approximately 15 to 30 degrees ("home view") images the mid-RA, tricuspid valve, right ventricle, and a short axis view of the aortic valve (Fig. 5-1). Large atrial septal aneurysms can sometimes be seen from the home view, as can many PFOs and secundum ASDs.
- The right ventricular outflow tract and pulmonic valve can be brought into view at 30 to 40 degrees of axial rotation ("right ventricular outflow tract [RVOT] view") (Fig. 5-2).
- At 45 degrees of rotation ("left ventricular outflow tract [LVOT] view"), the left ventricle (LV) is seen in the oblique long axis, as well as a long axis view of the aortic valve. This view is often used for color Doppler evaluation of the aortic valve (Fig. 5-3) or when evaluating for a perimembranous ventricular septal defect.

TABLE 5-1 COMPARISON OF CURRENTLY AVAILABLE ICE CATHETERS AND THEIR ULTRASOUND SYSTEMS

	Boston Scientific Ultra ICE Catheter	Biosensense Webster AcuNav Diagnostic Ultrasound Catheter	St Jude Medical ViewFlex PLUS Catheter
Transducer Type	Radial/mechanical	Phased array	Phased array
Size	9 F	10 F 8 F	9 F
Useable Length	110 cm	90 cm (10 F) 110 cm (8 F)	NA
Ultrasound Frequencies	9 MHz	5.0–10.0 MHz (depends on system)	4.5–8.5 MHz
Ultrasound Modes	2D	2D M-mode Spectral Doppler Color Doppler Tissue Doppler	2D M-mode Spectral Doppler Color Doppler
Penetration Depth	~8 cm	~15 cm	~12–15 cm
Compatible Ultrasound System	Boston Scientific iLab System	Siemens GE	St Jude View Mate Z
System Versatility	IVUS and ICE	Variable	Variable
Insertion Technique	Guidewire and 10F long guiding sheath extends into right atrium	11F or 8–9F vascular access, echo and fluoroscopy guidance to imaging target	10F vascular access sheath, echo and fluoroscopy guidance to imaging target
Advantages	Lowest cost ($800), excellent near field resolution	Full echo Doppler capabilities, four-way steering, adjustable frequency, depth of penetration	Full echo Doppler capabilities, simplified user interface, depth of penetration
Disadvantages	2D only, limited depth, no steering	Cost	Cost, two-way steering

NA, not applicable

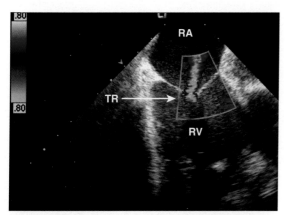

Figure 5-1. The home view. The mid-right atrium (RA), tricuspid valve (*arrow*) with color Doppler demonstrating tricuspid regurgitation (TR), and right ventricle (RV) are seen.

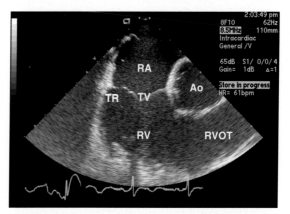

Figure 5-2. The right ventricular outflow tract view. From the home view, rotate slightly more clockwise to approximately 30 to 40 degrees. This angle brings the pulmonic valve (pulmV) into view. The mid-RA, tricuspid valve (not labeled), RV, and short axis view of the aortic valve (AV) are seen.

• Then the catheter may be inserted more superiorly into the RA, and clockwise rotated to 60 to 70 degrees ("left atrial appendage [LAA] view" or "lower interatrial septal view") (Figs. 5-4 and 5-5). The lower interatrial septum, left atrium (LA), left atrial appendage, MV, and an oblique view of the LV are seen in this view. This view is used for Doppler interrogation of the MV and guidance of balloon mitral valvuloplasty. If the LAA is well seen, then it may be possible to visualize medium to large thrombi.

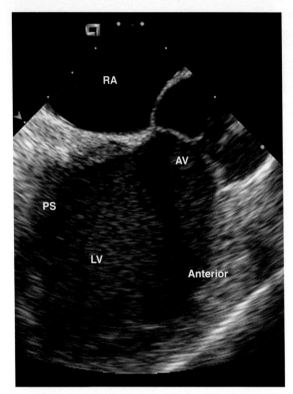

Figure 5-3. The left ventricular outflow tract (LVOT) view. This view brings the left ventricle (LV) into view in the oblique long axis. The anterior and posterior septal (PS) walls of the LV, the LVOT (not labeled), and the long axis view of the AV are seen. A portion of the RA is visualized. This view is best for color Doppler evaluation of the AV.

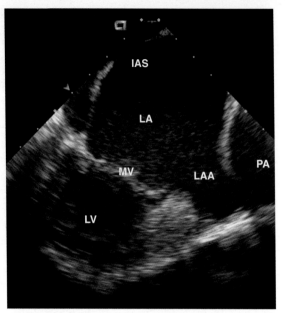

Figure 5-4. The lower interatrial septal and left atrial appendage view. These closely related views are obtained by advancing the catheter superiorly into the RA and rotating clockwise. A small left degree of anterior flexion may be required to direct the ultrasound beam toward the apex of the LV. This view is best for imaging the inferior portion of the interatrial septum (IAS), left atrium (LA), left atrial appendage (LAA), and mitral valve (MV). Color Doppler interrogation of the MV may be performed in this view, and thrombus or smoke in the LA can be evaluated. A four-chamber view can be obtained from this position by tilting the catheter to the right. The pulmonary artery (PA) is seen anteriorly.

- Typically, we enter the pulmonary artery to image the LAA when thrombus needs to be excluded definitively.
- Rotating to 90 to 100 degrees ("left pulmonary veins view") demonstrates the left inferior and left superior pulmonary veins in long axis (Fig. 5-6A). They extend from the LA with the interatrial septum at the top of the image, an ideal view for ICE-guided pulmonary vein isolation.
- The catheter may then be flexed posteriorly and rightward to obtain the "interatrial septal long axis view" (see Fig. 5-6B). This view is ideal for ASD and PFO closure, or transseptal puncture.
- Rotating and further posterior flexing the catheter results in the "septal short axis view" (Fig. 5-7). This view demonstrates the aortic valve in short axis and the upper interatrial septum, dividing the RA and LA. The pulmonic valve is also seen. This view is comparable with the short axis view of the septum and aortic valve seen on TEE.

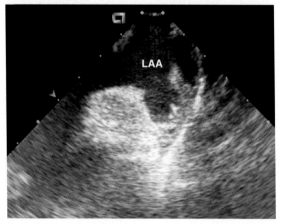

Figure 5-5. A zoomed image of the LAA from this view. Please note that imaging from the RA does not allow sufficient visualization to exclude small thrombus in the LAA.

- With the catheter returned to neutral, it is then further clockwise rotated to produce the "right pulmonary veins view" (Fig. 5-8). Here the short axis of the right inferior and superior pulmonary veins are visualized.

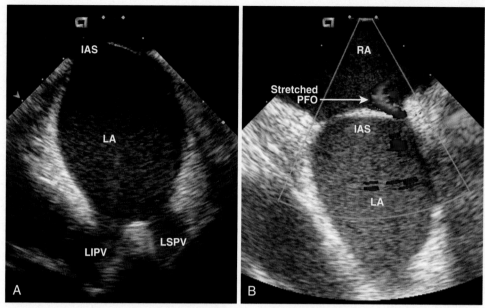

Figure 5-6. **A,** 90 to 100 degrees (left pulmonary veins view). This view demonstrates the IAS, LA, and long axis of the left inferior and left superior pulmonary veins (LIPV and LSPV, respectively). **B,** interatrial septal long axis view. This view is ideal for atrial septal defect (ASD) and patent foramen ovale (PFO) closure, or transseptal puncture. Pictured are the RA, IAS, LA, and color Doppler flow (*arrow*) from left to right through a stretched PFO.

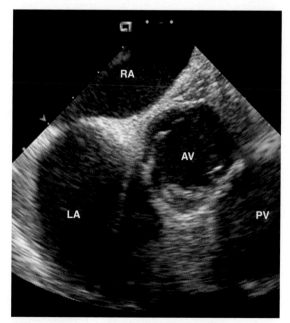

Figure 5-7. 100 to 150 degrees with posterior and rightward deflection (aortic or septal short axis view). This view demonstrates the AV in short axis and the upper IAS, dividing the RA and LA. The pulmonic valve is also seen. This view is comparable with the short axis view of the septum and AV seen on transesophageal echocardiography.

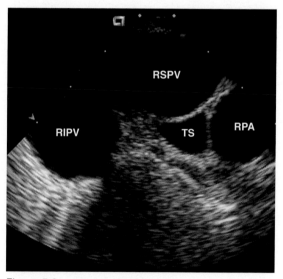

Figure 5-8. 150 to 180 degrees (right pulmonary veins view). This view demonstrates a short axis view of the right inferior and right superior pulmonary veins (RIPV and RSPV, respectively) and right pulmonary artery (RPA). The transverse sinus (TS) is often seen as well.

Atrial Septal Defect Closure

- Percutaneous closure of ASDs or PFO are common indications for ICE.
- Two of the most popular ASD and PFO closure devices are the Amplatzer PFO and ASD Occluders (AGA Medical Corp., Plymouth, MN, now merged with St. Jude, St. Paul, MN), and the Gore Helex device (W.L. Gore & Associates, Newark, DE). Numerous other devices are on the market or under investigation.
- The Amplatzer ASD Occluder consists of two nitinol self-expanding disks with polyester insert connected by a central waist of varying sizes.
  - The device is brought up inside a catheter, which is placed across the ASD (Figs. 5-9 through 5-12). The left atrial disk is deployed with a pushing motion, and then pulled up against the septum.
  - The right atrial disk is deployed in a similar fashion, and stability is checked by pushing and pulling the device against the septum.
  - The device delivery catheter must be unscrewed from the right atrial disk in order to release it. Color Doppler flow may be

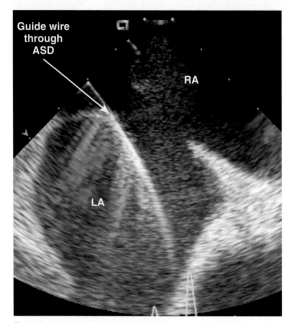

Figure 5-9. Guidewire crossing an ostium secundum ASD from the RA to the LA.

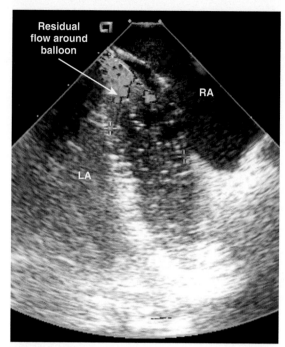

Figure 5-10. Demonstrates balloon sizing of an ASD prior to percutaneous closure. Color Doppler flow is used to demonstrate the maximal diameter where stoppage of flow is seen from the LA to the RA and the waist of the balloon as it crosses the ASD is measured. This frame demonstrates some residual flow around the balloon.

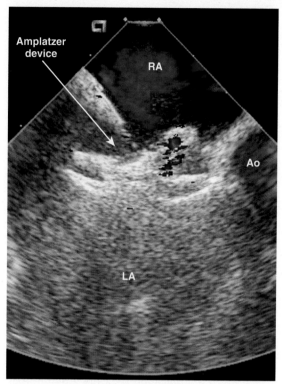

Figure 5-11. Placement of an Amplatzer ASD closure device in a secundum ASD. Shown is the LA, RA, device attached to the guiding cable (*arrow*), and aortic root (Ao). A small amount of residual color Doppler flow is seen as the device is pulled backward to ensure stability.

seen within the device until it endothelializes, but it should fully cover the defect and there should be no color jets around it.

- The Helex device (Gore Medical, Flagstaff, AZ) is made of an expanded polytetra-fluoroethylene (ePTFE) membrane stretched in a nitinol wire frame (Fig. 5-13).
  - Disks are formed against the septum by a "push, pinch, pull" technique in which the operator forms the left atrial then right atrial disks by extruding them from a catheter positioned across the septum.
- A "lock loop" pins the disks together. Both the Amplatzer and Helex devices are easily retrievable with snares even after withdrawing the device delivery catheters.
- ICE imaging for ASD closure involves quantifying the size and number of septal fenestrations, excluding anomalous pulmonary veins, measuring the septal rims for attaching the device, balloon sizing the defect, and assessing color Doppler flow pre- and postdeployment.
  - The septal rim of tissue, which is critical to be present for successful closure, is assessed in six quadrants—superior, anterosuperior, anteroinferior, inferior, posteroinferior, and

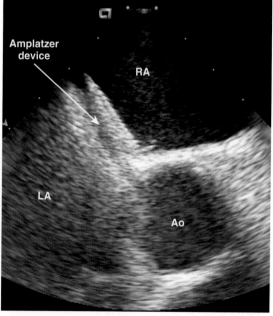

Figure 5-12. Final position of the ASD closure device after release from the guiding cable. Shown is the LA, RA, device attached to the guiding cable (*arrow*), and Ao.

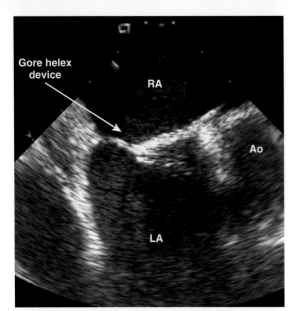

Gore helex device

RA

Ao

LA

Figure 5-13. Final position of a Gore Helex ASD closure device after release from the guiding cable. Shown is the LA, RA, device attached to the guiding cable (*arrow*), and Ao.

posterosuperior—and typically 4 to 5 mm of tissue around the defect is considered adequate. Numerous reports of successful closure exist with one area of rim deficiency, but numerous areas of inadequate rim may identify a patient who is not ideal for percutaneous transcatheter closure. The Helex device may be a better choice when there is deficient septal tissue along the aorta, as the ePTFE membrane is soft and conforming (see Fig. 5-13).

- For septal defect closure, ICE imaging begins in the home view. The tip is then flexed posteriorly and held in place by the locking mechanism.
- It should be pointed out that the lock merely holds the position, which then can be further adjusted against mild resistance.
- The interatrial septal long axis view is obtained by clockwise rotating to 90 to 100 degrees and flexing the catheter posteriorly. From this position, it is rotated clockwise to obtain the septal short axis view. This is an ideal working view for transcatheter closure.
- To see more of the superior aspect of the septum, the catheter may be advanced toward the superior vena cava to show the superior portion of the septum, then withdrawn into the inferior vena cava to show the inferior portion. In this regard, ICE is better suited than TEE to visualize the inferior septum.
- The operator or imager may need to switch to the lower interatrial septal/left atrial

appendage view at 60 to 70 degrees as needed to visualize additional parts of the septum.
- Repeat color Doppler imaging or agitated saline injection is typically performed prior to closure and at the end of the procedure after the device has been placed prior to its final release.

KEY POINTS

Best Views for Atrial Septal Defect and Patent Foramen Ovale Closure
- **15–30° (home view) with the tip flexed posteriorly and locked.** Scan the mid-right atrium, tricuspid valve, right ventricle, and aortic valve.
- **90–100° with posterior and rightward deflection (interatrial septal long axis view).** Examine the septum secundum and fossa ovalis.
- **100–150° with posterior and rightward deflection (aortic or septal short axis view).** This view shows the aortic valve in short axis and the upper septum. Be sure to look for deficient rim.
- **Take off flexion and advance in to the SVC in neutral.** Examine the superior septum.
- **Withdraw into the IVC** to show the inferior septum.
- **Reposition at 100–150° with posterior and rightward deflection (aortic short axis view),** the best working view to perform the procedure. Switch to the lower interatrial septal/left atrial appendage view at 60–70° as needed.

Transseptal Puncture

- Transseptal puncture is used for direct left atrial hemodynamics, device delivery to the left heart for percutaneous valve repair, and balloon stretching of interatrial septal defects when a sheath does not easily traverse the defect.
- The proper position for crossing the septum is at the mid-portion of the RA and posterior-inferior to the aortic valve.
- First obtain the interatrial septal long axis view by clockwise rotating to 90 to 100 degrees and aiming posteriorly, then rotating into the septal short axis view.
- Next, the Mullin sheath is brought into the RA and the Brockenbrough needle is advanced to the mid-septum until tenting is seen.
- The needle should go through at the level of the mid-septum. If the needle is directed too

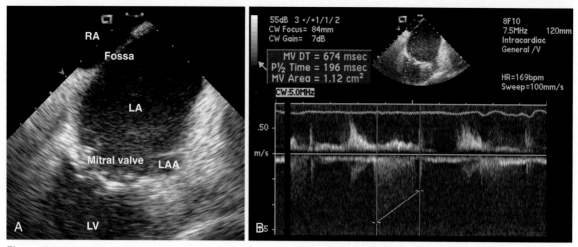

Figure 5-14. Lower septal view of patient with severe mitral stenosis. Shown is the LA, RA, fossa ovalis, MV, LV, and LAA. This view is used for obtaining continuous wave Doppler evaluation of mitral gradients and pressure half time estimation of the MV area, as is demonstrated in **B**.

low, it can potentially stitch both atria, risking bleeding into the pericardial space, and if the needle is directed too high, it can puncture the aorta.

KEY POINTS

Best Views for Transseptal Puncture
- **90–100° with posterior and rightward deflection (interatrial septal long axis view).** Examine the septum secundum and fossa ovalis.
- **100–150° with posterior and rightward deflection (aortic short axis view),** the best working view to perform the procedure. Be sure that the needle is in the mid-septum.

Mitral Valvuloplasty

- For balloon mitral valvuloplasty, ICE can be used to guide transseptal catheterization as described above, as well as monitor guidewire and balloon position, monitor during balloon inflation, and most importantly assess for mitral regurgitation after each inflation.
- ICE can be used for each of these steps.
- We typically start with the catheter mid-RA, and axially rotate approximately 60 to 70 degrees to the lower interatrial septal view. Often a small to moderate amount of anterior flexion is used to direct the beam caudad toward the valve. From this view, spectral Doppler can be performed to measure the mitral inflow deceleration slope and calculate the MV area by the pressure half-time

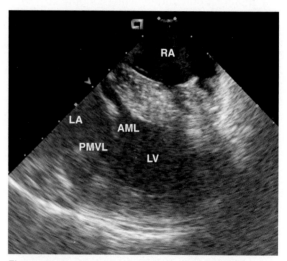

Figure 5-15. Advancing the ICE probe into the RV enables imaging of the MV leaflets and the LV in a long axis. Also pictured is the apex of the right ventricle (RV) and portion of the LA. AML, anterior mitral valve leaflet; PMVL, posterior mitral valve leaflet.

method. Peak and mean gradients can be measured using this view. Preprocedure mitral regurgitation is assessed by careful color Doppler evaluation (Fig. 5-14A and B).
- Additional views can be obtained of the LV, MV, and LA by advancing the catheter into the right ventricle and deflecting the catheter rightward to create an oblique long axis view of the LV. This is a good position to assess mitral regurgitation, mitral leaflet calcification, and subvalvular thickening (Fig. 5-15).
- After a careful baseline examination, the procedure begins by performing transseptal puncture with ICE guidance, as previously described.

- Once through the septum in the LA, the catheter is returned to the 15- to 30-degree home view and the guidewire and sheath are advanced into the LA under ICE guidance.
- After the wire is securely positioned in the LA, the catheter is rotated to the 60 to 70 degree left atrial appendage view/lower interatrial septal view to evaluate the MV and LV.
- A wire is placed across the MV over which the balloon is inflated. Once the balloon is pulled back, we typically repeat the spectral Doppler analysis, recalculate the MV area, and reassess mitral regurgitation.
- Once the valvuloplasty equipment is removed, the catheter may be returned back to the septal short axis view at 100 to 150 degrees to evaluate the small ASD created by the transseptal puncture on color Doppler.

> ## KEY POINTS
>
> **Best Views for Balloon Mitral Valvuloplasty**
> - **60–70° (lower interatrial septal view).**
> - **90–100° with posterior and rightward deflection (septal long axis view).** Examine the septum secundum and fossa ovalis.
> - **100–150° with posterior and rightward deflection (aortic short axis view),** the best working view to perform the transseptal portion of the procedure.
> - **15–30° (home view) with the tip flexed posteriorly.** Focus on wire and catheter passage into the mid-right atrium, then across into the left atrium.
> - **60–70° (lower interatrial septal view).** The lower interatrial septum, left atrium, left atrial appendage, and mitral valve are well seen. Focus on balloon inflation from this view. Color Doppler interrogation of the mitral valve is best in this view.
> - **100–150° with posterior and rightward deflection (aortic short axis view).** Return to this view after balloon mitral valvuloplasty is performed to examine the atrial septal defect created during the transseptal portion of the procedure.

Imaging of Complications

- The operator performing ICE should be prepared to evaluate for complications during and after ICE-guided procedures.
  - Thrombus formation on wires or devices, perforation of cardiac, arterial, or venous structures, and pericardial effusion are some

of the complications to be aware of and monitor for vigilantly.
- Views for imaging a pericardial effusion include the 15 to 30 degree home view, which shows the right ventricular free wall, and the 45 degree left ventricular outflow tract view, which shows the inferior wall of the LV. Occasionally, the ICE catheter is placed in the right ventricle to scan for effusion as well.
- Doppler interrogation to examine inflow variation across the tricuspid valve is best from the 15 to 30 degree home view and from the 60 to 70 degree lower interatrial septal view for the MV.
- Overall, ICE imaging should decrease the chance of having major complications.

Conclusion

- Intracardiac echocardiography is widely used to guide transcatheter interventions for structural heart disease to facilitate procedural success and minimize complications.
- Phased array transducers such as the AcuNav are popular because they produce images similar to those of TEE and may be performed solo by the interventionalist or electrophysiologist who is the primary operator of the procedure.
- Standard views and specific imaging protocols are helpful for interventions on the interatrial septum, transseptal puncture, and balloon mitral valvuloplasty.
- If 3D ICE transducers produce images of comparable quality to those of 3D TEE, it could become a favored imaging mode for newer, more complex interventional techniques, such as clipping of regurgitant MV leaflets, transcatheter aortic valve replacement, and left atrial appendage occlusion.

Suggested Reading
1. Silvestry FE, Kerber RE, Brook MM, et al. Echocardiography-guided interventions. *J Am Soc Echocardiogr.* 2009;22:213-231.
   This article is the ASE guidelines for the use of echocardiography in guiding interventions. It includes a discussion of intracardiac echocardiography.
2. Hudson PA, Eng MH, Kim MS, et al. A comparison of echocardiographic modalities to guide structural heart disease interventions. *J Interv Cardiol.* 2008; 21:535-546.
   This article provides a discussion of the advantages and disadvantages of ICE and TEE as tools to guide structural heart disease interventions.
3. Hijazi Z, Wang Z, Cao Q, et al. Transcatheter closure of atrial septal defects and patent foramen ovale under

intracardiac echocardiographic guidance: feasibility and comparison with transesophageal echocardiography. *Catheter Cardiovasc Interv.* 2001;52:194-199.
This paper reports the feasibility of using ICE to guide atrial septal device placement procedures and includes a discussion of the strengths and weaknesses of this approach vs. TEE.

4. Silvestry FE, Weigers SE, eds. *Intracardiac Echocardiography.* New York, NY: Taylor & Francis; 2006.
This textbook is a definitive reference for intracardiac echocardiography.

5. Sievert H, Qureshi SA, Wilson N, Hijazi ZM, eds. *Percutaneous Interventions for Congenital Heart Disease.* Oxon, United Kingdom: Informa Healthcare Books UK Ltd; 2007.
This book provides a discussion of closure devices for ASDs and PFOs and offers a background for understanding the selection of devices.

6. Bannan A, Herrmann HC. Transseptal catheterization in adults. In: Hijazi ZM, Feldman T, Cheatham JP, Sievert H, eds. *Complications of Percutaneous Intervention for Congenital and Structural Heart Disease.* New York: Informa Healthcare Books; 2009.
This chapter provides a discussion of transseptal catheterization and its complications.

7. Perk G, Lang RM, Garcia-Fernandez MA, et al. Use of real time three-dimensional transesophageal echocardiography in intracardiac catheter based interventions. *J Am Soc Echocardiogr.* 2009;22:865-882.
This paper illustrates the utility of 3D TEE for guiding a variety of catheter-based interventions.

8. Applebaum RM, Kasliwal RR, Kanojia A, et al. Utility of three-dimensional echocardiography during balloon mitral valvuloplasty. *J Am Coll Cardiol.* 1998;32:1405-1409.
This paper illustrates the utility of 3D TEE for guiding mitral balloon valvuloplasty. It provides a framework for considering the potential advantages of 3D ICE (when available).

Strain and Strain Rate Imaging

Thomas H. Marwick

6

Basic Principles

Assessment of Left Ventricular Function
- Assessment of left ventricular (LV) function is the most common indication for echocardiography.
- The most widely used parameter for this measurement is ejection fraction (EF). Although this measure is simple and intuitive, as well as being supported by a wealth of prognostic information, it has important limitations:
  - Image quality dependence
  - Geometric assumptions
  - Load dependence
  - Insensitivity to early disease
- There is an emphasis on moving from the diagnosis of late heart failure (advanced structural change, poor outcome) to early stage heart failure (limited structural change—more chance of reversal). Early myocardial disease is usually characterized by:
  - Disturbances of longitudinal function
  - Compensatory radial and circumferential function (and hence preserved EF)
- Recognition of longitudinal dysfunction is an important process in heart failure with normal EF.

Defining Strain
- Strain is a fundamental physical property of matter that reflects its deformation under an applied force.
- Strain can be expressed in any dimension—radial, longitudinal, or circumferential:
  - Longitudinal deformation has been the most widely assessed.
  - Speckle strain (see later discussion) can measure circumferential and radial strain more readily than tissue velocity

techniques, but radial strain is difficult to measure by any method.
- Potentially, shear stresses between these planes may be identified.
- Strain may be measured as Lagrangian or natural strain:
  - Lagrangian strain is defined on the basis of deformation from the original length (i.e., not subject to external forces):
    $e_L = \{L_t - L_{(t=0)}\}/L_{(t=0)}$
  - Natural strain is defined relative to a previous time instance but not original length: $e_N = \ln\{1 + e_t\}$
  - Natural strain is more relevant to cardiac imaging.
  - Lagrangian and natural strain are analogous at low strain (<10%), and one can be corrected to the other.
- In the tissue Doppler methodology, strain rate (SR) was derived from the gradient of velocity over a sampling distance, and strain obtained as the integral.
- Using speckle tracking, strain is derived from excursion of the speckles, and SR is derived from differentiation of the strain curve.
- By convention:
  - Shortening is described as negative strain (the main longitudinal waveform).
  - Lengthening is described by positive strain (the main radial component) (Fig. 6-1).
- Strain can be measured as:
  - a magnitude (i.e., the nadir of the strain signal)
  - a rate of change (SR)
  - a timing parameter (time to peak strain)
  - a mixture of magnitude and timing (SR, end-systolic strain)
- Potential magnitude parameters include:
  - Peak systolic SR
  - Peak isovolumic relaxation (IVR) SR (i.e.,

84

TABLE 6-1 NORMAL RANGES OF STRAIN AND SR HAVE BEEN DEFINED AT EACH PHASE OF THE CARDIAC CYCLE

	Septum	Lateral	Inferior	Anterior
Peak systolic wave (Ssr)				
Basal	0.99 ± 0.49	1.5 ± 0.74	0.88 ± 0.39	1.64 ± 0.9
Mid	1.25 ± 0.73	1.29 ± 0.58	0.95 ± 0.54	0.98 ± 0.68
Apical	1.15 ± 0.5	1.09 ± 0.59	1.38 ± 0.45	1.05 ± 0.63
Early diastolic wave (Esr)				
Basal	1.95 ± 0.89	1.92 ± 1.11	1.85 ± 0.89	2.03 ± 0.99
Mid	1.94 ± 0.97	1.71 ± 0.66	1.92 ± 1.2	1.7 ± 0.82
Apical	1.91 ± 0.66	1.81 ± 0.87	2.29 ± 0.88	1.76 ± 0.98
Late diastolic wave (Asr)				
Basal	1.54 ± 0.93	0.93 ± 0.59	1.18 ± 0.78	1.49 ± 0.96
Mid	1.29 ± 0.86	1.48 ± 0.77	0.78 ± 0.62	1.04 ± 0.57
Apical	0.95 ± 0.54	1.07 ± 0.68	1.68 ± 0.76	0.68 ± 0.65
Displacement (D)				
Basal	1.2 ± 0.19	0.93 ± 0.22	1.33 ± 0.22	1.05 ± 0.27
Mid	1.13 ± 0.27	0.91 ± 0.18	0.62 ± 0.22	1.04 ± 0.19
Apical	0.65 ± 0.24	0.82 ± 0.27	0.55 ± 0.18	0.41 ± 0.25
Systolic strain (E)				
Basal	17.5 ± 5.32	18.22 ± 6.79	14.97 ± 5.74	22.19 ± 7.75
Mid	18.27 ± 6.96	18.83 ± 5.29	14.2 ± 5.14	17.95 ± 5.53
Apical	19.31 ± 6.07	17.56 ± 5.85	23.6 ± 5.17	13.17 ± 5.83

Displacement shown in centimeters. Systolic strain shown in percent.
Peak systolic (Ssr), early (Esr), and late (Asr) diastolic strain rates shown in 1/s.

peak SR between aortic valve closure [AVC] and mitral valve opening [MVO])
- Peak early diastolic SR
- Peak systolic strain
- End-systolic strain
- Maximum strain
- Postsystolic thickening (maximum strain after AVC minus end-systolic strain)
- Potential timing parameters include:
  - Time to relaxation (i.e., time to SR crossover at middle of cycle)
  - Time to contraction (i.e., time to SR crossover at start of cycle)
  - Time to peak SR
- Normal ranges of strain and SR have been described (Table 6-1). SR and strain may be expressed as curves relating to measures at one site (see Fig. 6-1) or in a parametric map (Fig. 6-2) where colors express magnitudes at various sites.
- There are minor differences between strain measurements provided by vendors. Nonetheless, strain and SR on all commercial systems have been extensively validated:

- Clinical validations have been performed on the basis of comparison with tagged magnetic resonance imaging (MRI) evidence of deformation. Unfortunately, this technique is imperfect.
- The most reliable validation is obtained in animal models using microcrystals to measure deformation.

Benefits of Strain
- Deformation offers four main benefits in comparison with other quantitative parameters: sensitivity, site specificity (i.e., independence from tethering), homogeneity, and physiologic significance (correlation with contractility):
- The *sensitivity* of the deformation techniques to identify subtle gradations in function is an important attribute, especially for identifying early-stage disease. This is dependent on both having a narrow enough standard deviation to readily separate normal from abnormal tissue, as well as being specific for the location of the abnormal tissue (see Fig. 6-2).

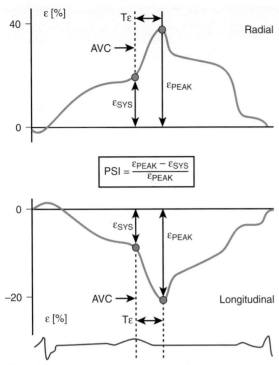

Figure 6-1. Morphology of radial (*above*) and longitudinal (*below*) strain curves. Systolic strain (measured at aortic valve closure, AVC), may be exceeded by peak strain, and the difference may be measured in timing or strain magnitude (postsystolic shortening), usually measured as postsystolic index (PSI).

$$PSI = \frac{\varepsilon_{PEAK} - \varepsilon_{SYS}}{\varepsilon_{PEAK}}$$

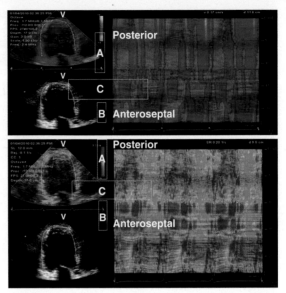

Figure 6-2. Parametric map of apical long axis in which colors express velocity (*above*) and strain rate magnitudes and timing (*below*) starting at the posterior and progressing to the anteroseptal wall. The example shows the relative sensitivity of strain rate imaging (SRI) to small regions of wall motion abnormality. An infarct in the posterior wall (zone A) is not detected by tissue velocity imaging, which shows a red color, consistent with movement toward the transducer. This is the same as the anterior wall (zone B) and reflects tethering by the remainder of the wall, causing translational movement within the infarct area (*upper panel*). Because of the site specificity of SRI, tethering does not alter the deformation of the risk area (zone A), which is identified correctly as infarcted (note the blue color in systole), and contrasts with the anterior wall (zone A), which shows a gold color, consistent with thickening (zone B). As this is a Doppler-based technique, the apex (zone C) is not well evaluated by either method.

- *Site specificity* implies that measurements obtained from within the sample volume truly reflect the performance of the tissue at this location rather than elsewhere in the wall. This is an inherent requirement for assessment of small areas of abnormal tissue, and techniques that are not site specific (e.g., tissue Doppler imaging or annular displacement) tend to average function along the length of the entire wall (see Fig. 6-2).
- The *homogeneity* of strain throughout the myocardium is relative rather than absolute, as there are minor variations of strain from apex to base. These variations are much less than the differences in tissue velocity within different parts of the heart (Fig. 6-3).
- The *physiologic correlates* of strain and SR have been sought in a number of experimental studies. Strain, which does not account for the time course of contraction, is analogous to regional EF. SR, a descriptor of the speed of contraction, is analogous to rate of change in pressure over time (*dP/dt*).

Disadvantages of Strain

- Measurement of myocardial deformation is a helpful but far from perfect technique for the assessment of regional or global LV function.
- Both tissue Doppler and speckle techniques are computationally complex.
- None of the methods is independent of user expertise, to the extent that a variety of artifacts need to be recognized and avoided, in order to prevent misleading results.
- The tissue velocity methodology is susceptible to artifact caused by angulation and works optimally when the direction of motion and the imaging access are as close as possible to parallel, and may be very misleading when angulation is major (Fig. 6-4).
- The speckle technique is very dependent on the quality.

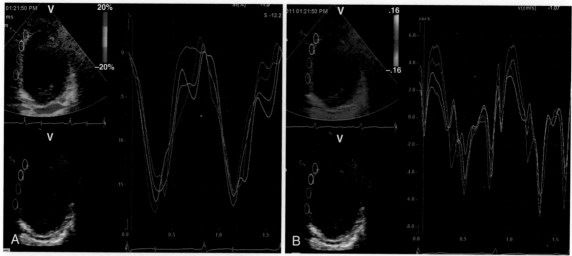

Figure 6-3. Regional variation of strain (**A**) and tissue velocity (**B**) in the septum. As the apex is fixed and the base moves away and toward this like a piston, there is a gradation of velocity from base (*green*) to apex (*turquoise*). In contrast, although there are minor regional variations of strain, strain values from apex and base are relatively uniform.

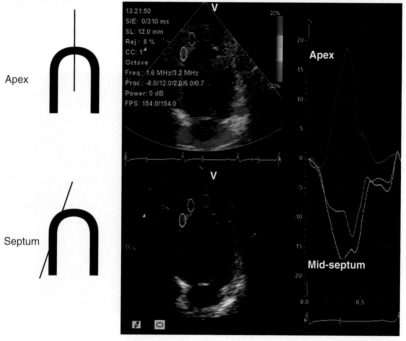

Figure 6-4. Impact of angulation on strain measurement. In the apical view, the mid-septum (*yellow*) is closest to parallel with the ultrasound beam. As the incident angle increases towards 45 degrees, apparent strain measurement decreases (*turquoise*). In the apex, the incident angle increases to 90 degrees, so radial strain is measured, the strain direction being opposite to that of longitudinal strain.

KEY POINTS

- LV EF is not an ideal measure of LV function because it depends on image quality, geometric assumptions, and loading conditions and is not sensitive for detection of early disease.
- Strain is defined as the change in myocardial length, relative either to original length or to length at a previous time, derived from excursion of speckles.

- SR is the rate of change in myocardial length (velocity), normalized to distance, and is the first derivative of the strain curve.
- SR and strain are displayed either as curves for one or more specific myocardial sites or as two-dimensional (2D)/three-dimensional (3D) maps of the left ventricle (LV) with color used to indicate magnitude over the entire LV.

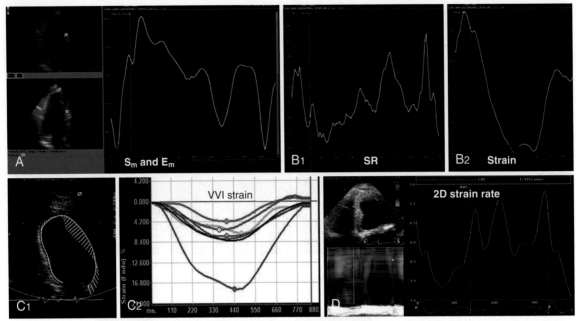

Figure 6-5. Myocardial imaging method. **A,** Tissue velocity imaging. **B,** Tissue velocity imaging (TVI)-based strain rate (SR) and strain. **C,** Speckle-based strain using velocity vector imaging. **D,** Speckle-based SR.

Methodologies

- A variety of approaches to strain are now available from equipment vendors.
- They differ fundamentally according to whether tissue velocity or speckle is used as the primary modality (Fig. 6-5).

Tissue Doppler-based Strain

- This was the initial echocardiographic approach to measurement of myocardial deformation.
- The technique is based on comparison of the gradient of tissue velocity over the rate of change in length over a sample volume to obtain SR ($\Delta V/\Delta r$). Strain is derived as the temporal integral of the spatial differential of velocity $\int(\Delta V/\Delta r)\delta t$.
- Steps in acquisition
  - Save three cycles (some equipment uses a minimum 1-s capture).
  - Optimize frame rate (>100 frames per second [fps]).
  - Check tissue velocity to avoid aliasing, and modify Nyquist accordingly.
  - Consider narrow sector acquisition to optimize spatial and temporal resolution, as long as whole LV is not required (e.g., stress or synchrony assessments).
- Interpretation steps
  - Define start and end of systole using electrocardiography (end of T wave), aortic

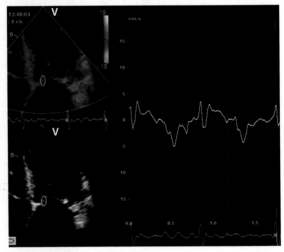

Figure 6-6. Definition of end systole from the isovolumic signal in the TVI waveform (*arrow*).

valve motion, color Doppler (isovolumic signal; Fig. 6-6) or LV outflow.
- Use a sample volume of 12×6 mm (note that data are gathered outside of this).
- Examine quality on the tissue Doppler; if there is artifact or aliasing, more complex analysis (i.e., strain) probably will not work.
- Track samples to the cardiac cycle.
- Move sample volume until a reproducible SR signal is obtained in the segment of interest and repeat in a reference segment. Measure peak systolic SR (Fig. 6-7).

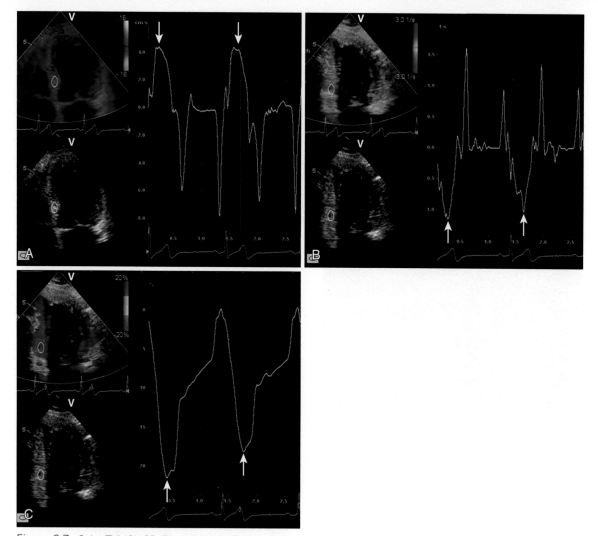

Figure 6-7. Color TVI (**A**), SR (**B**), and strain (**C**) from the same two cardiac cycles. Systolic deflections (*arrows*) are positive by tissue Doppler and negative by SR and strain.

- Change to strain, check timing, peak systolic strain, and postsystolic index.
- Limitations
  - The fundamental limitation of tissue Doppler-based strain is directional.
  - The motion that is measured should be parallel to the ultrasound beam, and generally this limits the application of the technique to apical images, although some work has been done in the anteroseptal and posterior walls from parasternal views.
  - This technique is somewhat dependent on image quality, but the signal-to-noise ratio of Doppler is higher than for gray scale imaging, meaning that pictures unsuitable for tracing endocardial borders can sometimes provide accurate tissue velocity-based strain.

- The requirement for high frame rate, particularly for SR imaging, may be difficult to reconcile with a wide imaging sector.
- Integration with contrast is difficult. While the signal usually appears reliable, some studies have shown discrepancies with noncontrast images.

Speckle-based Strain
- The application of 2D speckle technology on standard commercial machines is now more than 5 years old.
- How it works:
  - The ultrasound image is composed of a matrix of speckles that correspond to minute tissue structures.
  - A process of pattern recognition allows these to be tracked from frame to frame,

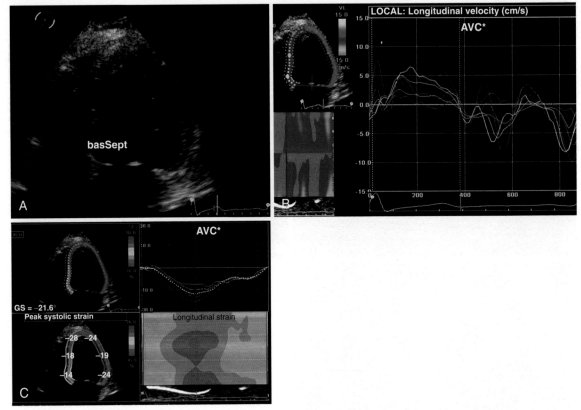

Figure 6-8. Processing of speckle tracking to obtain strain. A high frame-rate two-dimensional image is traced at end systole (**A**). The wall is automatically segmented to provide velocity (**B**) or strain (**C**). Curves show the course of development of velocity or strain over time.

allowing the assessment of strain in any direction. Speed of movement is identified on the basis of the degree of excursion from frame to frame.

- Acquisition frame rate is extremely important, and optimal rate is 60 to 80 fps. If too low, speckles risk traveling out of the image; if too fast, the excursion between frames will be too small to measure.

- The adequacy of tracking can be expressed as the correlation between images. This can be mapped, to give the reader an impression for the reliability of the data, but apart from a process of offering minor guidance about tracking by one manufacturer, this quality control measure is unexploited.

- Strain measurement on archived images can be performed using some software that will process data from all vendors. However, caution needs to be applied to using this on DICOM images or the gray scale image in the background of color tissue velocity imaging (TVI), as the temporal resolution of both are too low for speckle tracking.

- The primary data are acquired as strain. SR can be calculated as the derivative of strain

over time, but some constraints arise from acquisition frame rate (Fig. 6-8).

- Acquisition
  - Optimize frame rate (50–80 fps).
  - Optimize image—speckle is susceptible to artifact (e.g., ribs).

- Interpretation steps
  - Trace endocardial border or add guide points to permit segmentation of myocardium.
  - Define timing markers (end systole).
  - Check adequacy of tracking.

- Limitations
  - Dependent on image quality, this may pose particular problems in the far field.
  - Use after contrast left ventricular opacification is not feasible, presumably because of tracking contrast microbubbles in the myocardium.
  - SR analysis is somewhat limited by temporal resolution.

Speckle- versus TVI-based Strain

- The relevant features of TVI, speckle, and TVI strain are summarized in Table 6-2.
- Generally, the feasibility and angle independence of speckle strain have made

this the test of choice in the assessment of myocardial deformation.

- The relative simplicity of TVI means that this should be considered when there is no requirement for site specificity, especially if timing data are sought.
- TVI-based strain is preferable if assessment of deformation is sought at high heart rate (e.g., during stress) or there is a need to measure SR.

	TVI	Speckle Strain	TVI Strain
Easy to apply	+	+	±
Dependent on image quality	±	++	±
Feasibility of online assessment	+	–	–
High-resolution timing data	++	+	++
Conceptually simple	+	±	–
Quick to add	+	±	±
Impact of other variables (age, heart rate, etc.)	+	+	+
Clinical evidence	+	–	±

TABLE 6-2 COMPARISON OF CLINICALLY RELEVANT FEATURES OF TISSUE VELOCITY IMAGING, SPECKLE, AND TVI STRAIN

Global Strain

- Derivation
  - Global strain can be calculated directly by the software or manually by averaging all interpretable segments.
  - Because of the risk of being misled by artifactual measurements, review of segmental strain curves is desirable rather than treating the software as a "black box."
  - Global strain may be calculated as global longitudinal strain (GLS) or global circumferential strain (GCS).
- Benefits
  - Global strain is a reflection of the sum of myocardial motion.
  - Global strain is also an analog of EF. There is *not* complete correspondence as EF is a means of assessing endocardial motion, with limitations posed especially by LV hypertrophy (see Table 6-1).
  - One of the attractions of GLS and GCS (in addition to lacking geometric assumptions) is that they are automated (and hence reproducible) (Fig. 6-9).
- Applications: While the variability of EF that relates to inaccurate border tracing can potentially be avoided, the technique remains dependent on both loading conditions and image quality.
  - Global LV function: Whether this measure will eventually supersede EF is unproven. This seems unlikely in the context of the amount of prognostic material available for

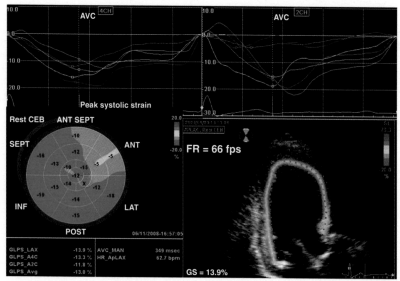

Figure 6-9. Calculation of global strain. Segmental strain is calculated in the three apical views (segmental strain in the apical four- and two-chamber views is illustrated at the top of the image) and then combined in a polar map.

EF, but GLS can certainly be used to approximate EF (Fig. 6-10).

- Subclinical dysfunction
- Sequential studies, where the superior test-retest reliability of global strain may be of value. Follow-up of patients after chemotherapy may constitute such a situation. Others, including assessing response to treatment in Fabry's disease, are discussed in the next section.

- Validation: There have been limited studies of outcome.
  - Stanton et al.[1] followed a group of 546 patients (91 of whom died over 5.2 ± 1.5 years) who underwent echocardiography to assess resting LV function. Clinical factors associated with outcome included age, diabetes, and hypertension. Addition of EF or wall motion score index added to predictive power, but GLS caused the greatest increment in model power. GLS provided incremental value in patients with EF greater than 35% and without wall motion abnormalities (WMA) (Fig. 6-11).
  - Cho studied 201 patients with heart failure (EF 34 ± 13%, ischemic in 55%), among whom 47 had events (heart failure 10%, death 13%) over 39 ± 17 months. GCS was an independent predictor of outcome, incremental to EF, filling pressure, and GLS.

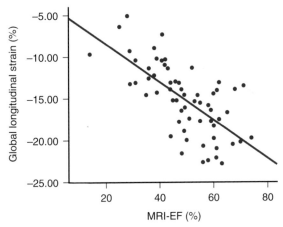

Figure 6-10. Relationship of global longitudinal strain to EF. *(From Brown J, Jenkins C, Marwick TH. Use of myocardial strain to assess global left ventricular function: a comparison with cardiac magnetic resonance and 3-dimensional echocardiography. Am Heart J. 2009;157: 102.e1-e5.)*

KEY POINTS

- Tissue Doppler-based strain measurements are based on myocardial velocities and thus only measure strain in the direction of the ultrasound beam.
- Speckle-based strain measurements are based on tracking the movement of individual points in the myocardium from frame to frame on the 2D or 3D images.
- Speckle strain measurements require a high frame rate (60–80 fps) for accuracy and depend on image quality, but speckle strain currently provides the best clinical approach.
- Global strain is a measure of overall myocardial motion, analogous to EF. A normal global strain is about −18 ± 2%; less negative numbers (<−14%) are abnormal.

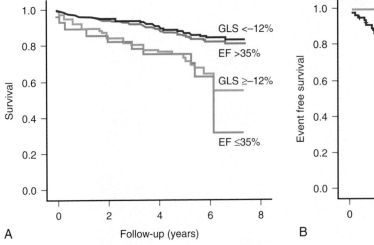

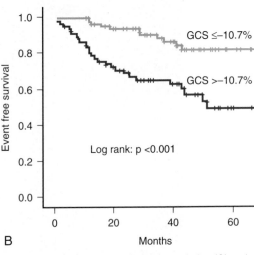

Figure 6-11. Association of longitudinal and circumferential strain with outcome in an unselected population (**A**) and patients with heart failure (**B**). *(Reprinted with permission from Stanton T, Leano R, Marwick TH. Prediction of all-cause mortality from global longitudinal speckle strain: comparison with ejection fraction and wall motion scoring. Circ Cardiovasc Imaging. 2009;2:356-364.)*

Subclinical Dysfunction

- Despite many therapeutic advances, patients presenting with symptoms and signs of heart failure continue to suffer an adverse prognosis and functional impairment.
- Improved identification and treatment of the early stages of heart failure may reduce later presentations with more advanced disease.
- Cardiac dysfunction has been identified in a variety of disease entities (Table 6-3). The most common and important are hypertrophy and infiltration, cardiotoxicity, early metabolic heart disease, and treatment response.
- Infiltrative heart diseases
  - While global strain should be considered as any other parameter of global LV function, in situations where the LV wall is thickened, strain may be a better marker of systolic function than EF.
  - The role of strain in patients with amyloid heart disease has been well studied. In a study of 93 patients with amyloid light chain (AL) amyloidosis, investigators divided the group into Group 1: No LV thickening (<12 mm); Group 2: LV thickened but no congestive heart failure (CHF); and Group 3: LV thickened and CHF. There were no differences in 2D echocardiography results between the groups (except LV thickness and left atrial [LA] diameter), but tissue Doppler E

wave at the basal septal mitral annulus (E_m), SR, and strain showed differences between Groups 1 and 2.
- Metabolic heart disease
  - Heart failure is the "forgotten complication" of diabetes, and the importance of this to the current epidemic of diabetes and obesity may exceed that of occult coronary artery disease (CAD).
  - A number of processes have been identified that may contribute to subclinical LV dysfunction in these patients, including fibrosis of the myocardium and vasculature, direct metabolic effects on the myocyte, autonomic neuropathy and microvascular disease.
  - If the appropriate treatment of this problem proves to be dependent on the balance of these mechanisms, myocardial tissue characterization with strain and other methods is likely to be important in patients with these metabolic disorders.
  - At present, it appears that diastolic markers are the most robust for tracking this process, but it is possible that fibrosis and other markers are best identified by different methods. More work is needed on this subject.
- Cardiotoxicity
  - Anthracycline-related cardiotoxicity is an established cause of heart failure, in which symptoms can be particularly intractable. It has largely been avoided by restricting dose.
  - The problem is increasing due to the concurrent use of not just anthracyclines but biological agents such as trastuzumab.
  - Prevalence is driven not only by changes in therapy, but also by increasing survival from cancer. Indeed, for many neoplasms, cardiac sequelae are more likely causes of death than recurrent cancer.
  - Current echocardiographic strategies for prevention of heart failure are based on surveillance of EF. This parameter is not very sensitive, and the 95% confidence limits are greater than 10% (implying changes of <10% to be of questionable relevance).
  - Strain measurements are quantitative and more sensitive than EF, and appear to precede EF changes (Fig. 6-12). Whether they merely identify subclinical disturbances that are not meaningful (i.e., they reverse) or represent a substrate that would benefit from treatment requires definition.

TABLE 6-3	EXAMPLES OF DISEASE ENTITIES WHERE STRAIN HAS BEEN USED IN THE DETECTION OF SUBCLINICAL LV DYSFUNCTION
Amyloidosis	Systolic ε/SR (not S' or E') identified subclinical disease[2]
Friedrich's	Reduction of LV (not RV), systolic ε/SR and diastolic SR proportionate to LVH[3]
LV hypertrophy	Systolic ε/SR reduced in LVH before abn filling,[4] Systolic ε distinguished HCM and HT-LVH[5]
Tetralogy	RV-S and ε/SR reduced,[6] IVA (not S' or SR) proportionate to PR severity[7]
Senning	Reduction of systolic ε/SR in the systemic RV[8]
Valvular disease	Subclinical LV dysfunction in asymptomatic MR[9]

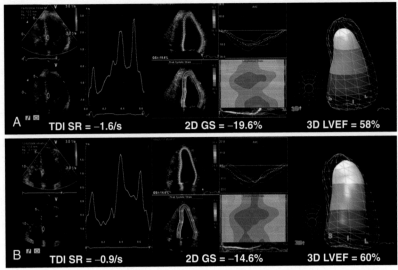

Figure 6-12. Reduction of strain in the presence of preserved EF. **A,** Normal average strain rate (SR) and global strain (GS) with normal 3D EF. **B,** Reduction of strain rate and strain with preserved 3D EF. *(From Hare JL, Brown JK, Leano R, et al. Use of myocardial deformation imaging to detect preclinical myocardial dysfunction before conventional measures in patients undergoing breast cancer treatment with trastuzumab. Am Heart J. 2009;158:294-301.)*

TABLE 6-4	EVIDENCE FOR USE OF DEFORMATION IMAGING IN TRACKING TREATMENT RESPONSE
Fabry's disease	Improved ε/SR with enzyme replacement Rx[10]
HT heart disease	Improved ε/SR with aldosterone antagonism[11]
Diabetes	Improved ε/SR with insulin[12]
Obesity	Improved ε/SR with lifestyle intervention[13]

- Response to treatment
  - Antineoplastic therapy is only one of several settings where repeat imaging may be used to guide therapy.
  - A number of conditions involving both overt and subclinical heart disease are looked upon as indications for repeat testing. Of these, deformation measurements appear to be most attractive in individuals with subclinical rather than overt disease (Table 6-4). The evidence base appears to be most mature for the follow-up of patients with Fabry's disease.

Ischemic Heart Disease

- Current qualitative methods depend on 2D image quality, training, and significant reading volume.

- The ability of strain to measure regional function could provide a reproducible, sensitive method with limited variation.
- The recognition of resting or stress-induced wall motion abnormalities is a very attractive indication for deformation imaging.

Resting Function

- An automated method for measurement of resting function could potentially improve the recognition of CAD at emergency room presentations with chest pain.
- Thresholds for diagnosis of CAD from resting imaging have been proposed, using cutoffs of 0.83/s for SR and 17.4% for strain.
- Although there is evidence that strain may be reduced as a manifestation of "ischemic memory," resting changes are more usually associated with prior scar. The challenge is to recognize reduced strain as being from an acute event rather than from the presence of scar, whether or not this is recognized as being due to previous infarction.
- Correlation with transmural extent of scar suggests that scar burden may be quantified by this method. Indeed, the comparison between longitudinal and circumferential or radial strain may offer indirect evidence of the transmural extent of scar. Additionally there have been efforts to measure this directly from subendocardial and subepicardial strain, although this remains a work in progress and radial strain measurement is probably not sufficiently robust to accomplish this.

- Resting deformation has been used to identify infarct size and predict remodeling and outcome.
- The problem with using this as an alternative to expert interpretation is that some expertise is required in order to recognize common artifacts.

Low-dose Dobutamine Response
- The augmentation of viable segments in response to dobutamine is subjective. Judging between degrees of hypokinesis in potentially tethered segments may be extremely difficult. There is now evidence that the dobutamine response of strain is able to provide quantitative data to support the diagnosis of viability.
- Experimental studies in closed chest porcine models have identified differences in deformation between acute and chronic reduction of coronary flow. Both *acute occlusion* and *chronic flow reduction* are associated with loss of systolic thickening and development of postsystolic thickening.
- A cycle of flow reduction and reperfusion leads to a model of stunning, during which dobutamine infusion leads to an increment of SR at low doses, exceeding baseline values at peak dose, while strain remains below baseline levels and increases only at peak dose.
- The dobutamine response of SR has been shown to correspond to viability as defined by positron emission tomographic (PET) imaging. This may be expressed using anatomical M-mode (Fig. 6-13). Segmental increases in SR and strain have also been used to predict functional recovery (Fig. 6-14).
- A problem remains with the use of speckle strain for this purpose. It appears to be less sensitive, especially in territories not of the left anterior descending artery, possibly reflecting the image quality limitations of the basal segments.

Strain During Ischemia
- The documentation of strain disturbances at peak stress is of critical importance to the role of deformation imaging for stress echocardiography.
- This is difficult, but there have been some encouraging steps:
  - Animal models have shown SR to have 81% sensitivity and 91% specificity for the recognition of reduced flow.
  - A human study showed an increment of both sensitivity and specificity by combination of SR data, and limited data

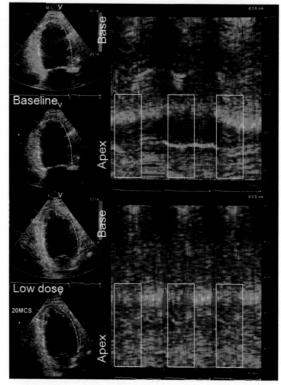

Figure 6-13. Improvement of anterolateral wall SR in response to dobutamine. The white boxes highlight systole in the anterolateral wall using the anatomic M-mode. At baseline, the predominant green and blue coloration indicates low strain rate and even paradoxical motion. In response to low-dose dobutamine, these change to orange and red, indicating thickening especially towards the apex. *(From Hoffmann R, Altiok E, Nowak B, et al. Strain rate measurement by Doppler echocardiography allows improved assessment of myocardial viability in patients with depressed left ventricular function. J Am Coll Cardiol. 2002;39:443-449.)*

have been obtained with speckle tracking using a hybrid technique of speckle and tissue velocity.
- However, there are problems:
  - The SR imaging approach is time consuming and subject to noise.
  - The most reliable marker of ischemia appears to be SR (this increases through stress while strain plateaus and falls in normal subjects), and this is difficult with speckle tracking, in part because of the limited frame rate, which becomes even more of a limitation during tachycardia.
  - Image quality remains a problem for speckle-based imaging. Indeed, a comparison of TVI and speckle strain has shown problems with the latter method, particularly in the posterior parts of the heart.

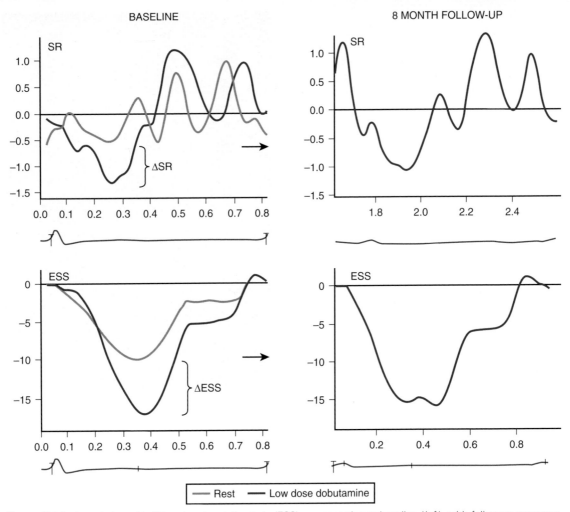

Figure 6-14. Association with SR and end-systolic strain (ESS) augmentation at baseline (*left*), with follow-up response after revascularization (*right*). *(Adapted from Hanekom L, Jenkins C, Jeffries L, et al. Incremental value of strain rate analysis as an adjunct to wall-motion scoring for assessment of myocardial viability by dobutamine echocardiography: a follow-up study after revascularization. Circulation. 2005;112:3892-3900.)*

- Stress echocardiography is very commonly performed as exercise echocardiography. Because of artifact and other reasons for compromised image quality, this poses a particular problem for strain analysis.
- An unresolved issue is the optimal parameter that should be used for quantitative analysis of ischemia. The peak strain and SR describe the magnitude of contraction (as discussed earlier, SR appears to be superior, at least on theoretical grounds). Delayed contraction is a sensitive marker of ischemia, but the segmental analysis of postsystolic index is time consuming. Anatomic M-mode displays may be a simpler means of expressing late contraction and offer spatial integration (Fig. 6-15).

Conclusions
- The promise of strain imaging for stress echocardiography is that it could overcome a number of the limitations of the standard practice of stress echocardiography, including the learning curve, variability between observers based on subjective interpretation, and difficulties inherent in judging gradations between degrees of hypokinesia, especially in the assessment of viability.
- The use of tissue Doppler imaging may overcome the dependence of stress echocardiography on image quality.
- However, we "aren't there yet" and our expectations need to be appropriate.

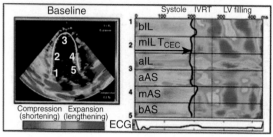

A

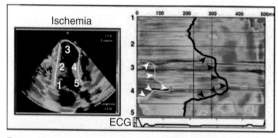

B

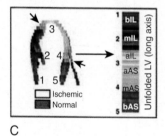

C

Figure 6-15. Strain rate maps at baseline and during ischemia, and corresponding perfusion-stained specimen, in apical long-axis view. **A,** Baseline strain rate imaging frame (*left image*) and the corresponding longitudinal M-mode strain rate map over one cardiac cycle (*right image*). Orange represents compression, blue expansion, and green low motion. The two vertical straight lines approximate the time of the aortic valve closure and of the mitral valve opening (identified from gray-scale two-dimensional loops). The compression/expansion crossover is indicated by the solid black line as the color transition from orange to blue. The time from the electrocardiographic peak R-wave to the compression/expansion crossover (T_{CEC}) is measured for each pixel line in the image. **B,** Ischemic strain rate maps from the same view. A prolonged compression pattern (*black arrows*) can be observed in the apical and mid anteroseptal segments (supplied by the occluded left anterior descending coronary artery), while the rest of segments have normal compression/relaxation pattern. Note also the delayed onset of systolic compression (*white arrows*) in the same ischemic segments. **C,** Computer reconstruction of the stained cardiac specimen at the same level in the heart. Myocardium at risk is represented by the white region (*arrows*), while the normally perfused myocardium is stained in red. The location of the apical postsystolic compression pattern in the strain-rate maps matches the location of the ischemic myocardium. (Segments are abbreviated: bIL, basal inferolateral; mIL, mid inferolateral; aIL, apical inferolateral; aAS, apical anteroseptal; mAS, mid anteroseptal; bAS, basal anteroseptal.) *(From Pislaru C, Belohlavek M, Bae RY, et al. Regional asynchrony during acute myocardial ischemia quantified by ultrasound strain rate imaging. J Am Coll Cardiol. 2001;37:1141-1148.)*

There may be limited room for an improvement in accuracy, and maybe strain's real gift will be in avoiding the limitations of an ischemia-based technique (diagnosis of single-vessel CAD, recognition of multivessel CAD, recognition of ischemia within areas of resting WMA).

KEY POINTS

- Strain and SR measurements indicate the presence of subclinical LV dysfunction (with a normal EF) in patients with many types of heart disease, including infiltrative cardiomyopathy, metabolic heart disease, and after cardiotoxic chemotherapy.
- LV myocardial strain measurements may improve early recognition of ischemic heart disease in patients presenting with chest pain and may provide more quantitative measures of regional function during echocardiographic stress testing.

Right Ventricular Strain

- The right ventricle (RV) is often described as the forgotten ventricle, for good reason. Quantification of both size and function have historically been challenging as this structure does not conform to a geometric shape.
- Recent recommendations from the American Society of Echocardiography have summarized the variety of measures using standard technology, including annular plane displacement of the tricuspid valve, fractional area change, and myocardial performance index.
- Strain has been used for RV measurements because of recognition that these parameters are imperfect. The following general observations are pertinent:
  - RV SR and strain values are less homogeneously distributed than in the LV. A reverse base-to-apex gradient is reported, with the highest values in the apical segments and outflow tract, reflecting the thickness and shape of the RV.

- Normal basal RV free wall strain is 25%, with normal SR of −4/s.
- Reduced deformation may reflect reduced RV contractility (due to myopathic processes, infiltration, or fibrosis), increased pulmonary pressure, or both (Fig. 6-16).
- Again, the selection is between tissue velocity or speckle-based strain:
  - Angle dependence of tissue velocity is potentially an issue and warrants careful acquisition and alignment with the RV free wall.
  - The high TVI frame rate may be helpful.

- TVI sample volume can be adjusted to assess RV myocardium alone.
- Speckle-based strain involves an assumption that the shapes that are applied to the LV are appropriate for strain analysis of the RV—this has not been validated and may be untrue.
- The ability to track speckles in RV myocardium of normal thickness can be problematic.
- While RV strain assessment is a promising tool for a significant ongoing problem, the position of the guidelines is that these data are insufficiently validated, with which this author concurs.

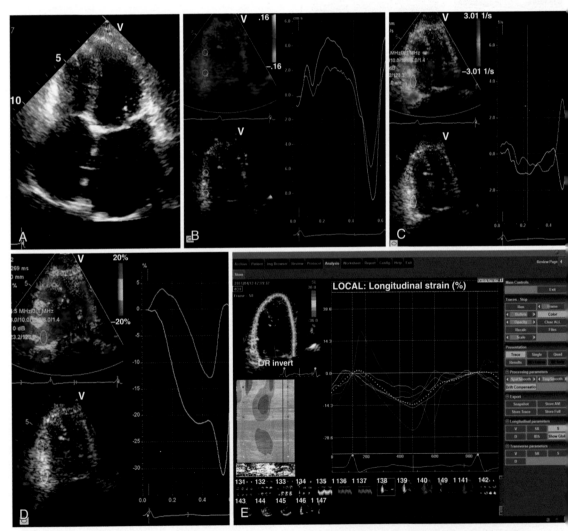

Figure 6-16. Myocardial imaging was used to facilitate evaluation of right ventricular (RV) function in this patient with tricuspid regurgitation and RV enlargement (**A**). Tissue velocity in the RV free wall was reduced below the normal range of greater than 10 cm/s at the annulus and greater than 5 cm/s in the mid-wall (**B**). Mid-RV tissue velocity-based longitudinal SR is reduced below the expected value of 1.5/s (**C**), and systolic strain is reduced to below the expected value of −20% (**D**). Reduction of speckle tracking-derived RV global strain (**E**) confirms the presence of RV impairment.

Atrial Strain ·

- Traditional Doppler and 2D echocardiographic measures of atrial function are affected by LV diastolic and systolic performance.
- Components of atrial function include reservoir, conduit, and active components.
- Changes in different LA phasic components may characterize different diseases and treatment responses:
  - Active LA contraction has been shown to demonstrate gradual recovery after cardioversion.
  - LA reservoir function rather than LA contractile function is the predictor of response to atrial fibrillation ablation and cardiac resynchronization therapy (CRT).
- Assessment of LA strain with 2D speckle tracking (Fig. 6-17) and Doppler strain (Fig. 6-18) may provide additional insight into LA myocardial mechanics:
  - LA reservoir function is portrayed by "total" strain (timed from the preceding QRS and reflecting LA filling from the minimum to the maximum LA volume).
  - LA contraction is represented by the "negative" strain following the start of the P wave.
- LA strain imaging is "not ready for prime time" due to:
  - Imaging challenges—thin LA wall, regional heterogeneity of contraction, imaging at depth, and lack of specific atrial software.
  - Neither of the current modalities is ideal— Doppler-based strain allows interrogation of limited walls (due to angle dependence) and the limited temporal resolution of 2D strain is very likely an impediment to accurate assessment of atrial contraction.

Strain in Electrophysiology

Indications

- Evaluation of LV dysfunction (determinant of risk, and hence CRT benefits). Global strain may be a possible substitute for EF.
- Use of deformation as a potential marker of viability, and hence optimal lead position as well as likelihood of response to CRT or ablation procedures.
- The other two indications focus on the ability of strain to measure dispersion of contraction, including in the assessment of dyssynchrony for CRT selection and optimization, as well as implantable cardioverter defibrillator (ICD) selection.

Left Ventricular Synchrony

- It is widely recognized that some patients with standard indications for CRT (New York Heart Association class III or IV, LV EF <35%, maximal medical therapy, and QRS width >120–150 ms) lack mechanical evidence of dyssynchrony, and these individuals may lack symptomatic or physiologic "response" to CRT.
- Mechanical evidence of dyssynchrony may occur in some patients with a narrow QRS.
- Promising results of single-center studies suggest a potential role for tissue Doppler imaging in the selection of patients for CRT. On the basis of these, it was hoped that the presence of synchrony could reduce implants by predicting nonresponders (30% by symptoms, 40% by volumes).
- There are a number of problems with this hypothesis:

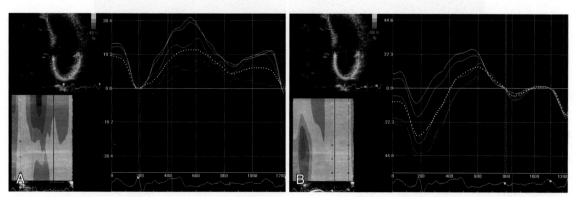

Figure 6-17. Speckle tracking-derived left atrial (LA) global strain can be shown with triggering on the QRS (**A**) or on the P wave (**B**). Use of the QRS is a good means for focusing on the total strain, reflecting total LA filling (RF, reservoir function), which is normally 38 ± 8%. Atrial contraction (AC) is easier to demonstrate by triggering on the P wave, and is normally −15 ± 5%. This patient has normal atrial function.

- Half of the published studies show a sensitivity of less than 90% and specificity of approximately 80%, implying that the use of contraction markers in patient selection would lead to some patients who are likely to benefit, being denied therapy.
- Issues related to observer variation. The PROSPECT (Predictors of Response to CRT) study showed an unacceptably wide variation of measurements between readers.[14]

- The lack of a single optimal parameter. The PROSPECT trial results showed that conventional markers of mechanical synchrony had limited predictive value for CRT response.
- This reflects both the limitations of tissue velocity imaging in being unable to distinguish active and passive movement, as well as issues related to spatial and temporal averaging.

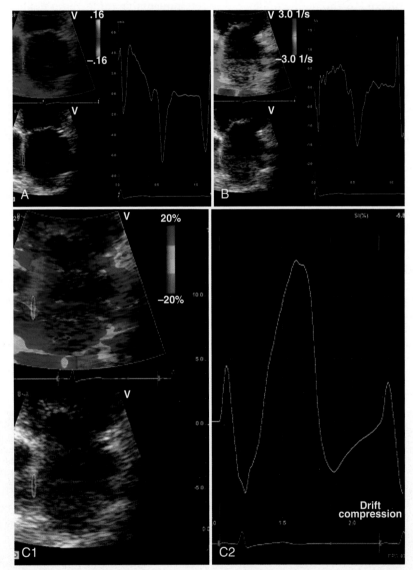

Figure 6-18. Left atrial function evaluation using tissue Doppler. A narrow sample volume is positioned in the mid-interatrial septum (this location offers the best stability and beam alignment). The tissue velocity signal (**A**) demonstrates systolic and diastolic motion analogous to LV longitudinal motion. TVI-derived LA SR (**B**) shows that the active contraction (after the P wave) is reduced below the lower limit (1.5/s). LA strain pertaining to AC, identified by initiating the SR integration from the P wave (**C**), is also reduced below the expected level of –20%. The upstroke of the subsequent positive wave during LV systole corresponds to LA RF, and its negative deflection reflects rapid emptying (RE).

- Strain has been used to address some of the limitations of Doppler:
  - It can combine regional contraction magnitude with timing
  - It imposes some spatial averaging
  - Although there are encouraging results, there are also negative findings. The use of strain is not a panacea for the limitations of Doppler, but there may be a role for dyssynchrony assessment in QRS of intermediate duration (QRS 120-149 ms).

ICD Selection

- In patients with impaired LV function (EF <35%), ICD implantation is associated with improved survival. Nonetheless, many patients who undergo implantation never receive a shock.
- Dispersion of mechanical activation correlates with cardiac events (cardiac arrest, documented arrhythmia, syncope) in patients with long QT syndrome. Prolonged myocardial contraction duration was associated with patients with genetically confirmed LQTS, and prolonged contraction duration better identified cardiac events compared with QTc in carriers, among whom dispersion of contraction was more pronounced in carriers with events. The putative mechanism is that the same fibrotic process that leads to rhythm disturbances is responsible for mechanical dispersion of LV contraction.

KEY POINTS

- The development of strain has provided clinicians a previously unavailable window on myocardial mechanics.
- Current realizable benefits of strain:
  - reduction of subjective interpretation
  - detection of subclinical heart disease
  - adjunctive test in detection of viable myocardium
- The detection of ischemia and use as a follow-up tool are potential contributions.
- Some disadvantages need to be resolved before the techniques enter routine practice.
- Urgent challenges include defining the balance of 2D strain relative to TVI strain and overcoming dependence on image quality.

References

1. Stanton T, Leano R, Marwick TH. Prediction of all-cause mortality from global longitudinal speckle strain: comparison with ejection fraction and wall motion scoring. *Circ Cardiovasc Imaging.* 2009;2:356-364.
2. Koyama J, Falk RH. Prognostic significance of strain Doppler imaging in light-chain amyloidosis. *JACC Cardiovasc Imaging.* 2010;3:333-342.
3. Weidemann F, Eyskens B, Mertens L, et al. Quantification of regional right and left ventricular function by ultrasonic strain rate and strain indexes in Friedreich's ataxia. *Am J Cardiol.* 2003;91:622-626.
4. Yuda S, Short L, Leano R, et al. Myocardial abnormalities in hypertensive patients with normal and abnormal left ventricular filling: a study of ultrasound tissue characterization and strain. *Clin Sci (Lond).* 2002;103:283-293.
5. Kato TS, Noda A, Izawa H, et al. Discrimination of nonobstructive hypertrophic cardiomyopathy from hypertensive left ventricular hypertrophy on the basis of strain rate imaging by tissue Doppler ultrasonography. *Circulation.* 2004;110:3808-3814.
6. Weidemann F, Eyskens B, Mertens L, et al. Quantification of regional right and left ventricular function by ultrasonic strain rate and strain indexes after surgical repair of tetralogy of Fallot. *Am J Cardiol.* 2002;90:133-138.
7. Frigola A, Redington AN, Cullen S, et al. Pulmonary regurgitation is an important determinant of right ventricular contractile dysfunction in patients with surgically repaired tetralogy of Fallot. *Circulation.* 2004;110:153-157.
8. Eyskens B, Weidemann F, Kowalski M, et al. Regional right and left ventricular function after the Senning operation: an ultrasonic study of strain rate and strain. *Cardiol Young.* 2004;14:255-264.
9. Lee R, Hanekom L, Marwick TH, et al. Prediction of subclinical left ventricular dysfunction with strain rate imaging in patients with asymptomatic severe mitral regurgitation. *Am J Cardiol.* 2004;94:1333-1337.
10. Weidemann F, Breunig F, Beer M, et al. Improvement of cardiac function during enzyme replacement therapy in patients with Fabry disease: a prospective strain rate imaging study. *Circulation.* 2003;108:1299-1301.
11. Mottram PM, Haluska B, Leano R, et al. Effect of aldosterone antagonism on myocardial dysfunction in hypertensive patients with diastolic heart failure. *Circulation.* 2004;110:558-565.
12. von Bibra H, Hansen A, Dounis V, et al. Augmented metabolic control improves myocardial diastolic function and perfusion in patients with non-insulin dependent diabetes. *Heart.* 2004;90:1483-1484.
13. Kosmala W, O'Moore-Sullivan T, Plaksej R, et al. Improvement of left ventricular function by lifestyle intervention in obesity: contributions of weight loss and reduced insulin resistance. *Diabetologia.* 2009;52:2306-2316.
14. Chung ARL, Tavazzi L, et al. Results of the Predictors of Response to CRT (PROSPECT) trial. *Circulation.* 2008;117:2608-2616.

Suggested Reading

1. Mor-Avi V, Lang RM, Badano LP, et al. Current and evolving echocardiographic techniques for the quantitative evaluation of cardiac mechanics: ASE/EAE consensus statement on methodology and indications endorsed by the Japanese Society of Echocardiography. *J Am Soc Echocardiogr.* 2011;24:277-313.
   Very detailed and current review of strain by the American Society of Echocardiography and European Association of Echocardiography (EAE). The sections on instrumentation and applications of strain imaging are especially valuable. Also well referenced.
2. Armstrong G, Pasquet A, Fukamachi K, et al. Use of peak systolic strain as an index of regional left ventricular function: comparison with tissue Doppler velocity during dobutamine stress and myocardial ischemia. *J Am Soc Echocardiogr.* 2000;13:731-737.

One of several papers emphasizing the superior sensitivity of strain, which arises from site specificity. In an animal model of infarction, strain identified functional changes before tissue velocity.

3. La Gerche A, Jurcut R, Voigt JU. Right ventricular function by strain echocardiography. *Curr Opin Cardiol.* 2010;25:430-436.
   Nice, current overview of application of strain to right ventricular evaluation from a group of experts in this area.

4. Tops LF, Delgado V, Bax JJ. The role of speckle tracking strain imaging in cardiac pacing. *Echocardiography.* 2009;26:315-323.
   Summary of myocardial imaging indications with pacing.

5. Marwick TH, Leano RL, Brown J, et al. Myocardial strain measurement with 2-dimensional speckle-tracking echocardiography: definition of normal range. *JACC Cardiovasc Imaging.* 2009;2:80-84.
   Normal range study involving definitively normal subjects from the community.

6. Haugaa KH, Smedsrud MK, Steen T, et al. Mechanical dispersion assessed by myocardial strain in patients after myocardial infarction for risk prediction of ventricular arrhythmia. *JACC Cardiovasc Imaging.* 2010;3:247-256.
   This landmark paper from a prominent Norwegian group emphasizes the association of mechanical dispersion with ventricular arrhythmias. Given the limited predictive value of ejection fraction, in the future strain may play an important role in risk evaluation for implantable defibrillator insertion.

7. Ho E, Brown A, Barrett P, et al. Subclinical anthracycline- and trastuzumab-induced cardiotoxicity in the long-term follow-up of asymptomatic breast cancer survivors: a speckle tracking echocardiographic study. *Heart.* 2010;96:701-707.
   One of about a dozen published studies emphasizing the use of strain to identify subclinical left ventricular dysfunction in patients treated with chemotherapy. This may prove to be an important application for strain imaging.

8. Stanton T, Leano R, Marwick TH. Prediction of all-cause mortality from global longitudinal speckle strain: comparison with ejection fraction and wall motion scoring. *Circ Cardiovasc Imaging.* 2009;2:356-364.
   This was the initial study that emphasized the predictive value of strain. Interestingly, this was noted in patients with relatively preserved left ventricular function. This is a setting where ejection fraction does not perform well, suggesting a potential role for the application of strain. Another circumstance is left ventricular hypertrophy, in which ejection fraction shows limitations as a marker of endocardial shortening, where mid-wall shortening (analogous to strain) may be a better marker of dysfunction.

9. Weidemann F, Niemann M, Breunig F, et al. Long-term effects of enzyme replacement therapy on Fabry cardiomyopathy: evidence for a better outcome with early treatment. *Circulation.* 2009;119:524-529.
   This study, which emphasizes the importance of intervention before the development of fibrosis (identified by contrast MRI), uses strain rate as the functional parameter of choice for follow-up.

10. Marwick TH. Consistency of myocardial deformation imaging between vendors. *Eur J Echocardiogr.* 2010;11:414-416.
    This editorial summarizes the very troubling evidence that "strain is not strain." Variability from one examination to the next depends not only on functional change and hemodynamics but also on which manufacturer's machine is being used. Until this is resolved, the implication is that the same device should be used for baseline and follow-up scans.

Assessing Twist and Torsion

Sherif F. Nagueh

7

Background

Left Ventricular Systole
- Left ventricular (LV) systole begins with a rapid rise in LV pressure.
- During the isovolumic contraction (IVC) period, pressure increases while LV volume is unchanged.
- During the ejection period, LV volume decreases until it reaches its lowest value at end systole.
- Invasive parameters of LV systolic function during the IVC period include rate of change in pressure over time (dP/dt).
- LV stroke volume, ejection fraction (EF), and stroke work can be used to assess LV systolic function during the ejection phase.
- LV rotation is another marker of LV systolic function during ejection.
- Apical rotation starts by an initial clockwise rotation during the IVC period, but the major rotation occurs during the ejection phase in a counterclockwise direction.
- Basal rotation starts by an initial counterclockwise rotation during the IVC period, but the major rotation occurs during the ejection phase in a clockwise direction.

Left Ventricular Diastole
- LV pressure declines rapidly during the isovolumetric relaxation (IVR) period.
- During IVR, untwisting or recoil takes place and precedes LV expansion in the longitudinal and radial directions.
- An intraventricular pressure gradient follows untwisting, which helps direct LV intracavitary flow to the LV apex.
- This is followed by LV long axis expansion and mitral annulus early diastolic recoil velocity (e').
- When the left atrial (LA) pressure exceeds LV diastolic pressure, the mitral valve opens and transmitral early diastolic velocity (E) is recorded.

- Therefore, LV untwisting is the earliest mechanical event during diastole.

Relation of Torsion to Cardiac Fiber Orientation
- Myocardial fibers are arranged in a helical structure.
- The subendocardial fibers are arranged in a right-handed helix.
- The subepicardial fibers are arranged in a left-handed helix.
- Earlier activation of subendocardial fibers accounts for the apical clockwise rotation during IVC.
- The later contraction of the subepicardial fibers accounts for apical counterclockwise rotation during ejection. This is due to the larger radius of subepicardial fibers.

Definitions of Twist and Torsion
- Direction of rotation is determined by looking at the heart from the apex.
- Apical rotation starts with an initial clockwise movement followed by a net counterclockwise direction (positive sign) in normal hearts (Fig. 7-1).
- Basal rotation starts with an initial counterclockwise movement followed by a net clockwise direction (negative sign) in normal hearts (Fig. 7-2).
- Twist is the net difference between apical and basal rotations (algebraic difference).
- Twist is normally around 7 to 9 ± 3 to 4 degrees.
- Twist varies with age and some studies have shown that it is higher in elderly subjects (>60 years).
- Torsion is the twist in degrees divided by LV long axis (distance between basal and apical segments).
- A better account of cardiac size is possible by calculating torsion as: Twist multiplied by average value of the radii of LV apical and basal cross sections divided by length.

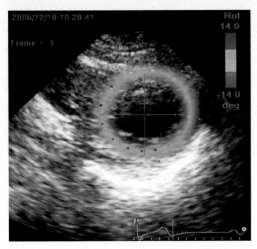
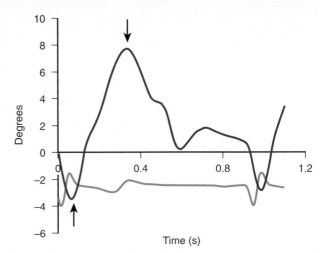

Figure 7-1. Apical rotation in degrees of rotation (*y* axis) versus time in seconds (*x* axis). Notice the presence of an initial small clockwise rotation (deflection below baseline, *arrow*), followed by counterclockwise rotation (about 8 degrees, *arrow*). The rotation curve is shown in blue. The electrocardiogram is shown in green.

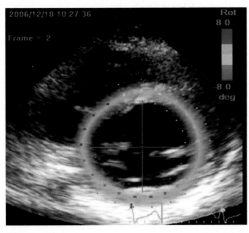
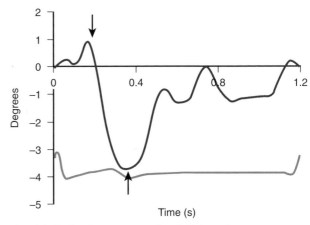

Figure 7-2. Basal rotation in degrees (*y* axis) versus time (*x* axis). Notice the presence of an initial small counterclockwise rotation (deflection above baseline, *arrow*), followed by clockwise rotation (about 3.5 degrees, *arrow*). Twist in this example is 8 − (−3.5) = 11.5 degrees.

- The above expression can allow comparison of rotational deformation between hearts of different sizes.

Definition of Untwisting
- Untwisting or recoil occurs during the isovolumetric relaxation time (IVRT) and early LV filling period.
- It occurs in a direction opposite to that of twisting.
- Untwisting can be expressed as the amount of recoil during IVRT.
- Peak untwisting velocity is usually measured and used to reflect the direction and speed of recoil.

- Untwisting rate during IVRT only can be measured as well.
- Aside from peak untwisting velocity, the timing of peak untwisting provides additional information.
- Normally, peak untwisting precedes LV expansion and mitral inflow.

Hemodynamic Determinants of Twist/Torsion
- An increase in LV contractility leads to an increase in torsion (Figs. 7-3 and 7-4). A direct positive correlation exists between torsion and LV EF, stroke volume, and *dP/dt*.

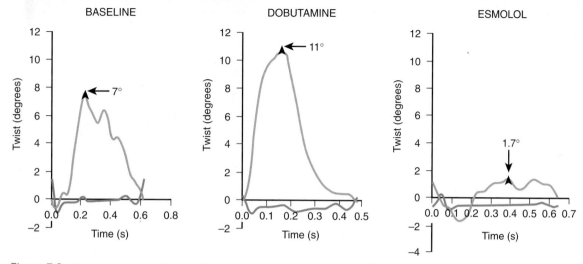

Figure 7-3. Changes in twist with alterations in left ventricular (LV) contractility from a dog with normal LV function. When contractility increased with dobutamine, twist increased from 7 to 11 degrees. When contractility was depressed with esmolol, twist decreased to 1.7 degrees.

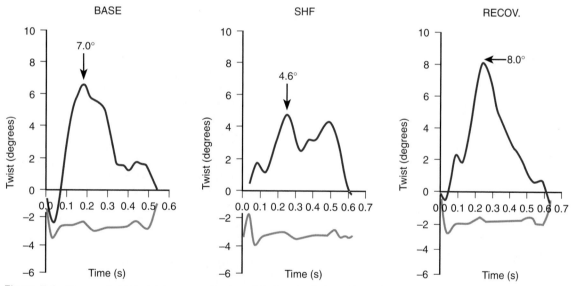

Figure 7-4. Changes in LV twist from an animal model of pacing-induced heart failure. When heart failure was induced by rapid pacing for several weeks, LV twist decreased from 7 to 4.6 degrees. Pacing was then stopped and LV function improved with time. At recovery twist was back to normal at 8 degrees.

- Some animal studies have shown that an increase in heart rate increases twist.
- Increased afterload with unchanged preload leads to a decrease in twist.
- In normal humans, increased preload can lead to an increase in twist.
- In patients, simultaneous changes in load and contractility often occur and limit the clinical application of twist as a pure index of LV contractility.

Hemodynamic Determinants of Peak Untwisting Velocity

- An increase in LV twist leads to an increase in untwisting. This positive correlation occurs in normal and diseased hearts.
- The positive association between twist and untwisting was shown in animal experiments and human studies.
- A faster decline in LV pressure during IVRT, in the absence of a change in loading

conditions, leads to an increase in LV peak untwisting velocity.
- In animal studies, dobutamine infusion was accompanied by shortening of tau and an increase in peak untwisting velocity.
- In animal studies, esmolol infusion was accompanied by prolongation of tau and a decrease in peak untwisting velocity.
- In animal studies, increased afterload was associated with reduced untwisting.
- In human studies, increased LV afterload leads to reduced and delayed untwisting.
- The impact of afterload on timing of untwisting was noted in patients with hypertrophic obstructive cardiomyopathy (HOCM).
- HOCM patients had delayed untwisting that occurred earlier after relief of dynamic obstruction.
- In animal models, an acute increase in LV end-systolic volume leads to a decrease in untwisting velocity, despite unchanged LV relaxation. Conversely, an acute decrease in LV end-systolic volume leads to an increase in peak untwisting velocity in the absence of changes in LV relaxation (Fig. 7-5).
- In normal animals where load and contractility are both altered, peak untwisting velocity tracks best the changes in LV end-systolic volume.
- In patients with systolic heart failure, LV twist, time constant of LV relaxation, and LV end-systolic volume are the hemodynamic determinants of peak untwisting velocity.
- In patients with diastolic heart failure (DHF), LV twist and LV end-systolic volume (but not the time constant of LV relaxation) are the hemodynamic determinants of peak untwisting velocity.

Relation of Peak Untwisting to Left Ventricular Filling
- The following sequence of events occurs during diastole in the normal heart:
  - LV untwisting.
  - Basal to apical intraventricular pressure gradient.
  - LV expansion in longitudinal and radial directions.
  - Mitral valve opening followed by LV filling during early diastole.
- The above normal sequence is preserved in normal hearts with exercise, which leads to earlier onset of LV untwisting and therefore adequate LV filling despite higher heart rate and shorter diastolic filling time.

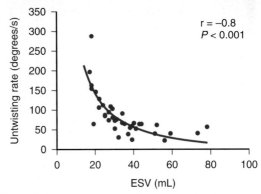

Figure 7-5. Regression plot (*y* versus 1/*x*) between LV untwisting rate and LV end-systolic volume (ESV) in animal experiments with LV volumes altered by inferior vena cava occlusion and esmolol infusion. There was no significant change in tau with changes in LV ESV. *(Data from Wang J, Khoury DS, Yue Y, et al. Left ventricular untwisting rate by speckle tracking echocardiography.* Circulation. *2007;116: 2580–2586.)*

- With cardiovascular disease, the above sequence is disturbed such that peak LV untwisting can be delayed and may even follow mitral valve opening. This deprives the ventricle from the beneficial effects of untwisting on LV filling, which is maintained in these hearts by increased LA pressure.
- In patients with abnormal myocardial function, delayed untwisting is associated with increased LV filling pressures.
- Patients with DHF and delayed untwisting have larger LA volumes and higher pulmonary artery pressures than patients without delayed untwisting.

Effects of Exercise on Left Ventricular Twist Mechanics
- In normal subjects, twist/torsion and untwisting velocity all generally increase with exercise.
- There are variations based on exercise type, intensity and duration, and whether measurements are obtained from elite athletes or not.
- LV untwisting occurs earlier with exercise and precedes mitral valve opening.
- Short-term high-intensity exercise is accompanied by increased torsion.
- After an ultra-long-distance triathlon, LV twist and untwisting can be reduced and delayed and accompanied by other indices of depressed LV systolic and diastolic function.

Echocardiographic Approach
(Table 7-1)

Acquisition

- Patients are imaged in the supine lateral position.
- Transducer frequency is 1.7 to 2 MHz; a higher frequency can be used in the absence of concerns for attenuation.

- Tissue Doppler (TD) has been used for measurement torsion and untwisting.
- TD has the advantage of high frame rate and superior temporal resolution.
- TD can be of value when imaging patients with rapid heart rates, as in children and during exercise.
- TD has the limitation of a low signal-to-noise ratio and is heavily dependent on the presence or absence of angulation between the ultrasound beam and the plane of motion.
- The above limitations of TD have limited its application for the objective of measuring torsion and untwisting.
- Speckle tracking echocardiography (STE) is the most practical technique to measure torsion at this time.
- Images are obtained from parasternal short axis views acquired using a frame rate of around 80/s.
- A basal short axis view is acquired at the mitral valve level. This is identified by noting mitral valve leaflets in the middle of the view.
- A basal short axis view at the apex level is acquired just above the level of cavity obliteration.
- Three cardiac cycles (excluding premature beats) are digitally captured for use in analysis.

Analysis

- Analysis is performed off-line using commercially available software.
- Region of interest is located in the mid-myocardia region, closer to the subendocardial location.
- LV rotation is computed from the angular displacement of six segments in the basal and apical short axis views.
- Analysts need to confirm adequate tracking for each of the six segments at basal and apical levels.

TABLE 7-1 TECHNICAL DETAILS TO AVOID PITFALLS IN TORSION MEASUREMENTS BY STE	
Transducer frequency and focus	Selected to allow most optimum temporal and spatial resolution
Frame rate	80–100/s to reduce the extent of missing speckles due to out-of-plane motion
Image optimization	Avoid artifacts, particularly reverberation artifacts, which disrupt the correlation between speckle patterns in different frames.
Short axis views	Ideally circular
Anatomic landmarks	The basal level has the mitral valve at its center. The apical level is the one where the cavity is still seen and is located just proximal to the plane without a lumen.
Adequate tracking	Regions of interest should be placed in the mid-myocardial level and correct tracking verified frame by frame.

- The analysis package will automatically display and compute torsion and its first derivative (twisting and untwisting rates).

Twist Mechanics in Cardiac Diseases

Systolic Heart Failure
Systolic Function
- Patients with systolic heart failure have depressed LV contractility usually as a result of coronary artery disease (CAD) and previous myocardial infarction or dilated cardiomyopathy (Table 7-2).
- Depressed systolic function in this population is routinely quantified by LV EF.
- Compensatory changes include LV dilatation to maintain forward stroke volume.
- Due to the transmural extent of abnormal myocardial pathology/function in systolic heart failure, both endocardial and epicardial fibers are affected.
- The reduced contractility of epicardial fibers leads to a decrease in apical counterclockwise rotation and a decrease in LV torsion (Fig. 7-6).

Diastolic Function
- Patients with systolic heart failure have impaired LV relaxation and increased LV filling pressures to maintain LV filling and stroke volume.
- Peak untwisting velocity is markedly reduced in this population, and there are three main reasons for this abnormality:

- Reduced torsion: Given the positive effect of torsion on untwisting, the reduced torsion leads to a decrease in peak untwisting velocity.
- Slow LV relaxation: The reduced rate of decline of LV pressure during the IVR period leads to a reduction in peak untwisting velocity.
- Increased LV end-systolic volume: The increased end-systolic volume leads to reduced early diastolic recoil and decreased peak untwisting velocity.
- Peak untwisting velocity is also delayed.
- Both abnormalities in untwisting velocity (decreased and delayed peak velocity) are associated with diastolic dysfunction and increased LV filling pressures.
- Patients with systolic heart failure and higher wedge pressure usually have lower peak untwisting velocity.
- The above global changes in LV torsion and untwisting can be accompanied by regional abnormalities.
- Specifically, variable abnormalities can occur in apical rotation, which depends on whether CAD is the etiology or not and on the presence of ischemia/infarction.

Diastolic Heart Failure
Systolic Function
- Patients have DHF usually due to hypertension and/or diabetes mellitus.
- LV end-diastolic and end-systolic volumes and LV EF are normal.

TABLE 7-2   TORSION IN PATIENTS WITH CARDIOVASCULAR DISEASE

Cardiovascular Disease	Torsion and Untwisting
LV hypertrophy in hypertension	Torsion normal or reduced and untwisting velocity normal or reduced and delayed
Diastolic heart failure	Torsion normal or increased, untwisting velocity normal but delayed
Systolic heart failure	Torsion, twisting, and untwisting velocities reduced and delayed
AS	Torsion increased and normalizes after valve replacement
MR	Torsion and untwisting usually normal when EF is normal, and decrease with decline in systolic function
Hypertrophic cardiomyopathy	Torsion normal as a group finding. Peak untwisting velocity is delayed and related to exercise tolerance.
Amyloidosis	Early disease associated with normal torsion, which is reduced with progression
Dilated cardiomyopathy	Reduced twist and delayed and reduced untwisting
Noncompaction cardiomyopathy	Reduced rotation, cardiac base and apex rotate in the same direction
CAD	Abnormality related to extent of ischemia and infarction. Improvement occurs after revascularization of viable areas.
Constrictive pericarditis	Reduced twist

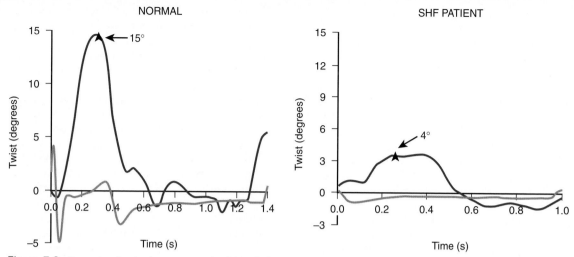

Figure 7-6. Example of twist from a normal subject (*left panel*) and from a patient in systolic heart failure (SHF; *right panel*). LV twist in the normal subject is 15 degrees, which is reduced to 4 degrees in the SHF patient. The abnormally reduced twist is concordant with the severely depressed EF (<30%).

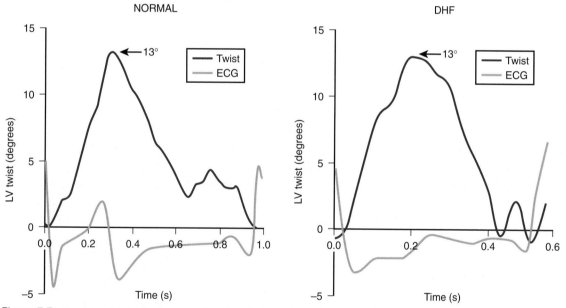

Figure 7-7. Example of twist from a normal subject (*left panel*) and from a patient in diastolic heart failure (DHF) (*right panel*). LV twist in both cases is normal at 13 degrees. LV peak twisting rate (first derivative of LV twist during systole) is 94 degrees/s in the normal subject and 121 degrees/s in the DHF patient.

- Patients usually have an abnormally reduced longitudinal function that can be quantified by longitudinal strain.
- Radial strain can also be reduced, though circumferential strain is often normal.
- Twist is usually preserved and can even be increased (Fig. 7-7).
- Abnormal endocardial function but preserved epicardial function account for the normal twist values in this population.

- Endocardial fibers are affected in patients with DHF, possibly due to fibrosis and abnormal coronary flow reserve. Accordingly, their action to produce clockwise rotation is limited.
- On the other hand, epicardial fibers have normal function and the major effect to produce counterclockwise rotation is unopposed, leading to increased apical counterclockwise rotation and LV twist.

- While twist is normal at rest, exercise is accompanied by small increments in torsion when DHF patients are compared with age-matched controls.

Diastolic Function
- Patients with DHF have impaired LV relaxation and increased LV filling pressures to maintain LV filling and stroke volume.
- Despite abnormal diastolic function, peak untwisting velocity is often preserved (Fig. 7-8).
- There are two main reasons for the latter observation:
  - Normal or increased torsion: Given the positive effect of torsion on untwisting, normal or increased torsion leads to a normal or increased peak untwisting velocity.
  - Normal LV end-systolic volume: Normal or even reduced LV end-systolic volume in patients with a hyperdynamic EF leads to

increased early diastolic LV recoil with preserved suction and normal or increased peak untwisting velocity.
- Thus, despite the slow LV relaxation, patients with DHF usually have a preserved peak untwisting velocity.
- In this population, no significant relation was observed between the time constant of LV relaxation (tau) and LV peak untwisting velocity.
- Although peak untwisting velocity is normal, it can be delayed in a number of patients.
- Importantly, the delay in peak untwisting velocity is associated with increased LV filling pressures.
- In addition, the delay of peak untwisting velocity is associated with larger LA volumes and increased pulmonary artery pressures in patients with DHF.
- In addition to the reduced twist reserve with exercise, patients in DHF have a reduced ability to augment untwisting with exercise in

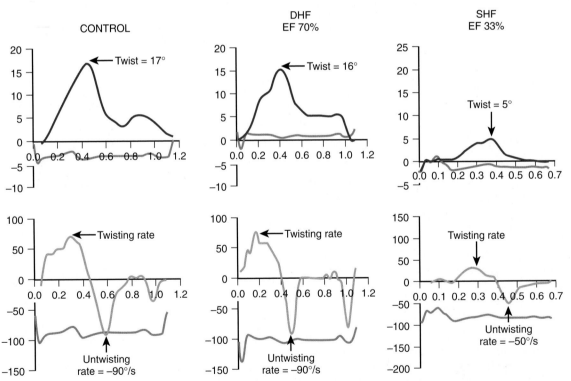

Figure 7-8. Examples of LV twist and the first derivative of twist versus time from three cases. *Upper panels,* Twist curves versus time (*y* axis = degrees of rotation and *x* axis = time in seconds). *Top left panel,* Twist curve from a normal subject (twist = 17 degrees). *Top middle panel,* Twist curve from a patient with DHF (16 degrees). *Top right panel,* Reduced twist from a patient with SHF (5 degrees). *Bottom panels,* Untwisting velocity (*y* axis = degrees/s) versus time (*x* axis = seconds). *Bottom left panel,* Untwisting velocity from a normal subject (untwisting rate, –90 degrees/s). *Bottom middle panel,* Untwisting velocity from a patient with diastolic heart failure and normal EF (untwisting rate = –90 degrees/s). *Bottom right panel,* Untwisting velocity from a patient with systolic dysfunction (untwisting rate = –50 degrees/s). (*Reprinted with permission from Wang J, Khoury DS, Yue Y, et al. Left ventricular untwisting rate by speckle tracking echocardiography. Circulation. 2007;116:2580–2586.*)

comparison with age-matched controls. This may account for their reduced exercise tolerance.

Coronary Artery Disease

- Abnormalities depend heavily on the presence or absence of ischemia at the time of imaging and the extent of ischemia.
- The presence, location, and extent of infarction also affect torsion in CAD.
- Accordingly, twist mechanics are affected by the location of coronary stenosis (Fig. 7-9).
- Torsion is affected by the presence and transmural extent of infarction.
- With apical transmural infarction, twist is reduced and its direction can change from normal (i.e., become net clockwise).
- With subendocardial infarction, apical rotation can be normal.
- Patients with acute anterior wall infarction have reduced apical rotation, largely due to reduced rotation of anterior and septal segments.
- Patients with proximal left anterior descending occlusion can have reduced basal rotation as well.

- In patients with acute anterior wall infarction, LV twist is inversely related to LV end-diastolic and end-systolic volumes but directly related to LV EF.
- LV peak untwisting velocity is reduced in acute anterior wall infarction when LV twist is reduced and LV end-systolic volume is increased.
- With successful revascularization of viable myocardium, LV twist can improve.
- With postinfarction cardiomyopathy and depressed EF, twist and peak untwisting velocity are reduced.
- There are limited data on the changes of torsion with stress echocardiography.
- One report with dobutamine and speckle tracking noted no difference in torsion between patients with anteroapical and inferoposterior infarction. Torsion was most impaired in patients with multiple areas of myocardial infarction.
- In one study, dobutamine-induced ischemia did not affect torsion. However, additional data are needed to draw meaningful conclusions regarding the effect of ischemia on torsion in humans.

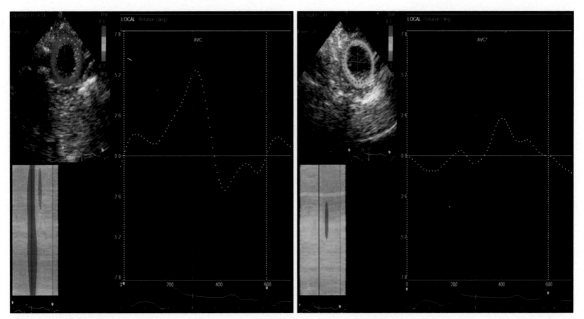

Figure 7-9. Changes in apical rotation after acute left anterior descending coronary artery occlusion. The two-dimensional image in the upper left region of each panel shows the LV short axis at the level of the apex. The color bar displays the color scale for rotation. The graphs show rotation in degrees (*y* axis) versus time in milliseconds (*x* axis). After occlusion, apical rotation is dramatically reduced from 5.2 degrees to 0.5 degrees.

Dilated Cardiomyopathy

- Twist is usually reduced in parallel with the magnitude of LV systolic dysfunction.
- Peak untwisting velocity is reduced and delayed.
- Treatment of dilated cardiomyopathy with biventricular pacing is associated with an increase in twist. This response can predict the occurrence of LV reverse remodeling after pacing.
- Patients with noncompaction cardiomyopathy can have solid body rotation with the base and apex rotating in the same direction during systole.

Hypertrophic Cardiomyopathy

- Twist is normal or increased in hypertrophic cardiomyopathy (HCM) patients as a group (Fig. 7-10), but it is reduced in some patients.
- Twist varies with pattern and extent of hypertrophy.
- Twist is also affected by preload and afterload in HCM.
- Patients with apical HCM frequently have reduced apical rotation and torsion.
- Abnormal rotation can be present in segments with normal thickness.

- Changes in torsion with disease progression are not yet known.
- A recent study with cardiac magnetic resonance (MR) reported that torsion was increased in mutation carriers who had normal wall thickness at a time when circumferential strain was reduced.
- Peak untwisting velocity is normal or increased in many but not all patients.
- There are studies that reported reduced untwisting velocity in HCM and linked it to abnormal LV filling.
- HCM patients with reduced untwisting have a more advanced grade of diastolic dysfunction.
- The delayed peak untwisting velocity is a more common abnormality than the decrease in peak untwisting velocity in HCM.
- The delayed peak untwisting velocity is present at rest and with exercise.
- The timing and amplitude of peak untwisting velocity are affected by afterload.
- Increased afterload is associated with a delay in peak untwisting velocity in HCM.
- HCM patients with dynamic obstruction have a longer delay in peak untwisting velocity than HCM patients without dynamic obstruction.
- Peak untwisting velocity occurs earlier after septal reduction therapy in patients with dynamic obstruction.

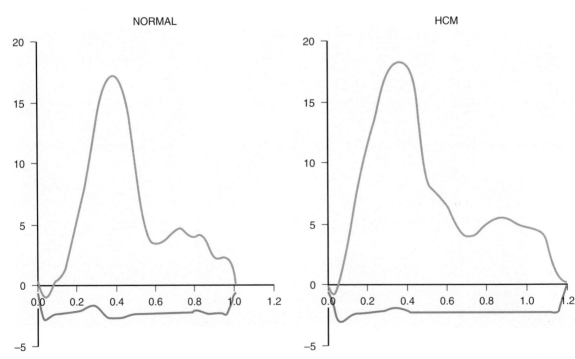

Figure 7-10. Example of twist from a normal subject (*left panel*) and from a patient with hypertrophic cardiomyopathy (HCM) (*right panel*). LV twist in both cases is preserved at 18 degrees.

- The delay in peak untwisting velocity is an important determinant of exercise tolerance in HCM patients with and without dynamic obstruction.
- The delay in peak untwisting velocity is directly related to LV diastolic pressures such that patients with the longer delay have higher LV filling pressures.
- The increase in LV torsion and peak untwisting with exercise are blunted in HCM patients.
- The earlier occurrence of peak untwisting velocity with exercise is also blunted and contributes to the symptoms of exertional dyspnea.

Cardiac Amyloidosis

- Few studies have evaluated twist mechanics in cardiac amyloidosis.
- In early disease, amyloid proteins are deposited in the subendocardium.
- Accordingly, longitudinal deformation is reduced but circumferential deformation is preserved.
- In early disease, twist and untwisting are normal.
- With advanced disease, amyloid deposits are more extensive.
- Accordingly, with late disease, circumferential deformation is affected and peak twist and untwisting rate are reduced.
- Reduced longitudinal strain has been shown to predict clinical events in patients with cardiac amyloidosis. However, it is unknown whether LV twist can also predict outcome in this population.

Aortic Stenosis

- Apical rotation is usually increased in patients with normal EF.
- Basal rotation can be normal or reduced in patients with normal EF.
- Accordingly, twist is usually increased in the presence of normal EF.
- In patients with aortic stenosis and depressed EF, LV twist is reduced.
- Torsion was inversely related to LV mass in some studies.
- Twist can be related to Doppler indices of aortic stenosis severity.
- Peak untwisting rate can be normal or increased in patients with aortic stenosis and normal EF.

- LV untwisting is usually delayed and prolonged in patients with aortic stenosis and normal EF.
- The delay to peak untwisting rate is related to the severity of diastolic dysfunction assessed by the E/e' ratio.
- Twist normalizes after aortic valve replacement.

Mitral Regurgitation

- There are changes in LV torsion and untwisting that accompany the development and the progression of MR.
- Twist mechanics depend on whether the regurgitation is acute or chronic and whether LV EF is normal or reduced.
- In general, MR progression with the development of LV systolic dysfunction is accompanied by a decrease in LV torsion.
- In an animal model, MR progression from an acute to a chronic lesion was accompanied by a decrease in early diastolic recoil.
- In an animal model of chronic MR, LV mass increased but torsion decreased.
- In patients with chronic MR and normal EF, LV twist and peak untwisting velocity are normal early in the disease course.
- In patients with chronic MR, similar to heart failure patients and animal models, peak untwisting velocity is inversely related to LV end-systolic dimension/volume.
- In patients with extensive LV remodeling due to chronic MR, LV twist and peak untwisting velocity decrease, and peak untwisting velocity is delayed.
- The above changes in LV mechanics may contribute to LV systolic and diastolic dysfunction in these patients.
- It remains to be seen whether the changes in LV torsion can help determine the timing of surgical repair.

Constrictive Pericarditis

- Diseases that cause pericardial pathology can also involve the epicardium.
- The involvement of the epicardial layer results in a reduction in circumferential deformation.
- Accordingly, LV twist and peak untwisting velocity are reduced with constriction.
- The presence of apical adhesions can also reduce apical rotation.
- The abnormal twist mechanics can help differentiate pericardial constriction from myocardial restriction.

- Additional studies are needed to evaluate the incremental role of twist mechanics in the diagnosis of constrictive pericarditis and its differentiation from restrictive cardiomyopathy.

KEY POINTS

- In systolic heart failure, twist and peak untwisting velocity are reduced.
- In DHF, twist and peak untwisting velocity are usually normal, though peak untwisting velocity can be delayed.
- In CAD, the abnormalities in twist mechanics depend on the presence and extent of myocardial ischemia and infarction.
- In dilated cardiomyopathy, twist and untwisting are reduced.
- In noncompaction cardiomyopathy, the LV apex and base can rotate in the same direction.
- In HCM, twist abnormalities are variable, but these patients often have normal torsion. Although peak untwisting velocity can be normal, it is often delayed.
- Aortic stenosis patients have increased twist, which normalizes after valve replacement.
- In mitral regurgitation with normal EF, twist and peak untwisting velocity are normal.
- Patients with constrictive pericarditis have impaired twist.

Alternate Approaches to the Assessment of Left Ventricular Systolic Function

- LV rotational deformation is not needed for the routine day-to-day evaluation of LV systolic function.
- Currently available measurements of LV global systolic function include EF, mitral annulus systolic ejection velocity, and global longitudinal strain.
- In patients with normal cardiac function, all of the above parameters and torsion are normal.
- In patients with depressed EF, torsion is reduced but does not appear to provide incremental information to standard parameters.
- In patients with DHF, EF is >50% but annular systolic velocity and global longitudinal strain may be reduced. However, torsion is usually preserved and provides additional insight into the assessment of LV systolic function in this setting.

Alternate Approaches to the Assessment of Left Ventricular Diastolic Function

- LV peak untwisting velocity is not a routine measurement at the present time.
- American Society of Echocardiography/ European Association of Echocardiography (ASE/EAE) guidelines for the assessment of LV diastolic function include mitral inflow velocities, pulmonary vein velocities, flow propagation velocity, and mitral annulus TD velocities with different algorithms based on LV EF.
- In patients with depressed EF, peak untwisting velocity is reduced and does not appear to provide incremental information.
- In patients with normal EF, peak untwisting velocity and its timing can be of potential value in identifying early stages of abnormal function when the velocity can be increased.
- During exercise, both torsion and untwisting velocity measurements can reveal the reduced inotropic and lusitropic reserves in patients with DHF. Additional studies are needed to address their clinical utility.
- TD mitral annulus velocities and respiratory variations in mitral and tricuspid inflow are recommended for the differentiation of pericardial constriction and restrictive cardiomyopathy.
- It is not yet known if reduced torsion is an early marker of myocardial disease. At the present time, TD velocities and strain can be considered for that objective.

Role of Torsion in the Setting of Cardiac Resynchronization Therapy

- Patients with LV remodeling in the setting of systolic heart failure have abnormal myocardial function in part due to dyssynchrony.
- In the presence of an advanced degree of intraventricular dyssynchrony, LV twist is markedly reduced with a direct relation between the two parameters (radial dyssynchrony and twist).
- The presence of dyssynchrony between apical and basal rotations further contributes to the abnormally reduced torsion.
- Acute improvement of LV systolic function after CRT is often accompanied by an improvement of LV twist.
- CRT responders show progressive improvement in twist that parallels the increase in LV EF.
- The ability of twist measurements to predict response to CRT was addressed in one study,

and its absolute change was the strongest predictor of reverse remodeling.

- While promising, this approach cannot be recommended at the present time due to paucity of data.

Cardiac Magnetic Resonance versus Speckle Tracking Echocardiography for Torsion Measurements

- Torsion measurements were first performed by cardiac magnetic resonance (CMR) in animal and human studies.
- CMR has the advantage of a high spatial resolution and is not affected by suboptimal images.
- STE has the advantage of a higher temporal resolution than CMR but is heavily affected by image quality.
- CMR measurements that are based on the analysis of tagged images are not affected by through plane motion, while STE is heavily affected by it.
- CMR is not performed in most patients with pacemakers/intracardiac defibrillators at the present time, whereas STE can be safely performed in these patients.
- Given the fact that echocardiography is often the initial imaging modality in many patients, STE is often the first modality to use for torsion measurements and CMR can be reserved for patients with technically challenging echocardiographic studies.

Suggested Reading

1. Buckberg G, Hoffman JIE, Mahajan A, et al. Cardiac mechanics revisited: The relationship of cardiac architecture to ventricular function. *Circulation.* 2008; 118:2571-2587.
   This review article describes the relation between cardiac motion and twisting with ventricular muscle architecture.
2. Geyer H, Caracciolo G, Abe H, et al. Assessment of myocardial mechanics using speckle tracking echocardiography: fundamentals and clinical applications. *J Am Soc Echocardiogr.* 2010;23:351-369.
   This review article summarizes the basic concepts behind the assessment of cardiac mechanics by STE as well as the emerging clinical applications.
3. Bertini M, Sengupta PP, Nucifora G, et al. Role of left ventricular twist mechanics in the assessment of cardiac dyssynchrony in heart failure. *JACC Cardiovasc Imaging.* 2009;2:1425-1435.
   The above review article addresses the role of twist in the evaluation of dyssynchrony and the prediction of reverse remodeling in heart failure patients.
4. Sengupta PP, Tajik AJ, Chandrasekaran K, Khandheria BK. Twist mechanics of the left ventricle: principles and application. *JACC Cardiovasc Imaging.* 2008;1:366-376.
   This review explains the theoretical basis of LV twist and its alterations under different experimental and clinical settings.
5. Notomi Y, Martin-Miklovic MG, Oryszak SJ, et al. Enhanced ventricular untwisting during exercise: A mechanistic manifestation of elastic recoil described by Doppler tissue imaging. *Circulation.* 2006;113:2524-2533.
   This article shows the relation of LV untwisting to cardiac filling at rest and with exercise in normal subjects and in patients with hypertrophic cardiomyopathy.
6. Notomi Y, Lysyansky P, Setser RM, et al. Measurement of ventricular torsion by two-dimensional ultrasound speckle tracking imaging. *J Am Coll Cardiol.* 2005;45:2034-2041.
   This article contains the validation results for twist measurements by STE against cardiac magnetic resonance as the gold standard.
7. Helle-Valle T, Crosby J, Edvardsen T, et al. New noninvasive method for assessment of left ventricular rotation: speckle tracking echocardiography. *Circulation.* 2005;112:3149-3156.
   This article contains the validation results for twist measurements by STE against sonomicrometry in animals and cardiac magnetic resonance in humans.
8. Bertini M, Nucifora G, Marsan NA, et al. Left ventricular rotational mechanics in acute myocardial infarction and in chronic (ischemic and nonischemic) heart failure patients. *Am J Cardiol.* 2009;103:1506-1512.
   The above article describes the changes in LV rotation in acute myocardial infarction and in patients with chronic heart failure.
9. Meluzin J, Spinarova L, Hude P, et al. Left ventricular mechanics in idiopathic dilated cardiomyopathy: systolic-diastolic coupling and torsion. *J Am Soc Echocardiogr.* 2009;22:486-493.
   This study shows the changes in LV torsion and the correlation between systolic and diastolic deformation in patients with dilated cardiomyopathy.

Echocardiographic Tools for Cardiac Resynchronization Therapy

8

Veronica Lea J. Dimaano, Kristian Eskesen, and Theodore P. Abraham

Background

- Cardiac resynchronization therapy (CRT) is a catheter-based therapy for patients with heart failure and evidence of left ventricular (LV) dyssynchrony.
- LV mechanical dyssynchrony is discoordinate (nonsimultaneous) ventricular contraction resulting from either an electrical timing delay or a functional abnormality.
- Atrial biventricular pacing addresses dyssynchrony at the atrio-, inter-, and intraventricular levels.
- There are two mechanisms of LV dyssynchrony:
  - LV dyssynchrony resulting from abnormal LV contraction caused by diffuse tissue damage or nonuniform wall structure (e.g., scar tissue from a previous myocardial infarction [MI]) that interferes with normal LV activation, which may not respond to CRT.
  - LV dyssynchrony resulting from discoordinated LV contraction caused by a regional delay in the electrical activation (electromechanical dyssynchrony), which is amenable to electrical resynchronization.
- In electromechanical dyssynchrony, infranodal conduction delay, most commonly in a left bundle branch pattern, results in a dyssynchronous LV contraction that is characterized by:
  - early activation of the inter-ventricular septum,
  - lateral wall prestretch,
  - delayed lateral wall contraction at higher stress,
  - further systolic stretch of the early activated septum.
- Early systolic contraction of the "early activated" septum results in forces that are unopposed by the contralateral quiescent lateral free wall.
- The conversion of the septal forces into prestretch of the inactive lateral wall mitigates any effect on LV chamber pressure, delaying intracavitary pressure rise (maximum rate of change in pressure over time [dP/dt max]).
- Through slow intramyocardial conduction, the lateral wall is activated in late systole with generation of peak force that occurs in early diastole after aortic valve closure (AVC).
- Delayed contraction and pressure development of the "late activated" lateral wall is unopposed by the now relaxing septum, which leads to end-systolic stretching of this region.
- The relaxing septum creates an energy "sink" for the late developing lateral forces, resulting in a reduced stroke volume and thus cardiac output, with an increase in left ventricular end-systolic volume (LVESV) (Fig. 8-1).
- In addition, late activation of the postero-lateral papillary muscle results in suboptimal mitral valve closure and mitral regurgitation, further decreasing forward cardiac output.

KEY POINTS

- LV dyssynchrony in heart failure patients results in ineffective LV systolic function and is associated with a worse prognosis.
- CRT addresses LV dyssynchrony at three levels: atrioventricular, interventricular, and intraventricular.
- The quantification of LV dyssynchrony is of key importance for optimum selection of patients for CRT because only those patients with severe mechanical dyssynchrony are likely to benefit from this therapy.

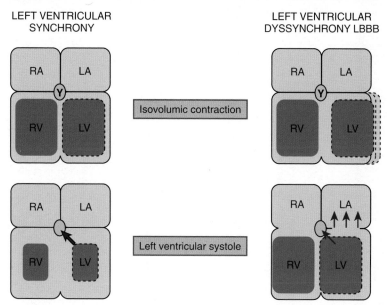

Figure 8-1. Schematic diagram illustrating pathophysiology of LV electromechanical dyssynchrony. *Left panel,* Effective recruitment of LV systolic forces from synchronous activation of the interventricular septum and the LV free wall. *Right panel, top,* In left bundle branch block (LBBB), earlier activation of the interventricular septum and the RV relative to the LV free wall results in a prestretch of the still quiescent LV free wall, thereby reducing the rate of pressure increase (*dP/dt* max) in the LV. *Right panel, bottom,* In LBBB, systolic forces generated by delayed LV free wall contraction are partly dissipated by late systolic stretching of the "early" relaxing septum. The late systolic septal stretch serves as a "sink" for blood volume that would otherwise be ejected, resulting in an increased end-systolic volume and reduced cardiac output. Moreover, discoordinated activation of the papillary muscles results in ineffective mitral valve closure and late systolic mitral regurgitation that further reduces effective forward flow.

Electrical Dyssynchrony

- Electrical dyssynchrony involves primary activation delay typically manifested by a widened QRS complex.
- Electrocardiography (ECG) is the simplest way to measure electrical dyssynchrony.
- While a prolonged QRS duration remains one of the criteria for the selection of patients for CRT, 30% to 40% of patients who fulfill this eligibility criteria do not show a symptomatic response or reverse remodeling.
- Hence, electrical dyssynchrony alone, as detected by ECG, may not be an optimal predictor of CRT response.

M-mode and Doppler Approaches to Quantifying Mechanical Dyssynchrony

- A wide range of imaging modalities have been used to measure mechanical dyssynchrony, with echocardiography having accumulated the largest pool of evidence and being used more frequently in selecting patients for CRT (Table 8-1).
- Strengths and weaknesses of the various echocardiographic techniques used in the assessment of mechanical dyssynchrony are summarized in Table 8-2.

M-Mode Echocardiography
Acquisition

- Using a parasternal long axis or a short axis view, the M-mode cursor is positioned at the mid-ventricular level (papillary muscle level).
- Color tissue Doppler (TD) can be activated if color TD M-mode is desired.
- Capture M-mode images at a sweep speed of 50 to 100 mm/s.

Data Analysis

- The time delay between the peak inward motions of the anterior septum and posterior wall is identified and measured (Fig. 8-2).
- A septal-to-posterior wall motion delay (SPWMD) of at least 130 ms has been shown to predict LV reverse remodeling and clinical outcome after CRT.

Pitfalls

- Complex septal dynamics may result in difficulties in detecting peak inward motion for timing.
- Can only assess anterior septum and posterior wall.

Text continued on page 120.

TABLE 8-1   ECHOCARDIOGRAPHIC TECHNIQUES IN QUANTIFYING MECHANICAL DYSSYNCHRONY

Echocardiographic Technique	Orientation of Dyssynchrony Measurement	Level of Dyssynchrony	Index of Dyssynchrony	Dyssynchrony Analysis	Cut-off Value
M-mode Routine M-mode	Radial	Intraventricular	Opposing wall motion delay Peak inward motion Septum and posterior wall	Time delay between the peak inward motions of the anterior septum and posterior wall	≥130 ms[a]
Color TD M-mode (adjunct to routine M-mode)	Radial	Intraventricular	Opposing wall motion delay Peak inward motion Septum and posterior wall	Time delay between the peak inward motions of the anterior septum and posterior wall	
Doppler Echocardiography	Not applicable	Interventricular	Pre-ejection period difference Time to onset of aortic and pulmonic flow LV and RV	Difference between the time to onset of aortic and pulmonic flows measured from the onset of the QRS complex on ECG	≥45 ms[b]
Tissue Doppler (TD) Color-coded TD velocity	Longitudinal	Intraventricular	Opposing wall time delay Time-to-peak systolic velocity (2-, 4-, 12-sites)	Time interval between systolic velocity peaks of two opposing walls in the same cine loop.	≥65 ms[c]
			Maximum time delay Time-to-peak systolic velocity (6 basal LV segments)	Difference between the longest and the shortest time-to-peak systolic velocities measured from the onset of QRS complex or peak of R wave among 12 LV segments (ejection phase and including post systolic shortening)	>110 ms[d]
			Maximum time delay Time-to-peak systolic velocity (12 LV segments)	Difference between the longest and the shortest time-to-peak systolic velocities measured from the onset of QRS complex or peak of R wave among 12 LV segments (ejection phase only)	≥100 ms[e]
			Dispersion of peak systolic velocity timing Time-to-peak systolic velocity (12 LV segments)	12-segment standard deviation of the time-to-peak systolic velocity measured from the onset of QRS complex or the peak of R wave	≥33 ms[f]
Pulsed TD velocity	Longitudinal	Intraventricular	Maximum time delay Time-to-onset of systolic velocity 4–6 basal LV segments	Difference between the longest and the shortest EMC time (measured from the onset of QRS complex to the onset of systolic velocity) wave among basal LV segments	NA

Method	Strain type	Parameter	Description	Value
	Interventricular	Maximum time delay Time to onset of systolic velocity RV and LV basal segments	Difference between the basal RV free wall EMC time and longest LV basal segment EMC	NA
	Composite intra- and interventricular		Sum of intra- and interventricular EMC time delay	≥100 ms[g]
TD-derived strain rate (SR)	Longitudinal	Delayed longitudinal contraction Systolic SR ending after AVC 12 LV segments	Percentage of segments with systolic SR ending after AVC	NA[h]
TD-derived strain	Longitudinal	Dispersion of peak longitudinal strain timing Time to peak longitudinal strain within the entire cardiac cycle 12 LV segments	12-segment SD of the time to peak longitudinal strain measured from the onset of QRS complex or the peak of R wave	NA[i]
	Radial	Opposing wall time delay Time to peak radial strain Anterior septum and posterior wall	Difference between peak positive (radial) strain timings in the anterior septum and posterior wall	≥130 ms[j]
Tissue synchronization imaging	Longitudinal	Dispersion of peak systolic velocity timing TSI-guided time-to-peak systolic velocity 12 LV segments	SD of time-to-peak systolic velocity (ejection phase)	>34 ms[k]
		Opposing wall time delay TSI-guided time-to-peak systolic velocity Anterior septum and posterior wall	Time interval between anterior septum and posterior wall systolic velocity peaks in the same cine loop	≥65 ms[l]
Speckle Tracking Strain Echocardiography	Longitudinal	Strain Delay Index End-systolic strain and peak negative (longitudinal) strain (entire cardiac cycle) 16 LV segments	Sum of the difference between the peak negative strain and end-systolic strain on 16 LV segments	≥25%[m]
		Strain Dyssynchrony Index Time to peak negative (longitudinal) strain (entire cardiac cycle) 12 LV segments	12-segment standard deviation of the time to peak negative strain within the entire cardiac cycle	NA[n]

Continued

TABLE 8-1 ECHOCARDIOGRAPHIC TECHNIQUES IN QUANTIFYING MECHANICAL DYSSYNCHRONY—cont'd

Echocardiographic Technique	Orientation of Dyssynchrony Measurement	Level of Dyssynchrony	Index of Dyssynchrony	Dyssynchrony Analysis	Cut-off Value
	Radial		Opposing wall time delay Peak positive strain Anterior septum and posterior wall	Difference between the anterior septum and posterior wall peak positive strain timing	≥130 ms[o]
Real time 3D	NA	Intraventricular	SDI or regional volumetric changes Time to minimum regional volume 16 LV segments	16-segment standard deviation of the time to minimum regional volume expressed as a percentage of the cardiac cycle	6.4% (6 months)[p]

NA, not applicable. AVC, aortic valve closure; EMC, electromechanical coupling; LV, left ventricle; RV, right ventricle; SD, standard deviation; SR, strain rate; TD, tissue Doppler; TSI, tissue synchronization imaging.

[a]Pitzalis MV, Iacoviello M, Romito R, et al. Ventricular asynchrony predicts a better outcome in patients with chronic heart failure receiving cardiac resynchronization therapy. JACC. 2005;45(1):65–69.

[b]Achilli A, Peraldo C, Sassarra M, et al. Prediction of response to cardiac resynchronization therapy: the Selection of Candidates for CRT (SCART) Study. PACE. 2006;29(Suppl 2):S11–S19.

[c]Bax JJ, Bleeker GB, Marwick TH, et al. Left ventricular dyssynchrony predicts response and prognosis after cardiac resynchronization therapy. JACC. 2004;44(9):1834–1840.

[d]Notabartolo D, Merlino J, Smith A, et al. Usefulness of the peak velocity difference by tissue Doppler imaging technique as an effective predictor of response to cardiac resynchronization therapy. Am J Cardiol. 2004;94:(6):817–820.

[e]Yu CM, Zhang Q, Chan YS, et al. Tissue Doppler imaging is superior to strain rate imaging and postsystolic shortening on the prediction of reverse remodeling in both ischemic and nonischemic heart failure after cardiac resynchronization therapy. Circulation. 2004;110(1):66–73.

[f]Yu CM, Chau E, Sanderson JE, et al. Tissue Doppler echocardiographic evidence of reverse remodeling and improved synchronicity by simultaneously delaying regional contraction after biventricular pacing therapy in heart failure. Circulation. 2002;105(4):438–445.

[g]Penicka M, Bartunek J, De Bruyne B, et al. Improvement of left ventricular function after cardiac resynchronization therapy is predicted by tissue Doppler imaging echocardiography. Circulation. 2004;109(8):978–983.

[h]Sogaard P, Egeblad H, Kim WY, et al. Tissue Doppler imaging predicts improved systolic performance and reversed left ventricular remodeling during long-term cardiac resynchronization therapy. JACC. 2002;40(4):723–730.

[i]Miyazaki C, Lin G, Powell BD, et al. Strain dyssynchrony index correlates with improvement in left ventricular volume after cardiac resynchronization therapy better than tissue velocity dyssynchrony indexes. Circ Cardiovasc Imaging. 2008;1(1):14–22.

[j]Dohi K, Suffoletto MS, Schwartzman D, et al. Utility of echocardiographic radial strain imaging to quantify left ventricular dyssynchrony and predict acute response to cardiac resynchronization therapy. AM J Cardiol. 2005;96(1):112–116.

[k]Yu CM, Zhang Q, Fung JWH, et al. A novel tool to assess systolic asynchrony and identify responders of cardiac resynchronization therapy by tissue synchronization imaging. JACC. 2005;45(5):677–684.

[l]Gorcsan J, Kanzaki H, Bazaz R, et al. Usefulness of echocardiographic tissue synchronization imaging to predict acute response to cardiac resynchronization therapy. Am J Cardiol. 2004;93(9):1178–1181.

[m]Lim P, Buakhamsri A, Popovic CV, et al. Longitudinal strain delay index by speckle tracking imaging: a new marker of response to cardiac resynchronization therapy. Circulation. 2008;118(11):1130–1137.

[n]Lim P, Mitchell-Heggs L, Buakhamsri A, et al. Impact of left ventricular size on tissue Doppler and longitudinal strain by speckle tracking for assessing wall motion and mechanical dyssynchrony in candidates for cardiac resynchronization therapy. J Am Soc Echocardiogr. 2009;22(6):695–701.

[o]Suffoletto MS, Dohi K, Cannesson M, et al. Novel speckle-tracking radial strain from routine black-and-white echocardiographic images to quantify dyssynchrony and predict response to cardiac resynchronization therapy. Circulation. 2006;113(7):960–968.

[p]Marsan NA, Breithardt OA, Delgado V, et al. Predicting response to CRT. The value of two- and three-dimensional echocardiography. Europace. 2008;10(Suppl):iii73–iii79.

TABLE 8-2 STRENGTHS AND WEAKNESSES OF DIFFERENT ECHOCARDIOGRAPHIC APPROACHES FOR ASSESSING PATIENTS FOR CARDIAC RESYNCHRONIZATION THERAPY

Echo Technique	Strengths	Weaknesses
M-mode	Simple and easy to measure Readily available on all echocardiographic systems Highly specialized training not required to perform analysis	Assesses only anterior septum and posterior wall Complex septal dynamics may result in difficulties in detecting peak inward motion Difficulty in detecting peak inward motion in cases of severe hypokinesis/akinesis in cases of infarction in the anterior septum or posterior wall Low prediction of responders/nonresponders
Color TD M-mode	A useful adjunct to M-mode determination of LV dyssynchrony Color changes in direction help identify the transition from inward to outward motion	Same as above
Doppler echocardiography	Readily available in all systems Requires no specialized training to perform analysis	Can only quantify interventricular dyssynchrony
Color-coded TDI	Can assess regional or segmental timing of myocardial contraction and relaxation A single view permits simultaneous comparison of the temporal profile of multiple segments by off-line analysis A highly comprehensive model of dyssynchrony can be provided by assessing the three apical views Useful in almost all patients	Requires dedicated hands-on training program Learning curve for offline dyssynchrony analysis Analysis in patients with atrial fibrillation is complex Presence of stationary artifacts or reverberations may alter the velocity plot and its postprocessing derivatives Largely affected by passive motion and tethering Malalignment of Doppler ROI increases as LV geometry becomes more globular Reproducibility of different echocardiographic indices has been challenged by PROSPECT trial results
Pulsed TDI	Available on most systems	Time consuming Susceptible to influences of breathing Requires manual transfer of the timing of the ejection interval Identification of peak velocity may be difficult Off-line analysis is not possible Affected by passive motion and tethering Prediction of response to CRT is less clearly studied
TDI-derived strain/strain rate/displacement	Theoretically translation and tethering independent (strain and strain rate)	Low signal-to-noise ratio and thus subject to error Angle dependent Can be influenced by reverberations and stationary artifacts Highly operator dependent
TDI-derived tissue synchronization imaging	Provides color-coded time-to-peak velocity data facilitating visualization of regional peak velocity timings Can be used to guide placement of ROI	Fundamental data are still TD velocity and therefore still require analysis of time-velocity curve for quantification of dyssynchrony

Continued

TABLE 8-2   STRENGTHS AND WEAKNESSES OF DIFFERENT ECHOCARDIOGRAPHIC APPROACHES FOR ASSESSING PATIENTS FOR CARDIAC RESYNCHRONIZATION THERAPY—cont'd

Echo Technique	Strengths	Weaknesses
Speckle tracking echocardiography	Routine gray scale images are used Can be used to assess dyssynchrony in longitudinal, radial, or circumferential direction	Image quality dependent Frame rate sensitive Requires training and experience in performing analysis May be time consuming as analysis is performed using one cardiac cycle at a time New technique with limited clinical documentation Only one tomographic plane is assessed
RT3DE	Allows evaluation of dyssynchrony by analyzing LV wall motion in multiple apical planes during the same cardiac cycle. Better spatial resolution than a single plane	Reduced temporal resolution Online image acquisition and off-line analysis of RT3D echocardiographic data are technically demanding Requires training to perform analysis Vendor-specific cut-off value

CRT, cardiac resynchronization therapy; ROI, region of interest; RT3DE, real-time three-dimensional echocardiography; TD, tissue Doppler; TDI, tissue Doppler imaging.

M-Mode   Color-coded tissue Doppler M-Mode

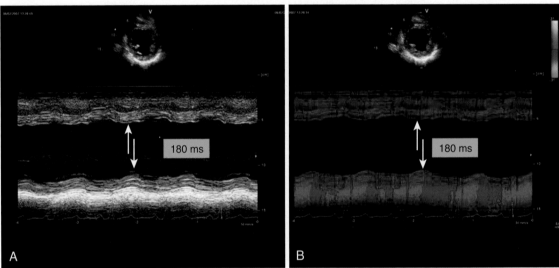

Figure 8-2. M-mode (**A**) at the mid-ventricular level and color-coded tissue Doppler M-mode (**B**) demonstrating septal-to-posterior wall motion delay (SPWMD) of 180 ms, consistent with significant mechanical dyssynchrony (>130 ms).

• Technical difficulty in detecting peak inward motion in severely hypokinetic or akinetic segments in patients with a previous history of MI involving either the septum or the posterior wall (Fig. 8-3).

Color Tissue Doppler M-mode
• A useful adjunct to M-mode determination of LV dyssynchrony is the addition of color TD M-mode.
• Color-coded changes in direction may aid in identifying the transition from inward

to outward motion in the septum and posterior wall.
• The same SPWMD of at least 130 ms is considered a significant dyssynchrony.
• This technique is affected by the similar limitations with routine M-mode.

Doppler Echocardiography
• Pulsed-wave Doppler flow velocities measured from the left ventricular outflow tract (LVOT) and the right ventricular outflow tract (RVOT)

M-Mode   Color tissue Doppler M-Mode

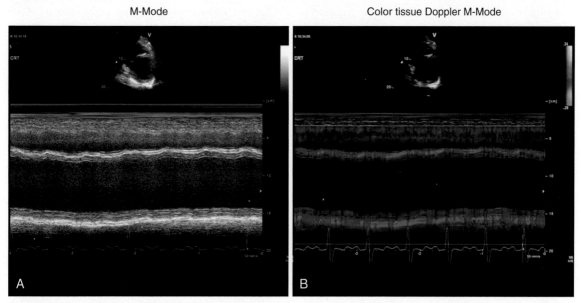

Figure 8-3. M-mode (**A**) at the mid-ventricular level and color-coded tissue Doppler M-mode (**B**) demonstrating severe hypokinesis to akinesis of the anterior septum and posterior wall. It is difficult to identify the maximum inward deflection of both walls, rendering assessment of mechanical dyssynchrony impossible.

Left ventricular pre-ejection period   Right ventricular pre-ejection period
(LV-PEP)   (RV-PEP)

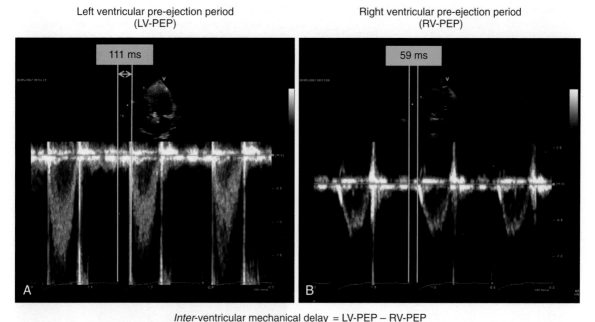

Inter-ventricular mechanical delay = LV-PEP − RV-PEP
                                   = 111 ms − 59 ms
                                   = 52 ms

Figure 8-4. Pulsed Doppler from the left ventricular outflow tract (LVOT) (**A**) and RVOT (**B**) demonstrating significant delay in LV ejection (>40 ms). PEP, pre-ejection period.

can provide information on both intra- and interventricular dyssynchrony.

- LV pre-ejection time, measured from the onset of the QRS complex to the onset of LVOT flow, is prolonged in patients with LV dyssynchrony.

- Interventricular delay is defined as the difference between the right ventricular (RV) pre-ejection time, measured from the onset of the QRS complex to the onset of the RVOT flow, and the LV pre-ejection time (Fig. 8-4).

- An interventricular delay of 45 ms or greater is considered significant.

Tissue Doppler Echocardiography for Quantifying Mechanical Dyssynchrony

- The assessment of the longitudinal LV shortening velocities using TD from apical windows constitutes the largest body of literature in the quantification of dyssynchrony and is the principal method currently in clinical use.
- There are two basic approaches to assess longitudinal TD velocities:
  - Color-coded TD.
  - Spectral pulsed TD.
- While both methods provide similar mechanical information, data obtained using each technique differ:
  - Pulsed TD has higher temporal resolution than color-coded TD.
  - Pulsed TD measures peak instantaneous velocity, while color-coded TD measures mean velocity.
  - Peak velocity measured by pulsed TD technique is 20% to 30% higher than the mean velocity obtained from color-coded TD.
- Postprocessing derivatives of color-coded TD velocity signals include strain, strain rate, displacement, and color-coded time-to-peak velocity data or tissue synchronization imaging (TSI).

Color-coded Tissue Doppler
Acquisition
- Ensure a good ECG tracing with a well-delineated QRS waveform.
- To ensure maximal apical-to-near field left atrial imaging, two-dimensional (2D) imaging is optimized by adjusting the gain settings and time gain control settings for clear myocardial definition.
- Position the LV cavity in the center of the sector and aligned as vertically as possible to allow for the optimal Doppler angle of incidence with LV longitudinal motion.
- Adjust the depth to include the level of the mitral annulus.
- Activate color TD and adjust the sector to include the entire LV with the goal of achieving high frame rates (usually >90 frames per second [fps]).
- To increase frame rates, decrease the depth and sector width to focus on LV as needed.
- Overall color gain is adjusted for clear delineation of the myocardium.

- Online color coding of time peak velocity data may be activated if available in the system.
- Capture three to five beats at end-expiration if the patient is able to suspend breathing transiently or at any phase where the image quality is optimal.
- Record in four standard imaging planes: apical four-chamber view, apical two-chamber view, apical long axis view, and parasternal short axis view at the level of the mid-LV.
- Determine LV ejection interval by recording the LV outflow tract pulsed Doppler velocity from an apical five-chamber or apical long axis view.

Data Analysis
- Using the ECG as a time marker, LV ejection timing is determined from the beginning (aortic valve opening [AVO]) to the end (AVC) of pulsed Doppler flow of the LVOT (Fig. 8-5).
- Timing for AVO to AVC is superimposed as the ejection interval on the subsequent time-velocity curve analysis.
- Place the region of interest (ROI), minimum of 5×10 mm to 7×15 mm, in the basal (~1 cm above the mitral annulus) and mid-regions of opposing LV walls to determine time-velocity plots (four segments for each view).
- Components of the velocity curve should be identified to check for physiologic signal quality (Fig. 8-6).
  - Systolic velocity (S wave) is represented by a positive deflection within the ejection

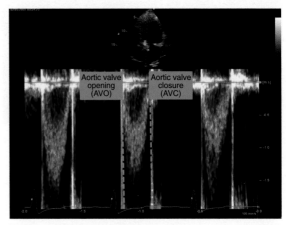

Figure 8-5. Determination of LV ejection interval. Before any TD or speckle tracking analysis is performed, LV ejection interval is determined using pulsed-wave Doppler spectral display of the LVOT. Event timing is the time to opening (AVO) or closure (AVC) of the aortic valve with reference to the ECG trigger markers. These event timings are superimposed on the images that are subsequently analyzed.

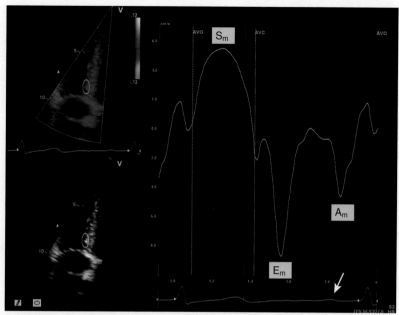

Figure 8-6. Components of a longitudinal tissue velocity data plot. A representative tracing of a tissue velocity data plot using a narrow sector image of the septum in a four-chamber view with the ROI (*yellow oval*) placed at its basal segment. Myocardial systolic velocity (S_m) is the positively deflected curve within the ejection period reflecting the movement of the specified ROI toward the transducer during systole. Normally, peak systolic velocity occurs during early to mid-systole. During diastole, the ROI moves away from the transducer and is represented in the data plot as a negatively deflected curve. The early diastolic velocity (E_m) occurs after AVC and before the p wave (*white arrow*) in the ECG tracing and corresponds to the LV relaxation phase that coincides with passive LV filling in diastole. The late diastolic velocity (A_m) is the negatively deflected curve after the p wave on ECG and corresponds to the LV relaxation phase that coincides with the active filling phase of diastole during atrial contraction.

period as the myocardium moves toward the transducer during systole.
- Early diastolic velocity (E wave) is represented by a negative deflection after AVC as the myocardium moves away from the transducer during passive LV filling.
- Late diastolic velocity (A wave) is represented by a negative deflection after the p wave in the ECG as the myocardium moves away from the transducer during atrial contraction.
- Identify the site where the peak velocity during ejection is most reproducible by manually adjusting the ROI within the segment horizontally and longitudinally within the LV wall.
  - In cases where the pre-ejection interval is severely prolonged, a very early peak may occur before the onset of LV ejection.
  - In cases where more than one peak systolic velocity is present, it is recommended that the first peak be taken.
- Measure the time-to-peak systolic velocity relative to the onset of the QRS complex (or the peak of the R wave) for each segment for a total of 12 segments.

- Alternatively, the time delay between opposing walls can be determined by measuring the time interval from the peak S wave of one wall to the peak S wave of the opposing wall in the same cine loop.
- Perform the measurements using three to five beats, and take the average to account for beat-to-beat variability.

Color-coded Tissue Doppler Approaches to Quantify Mechanical Dyssynchrony
- Opposing wall time delay technique:
  - The simplest method to quantify LV dyssynchrony uses the basal segments of the apical four-chamber view to determine the time delay between the septum and the lateral wall (septal-to-lateral delay) (Fig. 8-7A).
    - Alternatively, the apical long axis view can be used to determine the time delay between the anterior septum and posterior wall.
  - The four-segment model uses basal segments of the septum and the lateral,

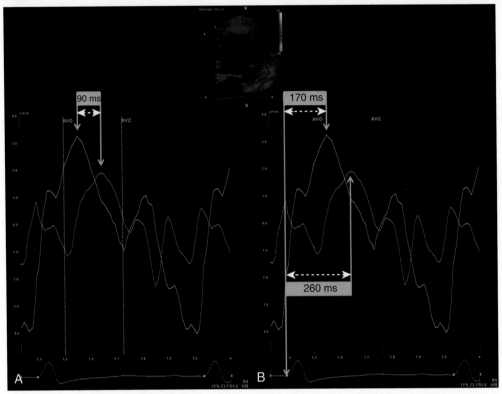

Figure 8-7. Color-coded TD time-velocity plot with sample volumes at the basal septum and basal lateral wall demonstrating septum (*yellow tracings*) to lateral wall (*green tracings*) time delay of 90 ms, consistent with significant dyssynchrony (65 ms). **A,** Opposite wall time delay is quantified by measuring the time interval between the peak systolic velocities of two opposing segments. **B,** To determine the temporal dispersion of LV peak velocity, time-to-peak systolic velocity is measured for each of the 12 LV segments relative to the onset of the QRS complex or peak of the R wave. This method can also be used to measure opposite wall time delay, if narrow-sectored single-wall images are collected for analysis.

inferior, and anterior walls to determine the time delay between two opposing walls.
- The 12-segment model uses basal and mid-LV segments of the three standard apical views. The maximum difference in the time-to-peak velocity values among the four segments in each of the three apical views is determined as the maximal opposing wall delay.
- An opposing wall time delay ≥65 ms has been found to predict both clinical and echocardiographic responses to CRT.
- Yu Index or the mechanical dyssynchrony index:
  - This index calculates the standard deviation (SD) of the time-to-peak systolic velocity in the ejection phase in the 12 basal and mid-LV segments (Fig. 8-7B).
  - A Yu index cut-off value ≥33 ms has been found to predict reverse remodeling, defined as a 15% or more decrease in LVESV after CRT.

- Maximum time delay technique:
  - Maximum time-to-peak systolic velocity difference among all 12 LV segments.
  - A cut-off value ≥100 ms was found to predict improvement after CRT.

Pitfalls
- Image acquisition is a critical determinant of analyzability and reproducibility for dyssynchrony assessment.
  - Signal noise is common.
  - Presence of stationary artifacts or reverberations may alter the velocity plot.
  - Malalignment of Doppler ROI increases as LV geometry becomes more globular.
  - Acquiring narrow-sectored single-wall images may improve wall alignment with the Doppler signals and therefore reduce the angle of insonation, but it precludes simultaneous comparison of opposing segments using the same cardiac cycle.

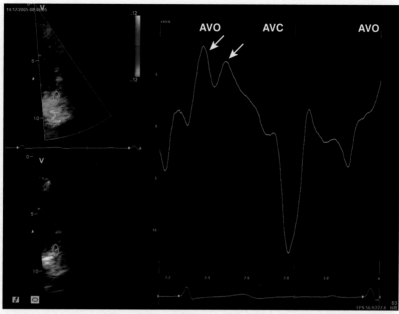

Figure 8-8. The presence of multiple systolic peaks (*white arrows*) is the most common pitfall in using tissue velocity–based quantification dyssynchrony. It has been recommended that the first peak be selected if moving the sample volume within the interrogated segment fails to define a single more reproducible peak.

- TD velocity cannot differentiate active thickening from passive translational or tethering movement.
- Presence of multiple peaks increases interobserver variability (Fig. 8-8).
- Moving the ROI within the segment under interrogation or increasing the ROI size may be performed to determine the most reproducible peak.
- The difference in the position of the ECG trigger markers between the LVOT pulsed Doppler spectral display and the TD images may produce relative disparity in LV ejection timing during analysis (Fig. 8-9).
  - Such error can be addressed by manually correcting the AVO and AVC timings to commence from the onset of the QRS complex and manually correcting the position of trigger markers in the TD images accordingly.

Spectral Pulsed Tissue Doppler
Acquisition
- The general approach to image acquisition follows that of color TD as previously described, with some modifications.
- Pulsed TD presets must be optimized on the system in order to provide a clean velocity tracing with minimal signal blurring and optimal delineation of systolic and diastolic components.

- Set the pulsed sample volume to 0.5 to 1 cm length.
- Set the velocity scale to maximize the time-velocity curve.
- Set the sweep speed to 50 to 100 mm/s.
- Moving the sample volume within the segment to search for a more reproducible time-velocity signal is performed on-line.

Data Analysis
- Analysis is performed on-line.
- The time interval between the onset of the QRS complex and the beginning of regional myocardial systolic shortening velocity is considered as a surrogate for regional electromechanical coupling (EMC) intervals (Fig. 8-10)
- LV dyssynchrony is measured as the difference between the longest and shortest EMC intervals in all the basal segments of the LV.
- Interventricular (LV-RV) dyssynchrony is quantified by the difference between EMC times in the basal lateral segment of the RV and in the most delayed LV segment.
- The sum of LV dyssynchrony and LV-RV dyssynchrony yields the combined index of intraventricular and interventricular mechanical dyssynchrony.
- A combined index of intra- and interventricular dyssynchrony ≥102 ms was found to predict the response to CRT.

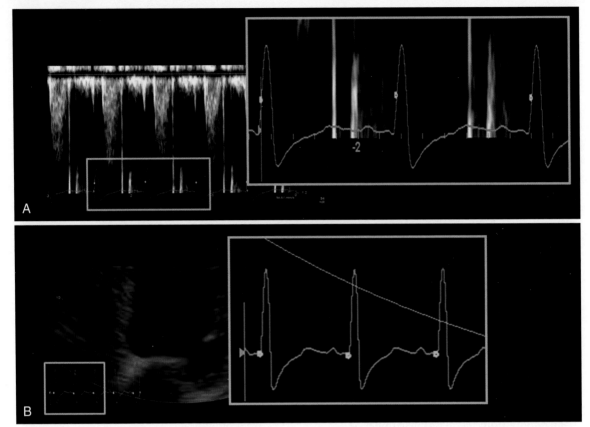

Figure 8-9. Discrepancies in the location of ECG trigger markers in (**A**) the LVOT Doppler spectral display and (**B**) images for analysis. Because the time to onset and cessation of aortic flow (LV ejection period) has its reference to the location of the ECG trigger markers in the LVOT Doppler spectral display, the event timing superimposed on the image being analyzed will likewise have its reference to the location of the ECG triggers in that specific image. The trigger markers (*yellow dots*) are located midway in the ascending arm of the QRS complex (**A inset**), while the trigger markers in the image to be analyzed are located at the onset of the QRS complex (**B inset**). If the event timing measured from **A** is super-imposed on the velocity data plot using the image in **B**, the AVO/AVC timing, which will now be referenced to the onset of the QRS complex rather than midway in the ascending portion of the QRS complex, will occur relatively early in the velocity plot data, resulting in possible inclusion of an isovolumic contraction wave in the analysis.

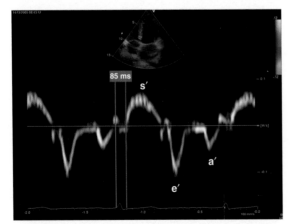

Figure 8-10. Pulsed-wave TD at the basal septum. The EMC interval is measured from the onset of the QRS complex on ECG to the onset of the tissue systolic velocity. In this example, the EMC interval at the basal septum measured 85 ms. s', systolic tissue velocity; e', early diastolic tissue velocity; a', late diastolic tissue velocity.

Pitfalls
- Time consuming:
  - Only one region can be interrogated at a time, precluding simultaneous comparisons of interrogated segments.
  - Off-line analysis is not possible.
- Spectral pulsed TD is susceptible to influences of breathing, patient movement, and alterations in heart rate.
- Correcting the measurements for the RR interval may minimize the influence of alteration in the heart rate.
- A broad spectral display with plateau during systole may render identification of peak velocity difficult.
  - This limitation can be overcome by lowering the gain setting during image acquisition and by measuring the time to onset of systolic velocity instead of using peak systolic velocity timing.

- It requires manual transfer of the timing of the ejection interval.
- Limited evidence of pulsed TD to predict response to CRT.

Tissue Doppler Longitudinal Strain/Strain Rate and Displacement Imaging
- Postprocessing of tissue velocity signals (color-coded TD) yields information on myocardial displacement and deformation (Fig. 8-11).
- Displacement mapping is the integration of myocardial velocity signals over time.
- Strain rate is the spatial derivation of tissue velocity data.
- Strain, the integration of myocardial strain rate over time, has the advantage of differentiating active deformation from passive translational motion.

Data Analysis
- Delayed longitudinal contraction (DLC) is calculated using strain rate analysis.
  - A segment is considered to present with DLC if the strain rate analysis demonstrates motion reflecting true contraction and if the end of the segmental contraction occurs after AVC.
  - Dyssynchrony is quantified by the number of segments demonstrating DLC, expressed as a percentage of the total number of segments evaluated.
- The strain-derived dyssynchrony index is the SD of the time-to-peak longitudinal (negative) strain within the entire cardiac cycle in the 12 segments of the LV.

Pitfalls
- Angle dependence.
- Low signal-to-noise ratio.
- Noise can be reduced by increasing the strain length or integrating strain rate signals to yield strain data.
- Because noise is included in the integration of strain rate signals, reference to the strain rate curve should be made when performing strain analysis (Fig. 8-12).
- Highly operator dependent.
- Although displacement mapping is inferior to TD velocities in predicting response to CRT, conflicting evidence exists for strain and strain rate analysis.

Tissue Doppler Radial Strain
Data Analysis
- Analysis is performed using the color-coded TD image of the short axis view at the mid-ventricular level.

- A 6×14 mm ROI is placed in the anterior septum and the posterior wall. Depending on the wall thickness, adjust the size of the ROI accordingly.
- Strain length is adjusted to include the entire thickness of the LV wall at its smallest diameter.
- Dyssynchrony is quantified by the time interval between the peak positive strain in the anterior septum and the posterior wall.
- An anterior septum to posterior wall delay of 130 ms has been found to predict response to CRT.

Tissue Synchronization Imaging
- Automated color coding of time-to-peak velocity data is another TD-derived approach to measure dyssynchrony.
- Color-coded temporal velocity data superimposed on routine B-mode images provide visual mechanical information on the anatomic regions.
- TSI is a signal processing of the TD data to automatically detect peak positive velocity color coding of the time-to-peak longitudinal velocities in the following spectrum: green for normal timing, yellow-orange for moderate delay, and red for severe delay.

Data Analysis
- Interval start time is manually set to begin with AVO to exclude isovolumic contraction time and extended to rapid filling (E-wave) to include post-systolic LV dyssynchrony.
- TSI color coding is used to guide the placement of oval ROI as with color TD in the basal and mid-segments from apical views.
- ROIs are placed where the color coding of timing is most representative for anatomic segment for time-velocity curve analysis.
- Time-velocity tracings are used to correctly identify the peak velocities for LV dyssynchrony analysis (Fig. 8-13).

Speckle Tracking Strain Echocardiography
- Speckle tracking strain echocardiography is an off-line computer processing technique utilizing routine B-mode gray scale images to determine the relative movement of speckle patterns within the LV wall. (See Chapter 6.)
- Compared with tissue Doppler echocardiography (TDE), speckle tracking technique:
  - Is relatively angle independent.
  - Requires a lower frame rate.
  - Has lower temporal resolution.
  - Uses strain as its fundamental data.

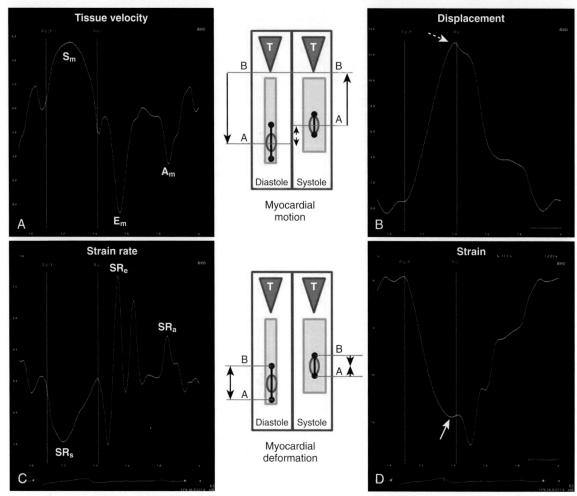

Figure 8-11. Schematic diagram illustrating the basic principles of longitudinal tissue velocity imaging and its postprocessing derivatives with corresponding tracings. *Upper middle panel,* As the myocardium contracts during systole, a specified ROI (*yellow oval, point A*) in a myocardial segment (*pink rectangle*) moves toward an external fixed reference (*point B*), that is, the transducer (*inverted blue triangle with T*). As the myocardium relaxes during diastole, the ROI moves away from the transducer. The rate by which the ROI moves toward/away from the transducer is known as tissue velocity, which is the fundamental data in TD echocardiography. The distance (*black broken double arrow*) traversed by the ROI during myocardial contraction/relaxation is known as displacement. **A,** Tissue velocity. As the ROI moves toward the transducer during systole, it registers a positively deflected curve, termed systolic velocity (S_m). As the ROI moves away from the transducer during diastole, it registers two negatively deflected curves: an early diastolic velocity corresponding to passive LV filling (E_m) and a late diastolic velocity corresponding to active LV filling during atrial contraction. **B,** Displacement. Temporal integration of tissue velocity data yields displacement. It registers a positively deflected curve (*white broken arrow*) that normally peaks near or at AVC (end-systole). The amplitude of the positive curve represents the amount of displacement (expressed in millimeters) the ROI has achieved during myocardial contraction. *Lower middle panel,* Along the Doppler line, there are two points that define the proximal (*point B*) and distal (*point A*) ends of the ROI (*yellow oval*) in relation to the transducer. Normally, the distal end has higher velocity compared with the proximal end as these points move toward/away from the transducer. This velocity gradient results in a reduction in the distance between points A and B (*dark blue line with rounded tips*) as the myocardium contracts during systole and vice versa. Strain rate is derived from the velocity gradient over the distance between points A and B at a given phase of the cardiac cycle. The change in the distance between points A and B relative to the original distance between them is known as myocardial deformation or myocardial strain. **C,** Strain rate is the spatial derivation of tissue velocity signals. Systolic strain rate (SR_s) is a negatively deflected curve during the ejection phase (from AVO to AVC). This is the rate by which the distance between two points in the myocardium is reduced when the myocardium shortens as it contracts. The early diastolic strain rate (SR_e) is a positively deflected curve after the AVC and reflects the rate by which the distance between the two points in the myocardium increases when the myocardium lengthens as it relaxes. The late diastolic strain rate (SR_a) is the positively deflected curve after the p wave and reflects the rate by which the distance between the points in the myocardium increases when the myocardium lengthens during atrial contraction. Postprocessing of tissue velocity signals can increase noise. In this particular SR curve, notice the presence of a negatively deflected curve after the AVC and a positively deflected curve immediately following the early diastolic peak, both of which may be regarded as a noise component. **D,** Strain, the temporal integration of strain rate, is represented by a negatively deflected curve (*white solid arrow*) that normally peaks near or at AVC. It represents how much shortening a myocardial segment has undergone during myocardial contraction relative to its original length. It is expressed in percent.

Strain rate   Strain

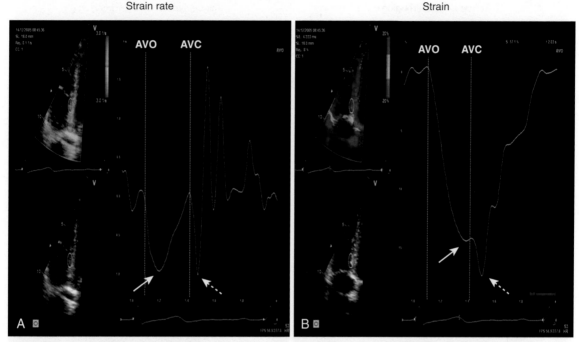

Figure 8-12. Differentiating noise from true peak strain. **A,** Longitudinal strain rate data plot illustrating systolic strain rate (*white solid arrow*), a negatively deflected curve during early to mid-systole, followed by another negatively deflected curve (*white broken arrow*), probably noise, and may not reflect true longitudinal contraction after AVC. **B,** Temporal integration of the strain rate data plot resulted in a strain curve with two discernible peaks: a less negative peak (*solid white arrow*) occurring near the AVC and a more negative peak (*broken arrow*) occurring after AVC. The second peak, although more negative in value, corresponds to the negatively deflected curve regarded as noise in **A** and therefore should not be taken as the peak longitudinal strain.

- Speckle tracking can assess strain in the longitudinal, circumferential, and radial directions.
  - Longitudinal strain analysis is performed using the standard apical views of the LV.
  - Circumferential and radial strain analyses are performed using the parasternal short axis view of the LV.

Acquisition
- Gain setting is optimized to ensure adequate delineation of endocardial borders because adequate image quality is a requirement for speckle tracking analysis.
- Section width is optimized to allow for complete myocardial visualization while maximizing frame rate.
- Frame rate should ideally be between 50 and 70 fps.

Data Analysis

Radial Strain Dyssynchrony
- Using the ECG as a time marker, LV ejection timing is determined from the beginning

(AVO) to the end (AVC) of pulsed Doppler flow of the LVOT.
- Analysis is performed using one cardiac cycle at a time.
- The ROI is manually traced on the endocardial cavity using a point-and-click approach.
- An outer border is automatically generated.
- The size of ROI is adjusted such that the outer border will be near the epicardium.
- Ensure adequate tracking for all the segments by visually assessing the ROI during cine loop playback and manually adjusting the ROI as needed.
- Segments with inadequate tracking are excluded from the analysis.
- Time delay between the anterior septum and posterior wall is determined by measuring the difference in the time-to-peak positive strain between the two opposing walls (Fig. 8-14).
- A cut-off value ≥130 ms has been found to predict response to CRT.

Longitudinal Strain Dyssynchrony
- The general approach to data analysis follows that of radial dyssynchrony analysis, with

Tissue Doppler imaging   Tissue synchronization imaging

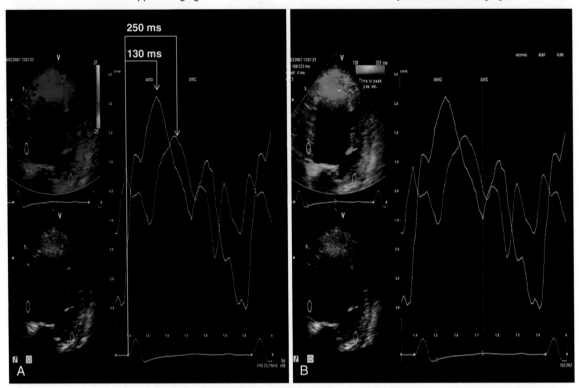

Figure 8-13. TSI is a postprocessing derivative of TDI. **A,** Representative time-velocity data plot from a four-chamber-view TD image with ROIs placed at the basal segment of the septum (*yellow oval*) and lateral wall (*green oval*). TD images color code the direction of myocardial motion with reference to the transducer: red for myocardial motion toward the transducer, blue for movement away from it. In this example, the time-to-peak systolic (positive) velocities in the septum and the lateral wall are measured at 130 ms and 250 ms, respectively. **B,** The same representative time-velocity data plot in **A** using TSI. With TSI, peak positive velocities from the different segments of the LV are automatically detected and the timing for each of these peak positive velocities is used to color code temporal velocity data that are superimposed on routine B-mode images. Time-to-peak velocities are color coded: green (20–150 ms) for normal timing, yellow-orange (150–300 ms) for moderate delay, and red (300–500 ms) for severe delays. Thus, TSI provides visual mechanical information that can be used to guide the placement of the ROIs in the region where the color-coded timing is most representative of the segment under interrogation. TDI and TSI yield the same time-velocity data curve. TSI uses tissue velocity–based methods of quantifying mechanical dyssynchrony.

some modifications in the dyssynchrony quantification.
- Strain Delay Index:
  - Global longitudinal strain is calculated from the average of the 16-segment regional strain curves normalized to the RR interval to account for variations in the heart rate and frame rate.
  - AVC or end-systolic timing is determined by measuring the time-to-peak global longitudinal strain.
  - For each of the 16 LV segments, the peak negative strain in the entire cardiac cycle and its corresponding timing relative to either the onset of the QRS complex or the peak of the R wave and the peak end-systolic strain values are generated.
  - The difference between the peak negative strain and the peak end-systolic strain

represents the "wasted" energy resulting from LV dyssynchrony.
  - The sum of the difference between the peak negative strain and peak end-systolic strain is the Strain Delay Index.
  - A Strain Delay Index cut-off value ≥25% was found to predict response to CRT in both ischemic and nonischemic patients with a wide QRS complex on ECG.
- The Strain Dyssynchrony Index is calculated from the SD of time-to-peak longitudinal strain within the entire cardiac cycle in 12 LV segments.

Pitfalls
- Poor image quality limits speckle tracking analysis.
- The quality of tracking is influenced by:

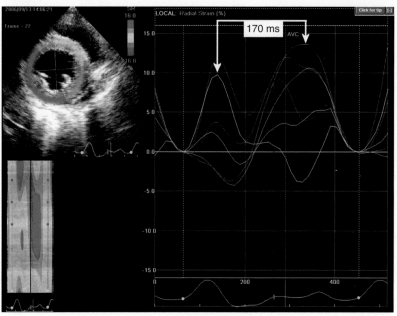

Figure 8-14. Speckle tracking strain analysis using a short axis view of the mid-LV demonstrating the presence of a significant mechanical dyssynchrony in the radial direction (130 ms).

- Low lateral resolution.
- Image drop-outs.
- Reverberations.
- Time-strain curve is greatly influenced by the placement and tracking of ROI.
  - This limitation can be overcome by retracing the ROI to generate a more reproducible time-strain curve.
- Speckle tracking is frame rate sensitive.
  - Frame rates that are too low or too high may result in poorer tracking.
- Differences in the position of the ECG trigger markers between the LVOT pulsed Doppler spectral display and the B-mode images may produce disparity in the LV ejection timing during analysis.
  - This error can be addressed by manually correcting the AVO and AVC timings to commence from the onset of the QRS complex and manually correcting the position of trigger markers in the B-mode images accordingly.

Alternative Approaches to Assessing Mechanical Dyssynchrony

- While the majority of clinical studies on LV dyssynchrony and prediction of response to CRT used echocardiography, the reproducibility of different echocardiographic

KEY POINTS

- There are several standard echocardiographic markers of LV dyssynchrony that have been found to predict response to CRT.
- Variation among these echocardiographic markers of LV dyssynchrony relates to:
  - The method of timing assessment.
  - The orientation of dyssynchrony measurements.
- Color-coded TD velocity currently remains the most commonly utilized echocardiographic modality to assess LV dyssynchrony in the clinical setting.
- Myocardial velocity is the fundamental data in TDE.
- Strain is the fundamental data being calculated in speckle tracking strain echocardiography.
- In mechanical dyssynchrony associated with delays in electrical activation pattern, time delay is usually greatest in the apical four-chamber and/or apical long axis views because they contain septum-free wall measurements.
- Timing is limited to the ejection interval to exclude post-systolic velocity peaks from analysis.
- Combining speckle tracking radial strain with TD longitudinal velocities has been reported to predict better response to CRT than either method alone.
- Presence of multiple peaks increases interobserver variability.

indices of mechanical dyssynchrony to predict response to CRT has been recently challenged by the Predictors of Response to CRT (PROSPECT) trial.

- The PROSPECT trial was a prospective, multicenter, nonrandomized trial that enrolled 498 subjects with standard indications for CRT.
- It evaluated the ability of 12 echocardiographic (conventional and tissue Doppler imaging [TDI]) indices of mechanical dyssynchrony to predict response to CRT using clinical composite score and LVESV reduction of 15% as end points.
  - Sensitivity of 6% to 74% and 9% to 77% for predicting post-CRT clinical improvement and LVESV reduction, respectively.
  - Specificity of 35% to 91% and 31% to 93% for predicting post-CRT clinical improvement and LVESV reduction, respectively.
  - High intraoperator and interobserver coefficient of variation for the different parameters of ventricular dyssynchrony.
- The study concluded that no single echocardiographic measures of ventricular mechanical dyssynchrony may be recommended to improve patient selection for CRT beyond current guidelines.
- The results of the PROSPECT trial can be interpreted in light of:
  - Limitations inherent to TDI.
    - Limitations of TDI can be overcome by speckle tracking strain imaging.
    - Speckle tracking strain imaging can be used either as a confirmatory or a complementary dyssynchrony analysis technique to TDI.
  - Adequacy of quantifying mechanical dyssynchrony in a longitudinal direction.
    - Consider mechanical dyssynchrony in the radial and circumferential directions.
  - Lack of a standardized method of analysis.
  - Level of training and expertise of the personnel performing the analysis.
  - Quality of the acquired images for analysis.
  - Variations in the echocardiographic platforms and equipment.
  - Contributing factors to nonresponse to CRT.
    - Lack of correctable mechanical dyssynchrony.
    - Extent and location of myocardial scars.
    - Suboptimal lead placement:
      - Suitability of coronary venous anatomy.
      - Site of latest activation.
      - Lead dislodgement.

- Suboptimal pacemaker setting:
  - Atrioventricular interval
  - Interventricular timing
- Other imaging modalities such as real-time three-dimensional echocardiography (RT3DE), cardiac magnetic resonance (CMR), and nuclear imaging are currently the focus of research in assessing mechanical dyssynchrony (Table 8-3).

Real-time Three-dimensional Echocardiography
Data Analysis
- Assessment of LV dyssynchrony is based on analysis of regional volumetric changes (Fig. 8-15).
- From the voxel-based three-dimensional (3D) dataset, a number of 2D slices are defined by the system.
- For each slice, the endocardial border is traced with semiautomated detection, creating an LV "cast" as a mathematical model that provides time-volume data for the entire cardiac cycle.
- The time-volume data are divided into pyramidal subvolumes around a nonfixed central point to gain an estimation of the time-volume data corresponding to each of the 16 standard myocardial segments as defined by the American Society of Echocardiography.
- The Systolic Dyssynchrony Index (SDI) can be derived from the dispersion of the time to minimum regional volume for all 16 LV segments.

Advantages
- Allows evaluation of dyssynchrony by analyzing LV wall motion in multiple apical planes during the same cardiac cycle.
- Offers better spatial resolution than a single plane.

Disadvantages
- Reduced temporal resolution.
- On-line image acquisition and off-line analysis of RT3DE data are technically more demanding.
- Manual editing of the endocardial border on suboptimal images may create an LV cast with irregular contour that may result in overestimation of dyssynchrony.
- Requires training to perform analysis.
- Variations in the algorithm of endocardial border detection and calculation of dyssynchrony between vendors result in different measured values and therefore different cut-off value.

TABLE 8-3   ADVANTAGES AND LIMITATIONS OF DIFFERENT MODALITIES IN ASSESSING PATIENTS FOR CARDIAC RESYNCHRONIZATION THERAPY

Technique	Advantages	Limitations
ECG	Easy to obtain and simple to interpret	Provides information on electrical dyssynchrony only Low specificity and sensitivity in prediction of response to CRT on its own
2D echocardiography	Readily available Can be used at any time-point in CRT and is useful for follow-up studies	Image quality dependent Requires skill and expertise in performing analysis Reproducibility of echocardiographic indices of mechanical dyssynchrony has been challenged by PROSPECT trial results
RT3DE	Better spatial resolution than 2D Allows dyssynchrony evaluation in multiple apical planes using the same cardiac cycle Can be used at any time-point in CRT and is useful for follow-up studies	Low temporal resolution Image acquisition and off-line analysis are technically demanding Requires training to perform analysis Image dependent Cut-off values are vendor specific Fewer studies on CRT patients compared to 2D echocardiography
CMR	Operator and patient independent High spatial resolution Provides 3D information, including circumferential mechanics	Low temporal resolution Cost Long procedural time Cut-off values not defined Incompatibility with implanted devices and therefore may not be used for follow-up studies Complex and long analysis time At present time only studies with very small sample sizes are available
Nuclear imaging	Potential for integrated evaluation of myocardial ischemia, infarction, viability, LV dysfunction, and dyssynchrony Potential to provide objective reproducible parameters on LV dyssynchrony	Low spatial resolution Limited availability of software for assessment Cut-off values not defined Limited data on its use in selection of CRT candidates

Cardiac Magnetic Resonance Imaging Techniques

- CMR techniques to assess dyssynchrony:
  - Strain analysis from magnetic resonance myocardial tagging.
  - Velocity-encoded CMR.
- There are three CMR-based indices used for measuring dyssynchrony:
  - Regional variance is determined from the variance of strain magnitude in 28 radially displaced segments for each short axis, or the number of segments with delayed shortening as a percent of total regions examined.
  - Regional variance vector is based on the product of a radial magnitude vector with a scalar representing time to maximal shortening.
  - Regional strain uniformity, based on regional strain differences at a given moment in time, yields the circumferential uniformity ratio estimate index.
- While CMR has the ability to obtain 3D information that includes circumferential mechanics, most studies are based on very small sample sizes.
- In the absence of larger studies in CRT patients from multiple experienced centers, the precise value of CMR in the assessment of LV dyssynchrony has yet to be determined.

Advantages
- High reproducibility.
- High spatial resolution.
- Ability to obtain 3D information, including circumferential mechanics.

Disadvantages
- Cost.
- Availability.

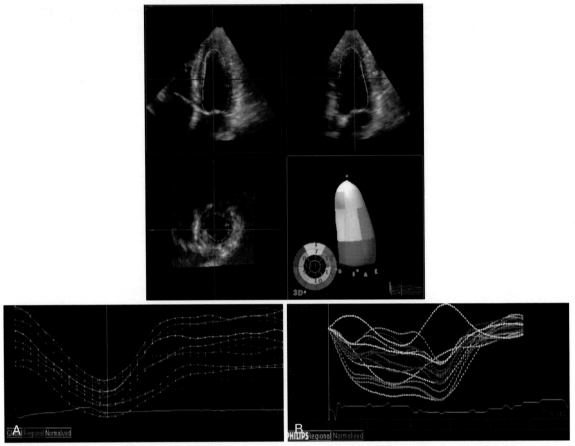

Figure 8-15. Three-dimensional echocardiography images illustrating analysis of regional volumetry to assess dyssynchrony. **A,** Synchronous LV contraction demonstrates homogeneous reduction in regional volume at or around end-systole. **B,** Heterogeneity in times to minimum volume characterizes LV dyssynchrony.

- Long imaging time.
- Complex and long analysis time.
- Incompatibility with implanted devices.

Nuclear Imaging

- In addition to LV dyssynchrony, assessment of viability and scar tissue is of prime importance in selecting patients for CRT since the location and extent of scar tissue is also predictive of nonresponse to the therapy.
- Nuclear imaging has been extensively used in heart failure patients to evaluate LV function and volumes, ischemia, viability, and scar tissue.
- Information from an ECG-gated single-photon emission computed tomography (SPECT) myocardial perfusion imaging (MPI) dataset can be derived to assess cardiac dyssynchrony.
- The technique relies on phase analysis of regional maximal LV count changes throughout the cardiac cycle, which tracks the onset of mechanical contraction.
- Uniformity/heterogeneity of the phase distribution over the entire LV represents LV synchrony/dyssynchrony.

Advantages

- Method is largely automatic.
- High reproducibility.
- High sensitivity and specificity for predicting response to CRT.

Disadvantages

- Low spatial resolution.
- Limited availability of software for assessment.
- Limited data are available for use of SPECT-MPI for selection of CRT candidates.
- Need for large, multicenter studies to define a clear role of SPECT-MPI in CRT.

Clinical Approach to Assessing Patients for Cardiac Resynchronization Therapy

- Current recommendation for CRT includes heart failure patients with:
  - New York Heart Association (NYHA) functional class III to IV.
  - Widened QRS of 120 ms.
  - LV ejection fraction of 35%.
- Approximately 30% of patients undergoing CRT do not respond favorably to the therapy.
- An echocardiography-based dyssynchrony study, specifically TDI, has been used in clinical practice to aid in identifying responders and nonresponders to CRT.
- Speckle tracking can be used to substantiate findings from TD-based dyssynchrony analysis.
- Information obtained from Doppler echocardiography such as LV pre-ejection interval and interventricular mechanical delay can also be used to supplement results of TDI analysis.
- While mechanical dyssynchrony, routinely identified by ECG as abnormal electrical activation, is a critical substrate for CRT efficacy, there are other factors that can influence a patient's response to this catheter-based therapy.
- The approach to evaluating patients for CRT entails a comprehensive evaluation that focuses not only on mechanical dyssynchrony but also on other factors that can influence response to CRT (Fig. 8-16).
  - Ensure optimal medical therapy.
  - Identify correctable causes of heart failure (hypertension, valvular heart disease, ischemic heart disease, etc.) and address them accordingly.

- Patients with ischemic cardiomyopathy were found to respond less favorably to CRT compared with their nonischemic counterparts.
  - Assess severity of ischemia.
  - Assess extent of myocardial viability.
  - Assess location and extent of myocardial scarring.
    - Myocardial scar located at the posterolateral LV is a predictor of nonresponse to CRT.
    - Higher percentage of nonviable myocardium is a predictor of nonresponse to CRT.
- The American Society of Echocardiography Dyssynchrony Writing Group does not recommend withholding CRT from patients who meet the accepted criteria for this therapy because of the results of echocardiographic Doppler dyssynchrony studies.
- The utility of echocardiographic dyssynchrony analysis as an adjunct to assist in clinical decision making for selection of patients for CRT can be best applied to patients with borderline inclusion criteria such as:
  - Borderline QRS duration (120–149 ms).
  - Borderline ejection fraction.
  - Ambiguous clinical history for functional class.
- If dyssynchrony echocardiography is clinically warranted/requested for these cases, several dyssynchrony parameters can be measured:
  - Tissue velocity–based parameters.
    - Septum-lateral wall or septum-posterior wall time delay of 65 ms is consistent with significant dyssynchrony.
    - 12-segment SD of time-to-peak systolic velocity (Yu index) of 33 ms is consistent with significant dyssynchrony.
      - When the timing of the ejection period is determined from the pulsed Doppler of LVOT, the time from the onset of the QRS complex to the onset of aortic flow (LV pre-ejection period) greater than 140 ms is indicative of intraventricular dyssynchrony.
      - When time-to-peak systolic velocity is measured in all 12 segments, the site with the most delayed activation can be identified.
- In nonischemic cardiomyopathy patients with suitable coronary venous anatomy, concordance between the site of LV lead placement and the site of most delayed activation in the LV (most commonly in the posterolateral region) has been found to yield a favorable response to CRT.

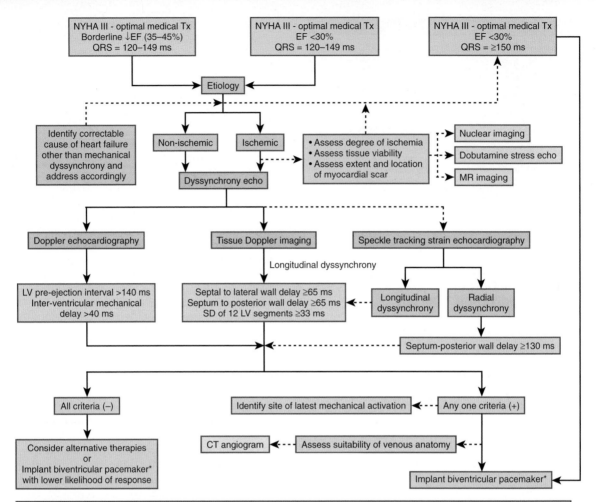

Figure 8-16. Comprehensive approach to evaluating patients for CRT. CRT is recommended for heart failure patients in NYHA functional class III to IV with reduced LV systolic function and intraventricular dyssynchrony manifested as a wide QRS complex on ECG. While echocardiography has been shown to be superior to ECG in predicting response to CRT, current guidelines have not included an echocardiographic dyssynchrony study for patient selection. The American Society of Echocardiography Dyssynchrony Writing Group does not recommend withholding CRT from patients who meet the accepted criteria for therapy based on the result of echocardiographic dyssynchrony analysis. The utility of an echocardiography-based dyssynchrony study as an adjunct to the clinical decision making for CRT is best applied in patients with borderline inclusion criteria such as borderline QRS duration. Tissue velocity–based parameters of longitudinal dyssynchrony, specifically septum-to-lateral wall delay, have been the most popular technique that is being used in many centers. Recognizing the limitations inherent to TDI, speckle tracking strain echocardiography can be used to confirm (longitudinal dyssynchrony) or supplement (radial dyssynchrony) TDI-based analysis. In these "borderline patients," dyssynchrony can also be confirmed by the presence of prolonged aortic pre-ejection interval and significant interventricular mechanical dyssynchrony using Doppler echocardiography. For all patients being considered for CRT regardless of the QRS duration, recommendation to implant biventricular pacemakers should be a clinical decision that is based on a comprehensive evaluation that takes into consideration other factors that may increase the likelihood of a favorable/unfavorable response to CRT aside from mechanical dyssynchrony.

- Speckle tracking strain-based parameters:
  - Longitudinal strain analysis can be performed to verify the presence of dyssynchrony in cases where there are multiple peaks in the time-velocity plot, or if results of tissue velocity analysis are deemed unreliable because of some limitations inherent to the technique.
  - Radial strain dyssynchrony (septum-to-posterior wall delay of 130 ms) can supplement tissue velocity dyssynchrony information.
- Doppler echocardiography:
  - In addition to the LV pre-ejection interval that is routinely measured when performing TDI or speckle tracking–based analysis, presence of significant interventricular dyssynchrony, that is LV-to-RV pre-ejection interval difference of 40 ms, can supplement the tissue velocity–based dyssynchrony analysis result.
- While several factors can influence patients' responses to CRT, it is crucial to determine the presence or absence of significant dyssynchrony in this "borderline" group of patients should CRT be contemplated:
  - CRT in the absence of true dyssynchrony can worsen heart failure.
  - Cost.
  - Complications associated with the procedure.
- Finally, recommendation for CRT should be a clinical decision based on a comprehensive assessment of the individual patient.

Suggested Reading

1. Kass DA. Cardiac resynchronization therapy. *J Cardiovasc Electrophysiol.* 2005;16(Suppl 1):S35-S41.
2. Cheng A, Helm RH, Abraham TP. Pathophysiological mechanisms underlying ventricular dyssynchrony. *Europace.* 2009;11:v10-v14.
3. Bax JJ, Abraham T, Barold SS, et al. Cardiac resynchronization therapy: Part 1-issues before device implantation. *J Am Coll Cardiol.* 2005;46:2153-2167.
4. Gorcsan J 3rd, Abraham T, Agler DA, et al, American Society of Echocardiography Dyssynchrony Writing Group. Echocardiography for cardiac resynchronization therapy: recommendations for performance and reporting—a report from the American Society of Echocardiography Dyssynchrony Writing Group endorsed by the Heart Rhythm Society. *J Am Soc Echocardiogr.* 2008;21:191-213.
5. Chung ES, Leon AR, Tavazzi L, et al. Results of the Predictors of Response to CRT (PROSPECT) trial. *Circulation.* 2008;117:2608-2616.
6. Yu CM, Bax JJ, Gorcsan J 3rd. Critical appraisal of methods to assess mechanical dyssynchrony. *Curr Opin Cardiol.* 2009;24:18-28.
7. Abraham T, Kass D, Tonti G, et al. Imaging cardiac resynchronization therapy. *JACC: Cardiovascular Imaging.* 2009;2:486-497.
8. Lardo AC, Abraham TP, Kass DA. Magnetic resonance imaging assessment of ventricular dyssynchrony: current and emerging concepts. *J Am Coll Cardiol.* 2005;46:2223-2228.
9. Abraham TP, Lardo AC, Kass DA. Myocardial dyssynchrony and resynchronization. *Heart Fail Clin.* 2006;2:179-192.
10. Chen J, Bax JJ, Henneman MM, et al. Is nuclear imaging a viable alternative technique to assess dyssynchrony? *Europace.* 2008;10:iii101-iii105.
11. Boogers MM, Chen J, Bax JJ. Role of nuclear imaging in cardiac resynchronization therapy. *Expert Review of Cardiovascular Therapy.* 2009;7:65-72.

Contrast Perfusion Echocardiography

9

Joan J. Olson, Feng Xie, and Thomas Porter

Background/Basic Principles

Ultrasound Contrast Agents

- The currently available ultrasound contrast agents (UCAs) in the United States are Optison (General Electric, Waukesha, WI) and Definity (Lantheus, N. Billerica, MA). In Europe, Sonovue (Bracco, Milan, IT) is an approved contrast agent.
- Contrast agents in the United States are currently approved only for left ventricular (LV) opacification. However, these agents can also be utilized to examine myocardial perfusion with perfusion imaging techniques (available on Philips [Andover, MA] and Siemens [Mountain View, CA] ultrasound scanners).
- Perfusion imaging adds incremental value to resting wall motion assessment. Following myocardial infarction, myocardial contrast enhancement within the risk area predicts recovery of function, independent of what resting wall motion is. In the evaluation of chronic coronary artery disease (CAD), the assessment of resting myocardial perfusion is also predictive of recovery of function following revascularization. Perfusion imaging adds incremental value to stress wall motion assessment. Perfusion imaging during dobutamine or exercise stress echo-cardiography detects abnormalities that antedate wall motion abnormalities and helps delineate subendocardial wall thickening abnormalities that are induced even when overall transmural wall thickening appears normal. Perfusion imaging may also help identify vascular masses.
- Myocardial perfusion imaging may be performed with real-time perfusion or triggered approaches.

KEY POINTS

- Contrast agents approved for LV opacification can also be used to assess perfusion, although this application is "off label."
- Perfusion imaging provides information that complements that obtained with resting and stress wall motion assessment.
- There are two approaches to perfusion imaging: real-time perfusion echocardiography (RTPE) and triggered perfusion imaging.

Approaches to Myocardial Perfusion Imaging

- Myocardial perfusion is typically examined during an infusion of microbubbles, during which a high mechanical index (MI) impulse (referred to as flash) is delivered to clear the capillaries of microbubbles. The rate of replenishment of myocardial contrast, and the plateau intensity, are subsequently examined either visually or quantitatively (Fig. 9-1).
- RTPE is a low-MI imaging technique that permits the real-time detection of myocardial contrast enhancement following either a small (0.1–0.2 mL) bolus injection or continuous infusion of UCA. Alternatively, since continuous higher MI imaging destroys microbubbles, myocardial perfusion may be assessed with high-MI imaging at triggered intervals (end-systolic frames), where contrast enhancement is visualized at progressively longer intervals after the bubbles have been destroyed by an initial high-MI impulse. The advantages and disadvantages of triggered perfusion imaging versus RTPE are outlined in Table 9-1.

Rest   Peak stress

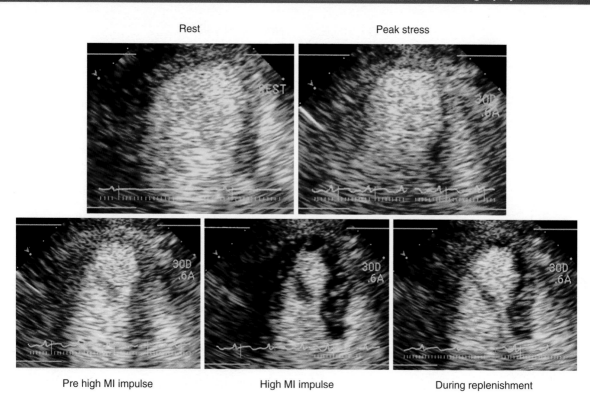

Pre high MI impulse   High MI impulse   During replenishment

Figure 9-1. Low-MI imaging in real-time using RTPE. These frames demonstrate that at low MI (<0.2), there are minimal to no signals from tissue, while contrast microbubbles can be delineated both in the LV cavity and myocardium.

TABLE 9-1	ADVANTAGES AND DISADVANTAGES OF LOW–MECHANICAL INDEX REAL-TIME PERFUSION ECHOCARDIOGRAPHY VERSUS HIGH–MECHANICAL INDEX TRIGGERED PERFUSION IMAGING	
	RTPE	**Triggered Perfusion Imaging**
Frame rate	20–25 Hz	Triggered end-systolic at incremental intervals
Sensitivity	Good	Excellent
Dynamic range	Low	High
Utility during exercise stress	Yes	Not feasible
Utility during dobutamine stress	Yes	Not feasible
Utility during vasodilator stress	Good	Excellent
Utility during resting perfusion assessment	Excellent	Excellent
Simultaneous analysis of wall motion/perfusion	Yes	No

Physiologic Basis for Examining Myocardial Perfusion with Ultrasound Contrast Agents

- Changes in myocardial blood flow can be analyzed by examining the replenishment of myocardial contrast following a high-MI impulse. This concept was developed by Wei et al.[1] and is demonstrated in Figure 9-2.
- The product of the rate of contrast replenishment (reflecting myocardial red blood cell velocity) and the plateau intensity (reflecting capillary cross sectional area) correlates with myocardial blood flow. By normalizing plateau intensity to adjacent LV cavity intensity, one can compute absolute myocardial blood flow.
- Most clinical applications analyze myocardial perfusion visually. A key concept is that under resting conditions with a typical diagnostic transducer having a 5-mm elevation plane,

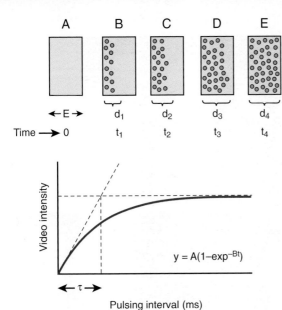

Figure 9-2. The schematic depiction of the 1-exponential curve that describes contrast replenishment following a high-MI impulse (**panel A**) during a continuous infusion of UCA.

normal myocardial contrast replenishment should be within 5 seconds, while under hyperemic conditions (exercise, dobutamine, vasodilator stress), replenishment should be within 2 seconds following the high-MI impulse.

KEY POINTS

- Real-time myocardial perfusion imaging uses continuous low-MI imaging.
- Triggered perfusion imaging uses intermittent (typically end-systolic) triggered high-MI imaging.
- Myocardial blood flow can be analyzed by examining the replenishment of myocardial contrast following a high-MI impulse.
- Normal resting myocardial contrast replenishment should be within 5 seconds.
- Normal stress myocardial contrast replenishment should be within 2 seconds.

Technical Considerations and Components

- The success of perfusion imaging is dependent on optimizing the gain, time gain compensation (TGC), and MI for imaging, as well as controlling the contrast infusion rate so as to obtain myocardial contrast enhancement without shadowing in the LV cavity.

Role of Physician

- The physician is responsible for the overall quality control of the procedure, which begins by ensuring that all personnel (cardiology fellows, nurses, sonographers) are adequately educated in the concepts of myocardial perfusion assessment with a continuous infusion of microbubble contrast. The physician needs to work with the lead sonographer and nursing team to develop a standard operating procedure to be followed whenever contrast is utilized to assess perfusion.
- Although RTPE during stress can be performed in a manner similar to standard stress procedures without contrast, the physician assigned to the laboratory needs to be Level III trained in echocardiography and have been trained in the performance and interpretation of at least 50 RTPE examinations before operating independently.

Roles of the Sonographer and Nurse

- Contrast is used to enhance images, improve border detection, and provide information on cardiac perfusion at rest and during functional stress echocardiographic studies.
- The contrast is administered by a registered nurse or other qualified medical personnel. A continuous infusion of Definity or Optison contrast is used both for resting, exercise, vasodilator, and dobutamine stress echocardiograms.
- The nurse will prepare the contrast solution prior to acquiring images.
- Definity is activated by agitating the vial for 45 seconds in the Vial Mix (Lantheus, Billerica, MA) (Fig. 9-3).
- Dilute 0.8 mL of Definity into 29 mL normal saline to make a total of approximately 30 mL, as demonstrated in Figure 9-3. One half of a vial of Optison can be diluted into 20 mL of saline if that is the agent desired.
- Do not mix until just prior to infusion. Two syringes should be made for stress echocardiograms. One syringe should be sufficient for resting echocardiograms. The infusion rate is approximately 4 mL/min by hand, watching the clock.
- The solution should be mixed back and forth periodically so that the contrast does not settle in the bottom of the syringe.
- The infusion is started when the sonographer is ready to capture resting images. The nurse will start the infusion and the sonographer will start to acquire the resting images.
- The infusion rate starts at 4 mL/min and can be increased or decreased if needed; this is

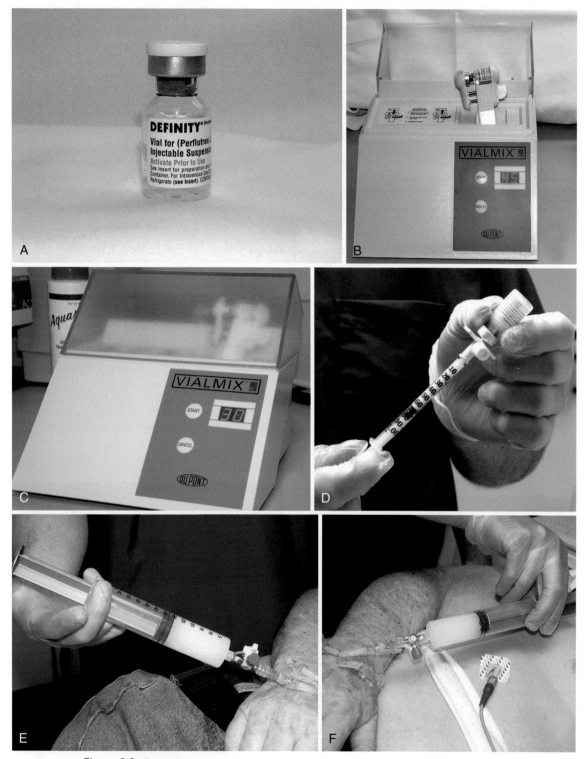

Figure 9-3. Essential components to preparing Definity UCA for a dilute contrast infusion.

dependent on the images. The sonographer will inform the nurse to increase or decrease the infusion rate as needed.

- One syringe of the mixture should be sufficient for a resting echocardiogram when looking for perfusion, LV function, wall motion abnormalities, and overall ejection fraction. This is also usually sufficient when examining for intracavitary thrombi or vascular tumors.
- The second half of the ultrasound contrast will be needed both for exercise and pharmacologic stress echocardiograms. In addition, any leftover diluted contrast from the syringe used to obtain resting images can be used for stress images as well. The range of solution left over from the resting images is from 0 to 20 mL for Definity, depending on the difficulty in obtaining the resting images.
- The second syringe is used for the stress images. In this setting, the infusion rate is usually lower because of the higher cardiac output (2–4 mL/min). The infusion rate should remain constant unless the sonographer indicates otherwise. It is important not to mix the second syringe until the sonographer is ready to capture the intermediate images for dobutamine stress echocardiography (DSE) and immediate post-stress images for exercise stress echocardiography.

resolution. This permits the detection of myocardial perfusion in real time along with regional function assessments. Despite this, SPECT and PET are the only techniques approved by the U.S. Food and Drug Administration (FDA) for examining myocardial perfusion.

- Myocardial perfusion imaging is also possible with magnetic resonance imaging (MRI). Although the spatial resolution of MRI is comparable with ultrasound, it is not currently capable of measuring myocardial blood flow and blood flow changes as is myocardial contrast echocardiography (MCE) (Table 9-2).

Acquisition of Perfusion Images

- The infusion rate must be adjusted so as to permit homogeneous myocardial opacification prior to application of high-MI impulses and analysis of contrast replenishment. This will usually require that TGC potentiometers be set to slightly higher in the near field to overcome automatic reductions that typically occur in the near field (Fig. 9-4).
- These settings must be such that a brief high-MI impulse (1.0–1.3 MI) results in clearance of signals from the myocardium.

KEY POINTS

- Dilute 0.8 mL of Definity into 29 mL normal saline to make a total of approximately 30 mL, or one half of a vial of Optison can be diluted into 20 mL of saline if that is the agent desired.
- Mix two syringes for stress echocardiograms and one syringe for resting studies.
- Do not mix until just prior to infusion.
- The infusion rate for resting starts at 4 mL/min and can be increased or decreased if needed.
- The infusion rate for post-stress imaging is 2–4 mL/min.

Advantages and Disadvantages of Using Real-time Perfusion Echocardiography versus Other Imaging Techniques

- Ultrasound has higher spatial resolution than either radionuclide imaging (single-photon emission computed tomography [SPECT] or positron emission tomography [PET]) techniques and provides greater temporal

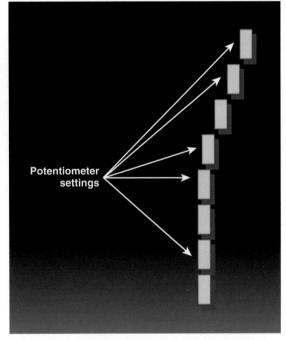

Figure 9-4. Typical time gain compensation (TGC) settings required to create homogeneous myocardial contrast during RTPE.

TABLE 9-2   PERFUSION IMAGING TECHNIQUES

	MCE	MRI	SPECT/PET
Resolution	< 2 mm	< 2 mm	10–15 mm
Subendocardial defects detected	Yes	Yes	No
Cost	Low	High	High
Portability	Yes	Not possible	Limited
Real-time perfusion	Yes	No	No
Availability	Extensive	Very limited	Limited
FDA-approved perfusion agent	Not approved	Not approved	Approved
Radiation exposure	None	None	>10 mSV*

*Higher radiation exposure for thallium- over technetium-based tracers; lower doses reported for D-SPECT imaging (Spectrum Dynamics, Danville, CA).

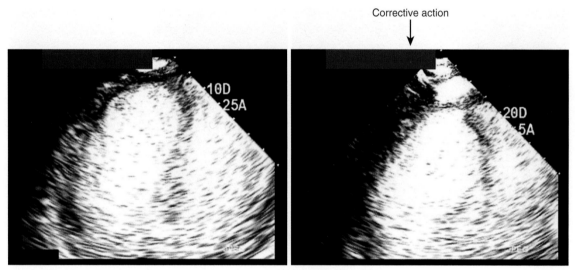

Figure 9-5. A TGC setting that is too low in the near field is manifested by the appearance of a pseudoapical perfusion defect. Slightly adjusting the TGCs higher in the near field prevents this artifactual perfusion defect. These adjustments should be made during the resting studies prior to stress imaging.

Figure 9-5 demonstrates how to adjust the TGCs to create homogeneous opacification. Figure 9-6 illustrates that occasionally the near-field TGCs must be adjusted back slightly to ensure that the post-high-MI impulse adequately clears the myocardium in all segments.

- The infusion rate of UCA must be adjusted so that the high-MI impulse only clears myocardial contrast and does not excessively destroy LV cavity contrast. This will result in a reduction of contrast entering the coronary circulation and create difficulties in analyzing myocardial contrast replenishment.
- Tissue Contrast Enhancement is available on the Philips iE33 and Sonos 5500/7500.

Real-time low-MI imaging is made possible with power modulation. This feature prolongs the contrast effect and provides real-time contrast visualization of perfusion using a low MI (<0.2). Therefore, both wall motion and myocardial contrast can be analyzed simultaneously.

- Cadence Contrast Pulse Sequencing technology is available on the Siemens Acuson Sequoia. This imaging technology provides low-MI imaging with tissue only, contrast only, or both. It recognizes and processes the unique nonlinear fundamental and higher order harmonic signals that are generated by the UCA. The nonlinear response is a result of the bubbles' asymmetric expansion and contraction with

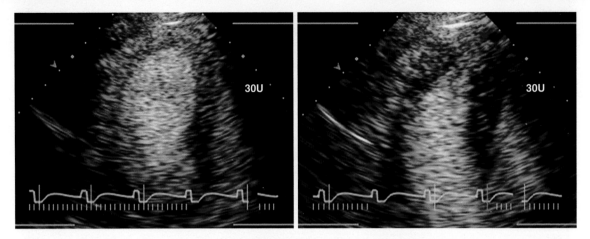

Corrective action: Turn down the near-field gain

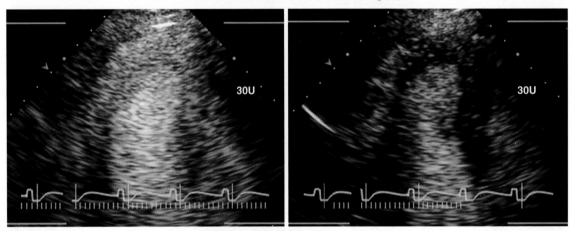

Figure 9-6. Conversely, TGCs that are too high in the near field (**top panels**) result in unwanted tissue signals appearing in the apex on the immediate post-high-MI image (**top right panel**), preventing one from adequately analyzing myocardial contrast replenishment in the apical segment. Corrective action is taken in the lower panels, where slightly lowering the TGCs in the near field results in a homogeneous absence of myocardial signals that will be adequate for analyzing replenishment. Note that TGCs in both the near and far fields are set to achieve both homogeneous myocardial opacification as well as ensure absence of signals from the myocardium immediately following the high-MI impulses.

an ultrasound pulse. The contrast signal is significantly increased with this new pulse sequencing scheme.

- Table 9-3 provides the recommended ultrasound settings and presets for both the Philips iE33 and the Acuson Sequoia™ when using RTPE.
- Low-MI contrast imaging (or RTPE) is dependent on the microbubbles resonating without disruption in the LV. The correct system adjustments are needed in order to have adequate bubble concentration in the LV cavity. Table 9-4 gives the definitions and concepts behind optimal settings for real-time perfusion imaging.

- Box 9-1 summarizes the key concepts in image set-up that are required to analyze resting or stress perfusion with RTPE.

KEY POINTS

- In order to perform perfusion imaging, machine settings and the contrast infusion rate must be optimized.
- Commercially available applications—Tissue Contrast Enhancement (Philips) and Cadence Contrast Pulse Sequencing (Siemens)—enable myocardial perfusion imaging.

TABLE 9-3 IMAGING SETTINGS/PRESETS FOR REAL-TIME PERFUSION IMAGING

	Presets for Philips iE33	Presets for Acuson Sequoia
Depth	140 mm	140 mm
Focus	Mitral valve level	Mitral valve level
Contrast option	Gen (1.5 MHz)	CPS (Cadence contrast agent imaging)
Gain/compression	60-68/50	CPS gain: –8 to –15
High-MI flash frame duration	2–5 frames at rest 5–20 frames during stress	2–5 frames at rest; 1–2 heartbeats during stress
Loop duration	10 s	10 s
High-MI setting	1.1	1.7
Features	XRes is on; gray map 2; chroma map 7	General H/V
Frame rate	22–25 Hz	22–25 Hz
TGCs	TGCs are set in the middle—hit iScan and adjust TGCs higher in the near field	TGCs are set in the middle and adjusted higher in the near field

TABLE 9-4 CONCEPTS BEHIND SYSTEM SETTINGS FOR REAL-TIME PERFUSION IMAGING

Key Concepts on System Settings	
Focus	Narrowest area of the beam with the greatest ultrasound intensity. Should be placed at the mitral valve level Allows greater resolution of the entire LV Helps to reduce "swirling" artifacts seen in the apex
Gain (overall)/ dynamic range	The overall gain amplifies intensity of the received echoes and uniformly increases or decreases the number of echoes displayed. Should be set higher in the near field for real-time perfusion imaging. The dynamic range boosts visibility of softer echoes from contrast. Both these do not effect microbubble destruction.
MI	MI set too high will cause too much bubble destruction. Should be around 0.1–0.2 MI. Should be >1.0 MI for brief destructive impulses to clear contrast from the myocardium.
Frame rate (FR)	The FR determines the repetition frequency at which pulses are received by microbubbles. Sector size, width, and imaging depth affect the FR. Too high an FR can disrupt microbubbles—should be around 20–25 Hz during low-MI perfusion imaging. Can be increased to 25–30 Hz during high heart rates (exercise or dobutamine stress).

BOX 9-1 Critical Parameters Utilized to Optimize Analysis of Perfusion

Key Set-up Points
- Optimize near field gain.
- Adjust contrast infusion to create homogeneous myocardial opacification without shadowing.
- Adjust duration of high MI impulses to minimize cavity destruction.
- Purposefully foreshorten images to analyze basal segment perfusion.

Physiologic Data Perfusion Imaging at Rest and During Stress

Intracardiac Masses: Thrombi and Vascular Tumors
Acquisition
- RTPE can be used for suspected abnormal intracardiac masses. This technique can be useful in determining whether the mass is vascular in nature. Perfusion images are

typically taken at the conclusion of the standard echocardiographic examination.

- The correct machine settings (see Table 9-3) for myocardial contrast imaging are selected, and the nurse starts the infusion of Definity or Optison. When homogeneous myocardial opacification is observed, the high-MI impulses are applied to destroy the microbubbles in the myocardium and in the mass.
- Images should be taken in the apical 4-, 2-, and 3-chamber views, respectively, if the intracardiac mass is closest to the transducer in these fields.
- If the intracardiac mass is closer to the transducer in the parasternal or subxiphoid views, then these should be utilized to analyze contrast replenishment.
- The flash duration should be set to around 3 to 10 frames and adjusted as needed depending on the destruction of the microbubbles in the myocardium and LV cavity. If too many bubbles are being destroyed in the LV cavity, then the flash duration needs to be reduced.
- As described above, the infusion rate is a continuous infusion of 29 mL of saline mixed with 0.8 mL of activated Definity. The infusion rate is approximately 4 mL/min. For Optison®, the vial can be mixed with a smaller volume of saline (20 mL), and infused at approximately the same rate.

Analysis
- Post-high-MI (flash) imaging of the mass will indicate whether it is vascular in nature. If there is an enhancement of contrast in the mass postflash, this indicates it is vascular (Fig. 9-7).
- If the mass remains dark postflash, this would suggest a thrombus or other nonvascular mass (Fig. 9-8).
- If the enhancement is similar to myocardial contrast enhancement, then metastatic tumor or capillary hemangioma should be suspected. Mild contrast enhancement (less than myocardial) is observed with stromal tumors.

Pitfalls
- All attempts should be made to place the mass or tumor as close as possible to the transducer. For example, avoid imaging atrial tumors in the four-chamber view. If it is an atrial tumor, examine in either the subxiphoid or parasternal views, or obtain very foreshortened apical windows.

KEY POINTS
• Contrast perfusion imaging may be used to assess the vascularity of intracardiac masses. • Views should be selected so that the mass is close to the transducer. • The perfusion protocol is similar to that for myocardial perfusion imaging.

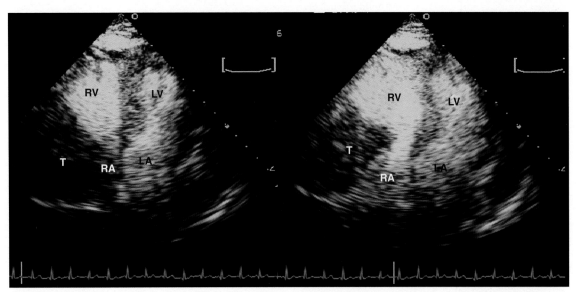

Figure 9-7. Images from an echocardiogram performed to evaluate a right atrial and ventricular mass noted in the four-chamber view (T). The immediate postflash image is shown on the left. The image obtained three to four cardiac cycles postflash on the right demonstrates contrast enhancement indicative of a vascular mass.

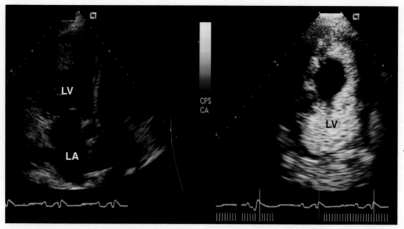

Figure 9-8. Resting echocardiogram on the left demonstrated severe global hypokinesis with an LV cavity mass. A contrast examination was performed during a continuous infusion of ultrasound contrast agent (UCA). The postflash impulses (2 seconds post-high-MI impulse) indicate that the mass is not vascular, most consistent with a thrombus.

Exercise Stress Real-time Perfusion

Acquisition

- A Bruce protocol is used, and images are taken at rest and immediately postexercise.
- The correct machine settings (see Table 9-3) and protocol for myocardial contrast imaging are selected and the nurse starts the infusion of either diluted Definity or Optison. Resting and immediate post-stress images are taken with the continuous infusion of contrast at approximately 4 mL/min for rest and 2 mL/min during stress.
- The myocardium should appear dark after the flash; however, the LV cavity should remain bright. If the LV cavity is dark, the infusion rate should be increased or the duration of the high-MI impulses should be adjusted.
- The myocardium should replenish within one to four heartbeats at rest and become bright again, while during stress replenishment should be less than 2 seconds.
- The high-MI (flash) duration at rest should be set at around five frames and adjusted as needed depending on the destruction of the microbubbles. If too many bubbles are being destroyed in the LV cavity, then the flash duration needs to be turned down. Because of the higher cardiac output and cardiac motion during stress, the high-MI duration may be increased to up to 12 to 15 frames (or one to two cardiac cycles on the Siemens system) for the stress images.
- When using the Philips iE33 scanner, the "iScan" button should only be used in the beginning when resting images are taken. For all systems, the frame rate should be around 22 to 25 Hz (it can be slightly higher with an increased heart rate). The MI should be set at around 0.18 and no higher than 0.20.
- For exercise stress, the full disclosure option is chosen, which indicates that each cardiac cycle is acquired after one pushes the "acquire" button. The flash is applied prior to acquiring the resting images. Once the flash is applied, wait a couple of heartbeats and then hit the "acquire" button. Choose the best two postflash images for each view.
- The nurse will need to start infusing the contrast prior to the patient getting off the treadmill for immediate post-stress images. The administration of contrast should start approximately 1 minute before the patient needs to terminate the test and get off the treadmill.
- Readjust the imaging parameters for exercise images. The flash duration should be increased to around 12 to 15 frames to account for the rise in blood volume postexercise. The overall gain can also be turned down if needed during image acquisition.

Analysis

- With RTPE, analysis of perfusion and wall motion occurs simultaneously. If you see an area of the myocardium that does not replenish (perfusion defect) after approximately two to three heartbeats after the high-MI flash following exercise, this indicates a stenosis (Figs. 9-9 and 9-10).
- Beware of segments that are often attenuated by rib or lung shadowing, such as the basal to mid-anterior and lateral segments. Purposely obtain some images in a foreshortened view to reduce attenuation of basal segments. As a tip

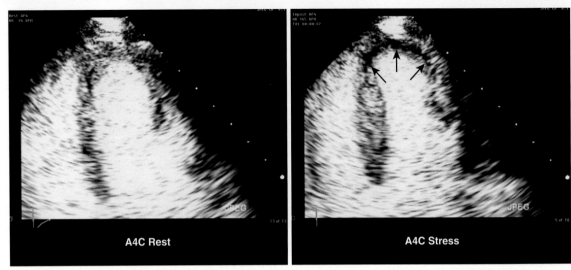

Figure 9-9. Images from an exercise stress echocardiogram. Using RTPE, a stress image obtained within 2 seconds following a flash impulse is shown on the right, while a rest image (obtained 4 seconds postflash) is shown on the left. Resting perfusion is normal, while the stress image demonstrates a transmural perfusion defect consistent with inducible ischemia.

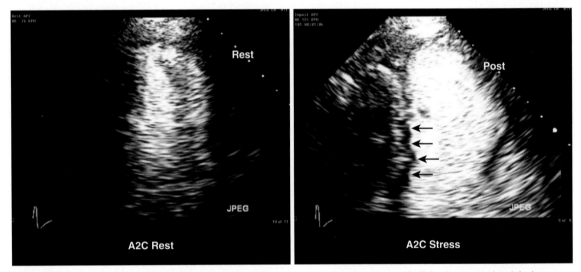

Figure 9-10. A rest image is demonstrated on the left, and a stress image post-treadmill is shown on the right in the apical two-chamber view (A2C) (Fig. 9-13). The rest image is normal. The arrows in the stress image delineate an inducible inferior perfusion defect.

to help identify attenuation, perfusion defects are often subendocardial, while attenuation tends to involve the entire transmural extent of the segment and involves areas outside the segment.

Pitfalls and Clinical Tips

- The image plane is very important. Moving the anterior/lateral wall to the middle of the sector can reduce wall filling dropout. One can purposefully foreshorten the apical windows to obtain views that will permit the analysis of replenishment and plateau contrast enhancement in the basal to middle segments.
- If there is not adequate filling of the LV with contrast, injecting at a faster rate may be needed.
- There should be some attenuation seen in the LV chamber to achieve maximum bubble response in the tissue. However, if there is an excessive amount of attenuation, reduce the administration of the contrast and wait for the attenuation to dissipate. The middle and basal

portions of the LV will be completely black if there is too much attenuation.

- Apical perfusion dropout is caused by lack of microbubbles in the apical myocardium of the LV. Possible technical causes are inadequate receiver gain in the near field; an MI that is set too high; suboptimal placement of the focus (repositioning the focus, sometimes moving it closer to the near field, can help to achieve better filling in the apex); and an infusion rate that is too low (see Fig. 9-4). The absence of microbubbles in the apex may also be due to hypoperfusion.
- The flash impulse is used to destroy contrast in the myocardium. The frames can be adjusted to control the duration of the impulse. If the myocardium is not dark enough after the impulse, the overall gain might need to be reduced or the number of flash frames might need to be increased. Having the patient inhale and hold his or her breath may also help in this situation.

KEY POINTS

- Exercise myocardial perfusion echocardiography is performed using real-time perfusion imaging since this permits the acquisition of wall motion and perfusion information.
- The contrast infusion is started 1 minute before the end of exercise.
- Additional nonstandard views (apically foreshortened) may be needed to image the basal and middle portions of the LV.
- Infusion rates and machine settings must be optimized for both rest and post-stress images.

Dobutamine Stress Real-time Perfusion
Acquisition

- A four-stage protocol is used and images are taken at rest, low dose (if a resting wall motion abnormality is present), intermediate stress, and peak stress. Images are only taken in the four-, two-, and three-chamber views.
- The nurse starts the infusion of Definity or Optison as described earlier. Once homogeneous myocardial opacification is achieved (adjusting gain settings and infusion rate), then hit the "acquire" button. Following this, a brief high-MI impulse (flash) is applied. The myocardium should appear dark after the flash; however, the LV cavity should remain

bright. If the LV cavity is dark, then you should increase the infusion rate or reduce the duration of the flash impulse. The myocardium should replenish within 5 seconds at rest. Once the myocardium is opacified postflash, then hit the "acquire" button again to end your acquisition.
- This same process is repeated for low-dose, intermediate stress (70% predicted maximum heart rate), and peak stress (>85% predicted maximum heart rate) images (Table 9-6).
- Low-dose dobutamine images are necessary mainly if a resting wall motion abnormality is present, to examine for wall motion recruitment as well as contrast replenishment in dobutamine-nonresponsive segments.
- The flash duration at rest should be set to around five frames and adjusted as needed depending on the destruction of the microbubbles. If too many bubbles are being destroyed in the LV cavity, then the flash duration should be reduced. This situation could occur if the patient's ejection fraction is low. It might be necessary to increase the flash at peak heart rate due to the increase in blood volume and cardiac output.
- The frame rate should be around 22–25 Hz (it can be slightly higher at higher heart rates).
- The MI should be set at around 0.18 and no higher than 0.20.

TABLE 9-5	ACQUISITION PARAMETERS FOR TWO-STAGE EXERCISE ECHOCARDIOGRAM (TYPICALLY THE BRUCE PROTOCOL)

Stage 1. Resting Images
Choose protocol (MCE)
Focus at the level of the MV
Set TGCs in the middle, hit iScan and then adjust your TGCs higher in the near field. The overall gain may need to be adjusted if the image is too bright.
Flash wait a couple of heart beats and then acquire the image.
Choose the best two images postflash for all views.

Stage 2. Immediate Post-stress Images
Increase flash duration to around 12–15 frames (or 1–2 cardiac cycles on the Siemens system).
Decrease the overall gain if needed.
Hit the timer button.
Hit "acquire" button and begin taking the postexercise images.
Hit the "Flash" for all apical views
Choose the images in sequence and create subloops. (The first one chosen for each apical view should be a preflash image.)

MV, mitral valve.

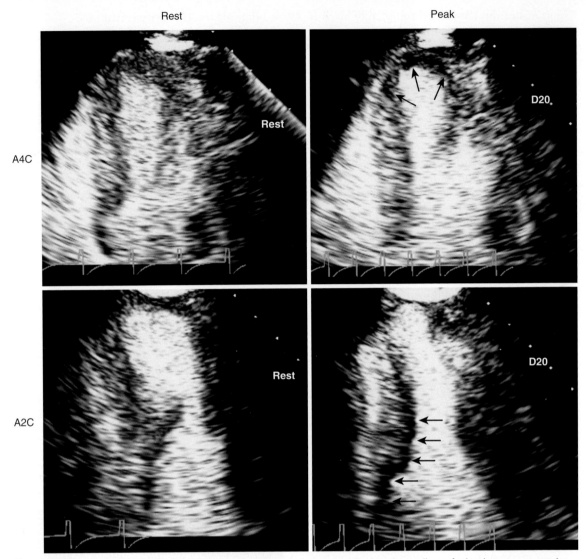

Figure 9-11. Images from perfusion imaging during dobutamine stress. Rest end-systolic perfusion images are on the left and stress images are on the right. Resting perfusion is normal. Stress images show inducible inferior and apical perfusion defects.

- Communication between the nurse and sonographer/physician is important to achieve the best results. The infusion rate may need to be altered to achieve adequate destruction of microbubbles in the myocardium. This optimal rate will vary from patient to patient and from rest to peak dobutamine stress. It is important to have adequate destruction of the bubbles in the myocardium postflash so that a perfusion defect can be confidently identified.
- An area of the myocardium that does not replenish (perfusion defect) after approximately two to three heartbeats post-high-MI flash could indicate a blockage (Fig. 9-11).

Analysis

- The physician will analyze the images after all four stages have been acquired. Note that if there is a resting wall motion abnormality and perfusion defect, the algorithm in Table 9-6 is changed to examine for myocardial viability (Fig. 9-12). In this instance, if attenuation has been ruled out as a cause of the resting defect, then images during a low-dose (5–10 µg/kg/min) dobutamine infusion should be examined for viability and used to compare with the intermediate and peak stress images.
- Overall, RTPE is more sensitive in detecting significant CAD than wall motion analysis

TABLE 9-6	**ACQUISITION PARAMETERS FOR FOUR-STAGE DOBUTAMINE STRESS ECHOCARDIOGRAPHY**
Acquisition Philips iE33 Four-stage Dobutamine	**Acquisition Acuson Sequoia™ Four-stage Dobutamine**
Stage 1. Rest Images Choose protocol (MCE). Focus at the level of the MV. Set TGCs in the middle, hit iScan and then adjust your TGCs higher in the near field. You may have to adjust your overall gain if the image is too bright. If resting wall motion abnormality, then low dose dobutamine needed to assess for recruitment and contrast replenishment.	**Stage 1. Rest Images** Choose protocol (MCE). Cadence turned on. Focus at the level of the MV. Triggers are turned on. Set TGCs in the middle, and adjust them in the near field as needed. You may have to adjust your CPS gain (overall) if the image is too bright. If resting wall motion abnormality, then low dose dobutamine needed to assess for recruitment and contrast replenishment.
Next Stage. Heart Rate Has Achieved 70% Repeat your images following the same protocol used for resting images. Accept your images.	**Next Stage. Heart Rate Has Achieved 70%** Repeat your images following the same protocol used for resting images. Clip store your images and review/label images. Advance protocol to peak stress.
Final Stage. Heart Rate Has Achieved 85% Repeat your images following the same protocol and accept your images. You may want to increase your flash duration during peak stress because of the increase in blood volume. It will take a higher flash duration to destroy the bubbles in the myocardium.	**Final Stage. Heart Rate Has Achieved 85%** Repeat your images following the same protocol. Clip store your images and review/label images. Make sure you adjust your frame rate with a higher heart rate before you capture your images. You may also want to increase your flash duration during peak stress because of the increase in blood volume. It will take a higher flash duration to destroy the bubbles in the myocardium.
If no low-dose dobutamine images obtained, an additional acquisition can be obtained at peak stress or following heart rate recovery.	If no low-dose dobutamine images obtained, an addition acquisition can be obtained at peak stress or following heart rate recovery.

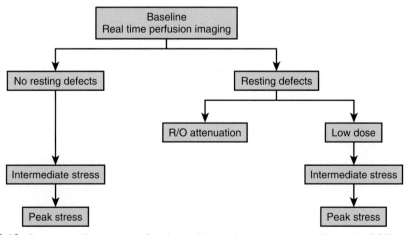

Figure 9-12. Sequence of steps in performing a dobutamine stress echocardiography (DSE) with RTPE.

(WMA) alone and provides better prognostic data.

Pitfalls and Clinical Tips
- Imaging planes are very important. Moving the anterior/lateral wall to the middle of the sector can reduce dropout. Purposefully foreshortening the apical windows can

improve visualization of wall motion and perfusion in the basal to middle segments.
- If there is not adequate filling of the LV with contrast, infusion at a faster rate may be needed.
- There may be some mild attenuation in the LV chamber if maximum myocardial opacification is to be achieved. However,

if there is an excessive amount of attenuation, complete myocardial microbubble destruction will be prevented, and analysis of basal segments will be almost impossible. If attenuation of the LV cavity is visually apparent, reduce the administration of the contrast and wait for the attenuation to dissipate.

- Apical dropout (absence of apical myocardial opacification despite opacification of basal and middle segments) is most often caused by inadequate TGC in the near field. The potentiometers should be adjusted as displayed in Figure 9-4. Other possibilities are that the MI may be set too high, causing near-field destruction, or that the focus needs to be repositioned to the near field.
- The flash impulse is used to destroy contrast in the myocardium. The frames can be adjusted to control the duration of the impulse. If the myocardium is not dark enough after the impulse, the overall gain may need to be reduced, the number of frames for the flash should be increased, or it may be helpful to have the patient hold his or her breath on inspiration.

KEY POINTS

- Dobutamine myocardial perfusion echocardiography is performed using real-time perfusion imaging since this permits the acquisition of wall motion and perfusion information.
- In addition to providing information about inducible ischemia, the test may be used to assess viability in the presence of resting wall motion abnormalities.
- Additional nonstandard views (apically foreshortened) may be needed to image the basal and middle portions of the LV.
- Infusion rates and machine settings must be optimized for both rest and stress images.

Vasodilator Stress Myocardial Perfusion Imaging
Acquisition

- A two-stage protocol is used and images are taken at rest and postinfusion of the vasodilator agent.
- Imaging can be with RTPE or with triggered end-systolic images at a high MI. If using triggered high-MI imaging, then one typically obtains the triggered images at one, two, and four cardiac cycles to analyze replenishment both at rest and during vasodilator stress.

- The correct machine setting and protocol for myocardial contrast imaging are selected, and the nurse starts the infusion of either diluted Definity or Optison.
- Rest apical images are taken with the continuous infusion of contrast at approximately 4 mL/min and adjusted as necessary to achieve myocardial opacification without cavity attenuation.
- The post-stress images are taken during the infusion of dipyridamole or adenosine, and immediately following the 400-µg bolus of Regadenoson (Astellas Pharmaceuticals, Deerfield, IL) (Table 9-7).
- The myocardium should appear dark after the flash; however, the LV cavity should remain bright. If the LV cavity is dark, the infusion rate should be increased or the duration (or MI) of the flash should be decreased. The myocardium should replenish within 5 seconds at rest. During vasodilator-induced hyperemia, the normal time for replenishment is short (<2 s). Once the myocardium is opacified postflash, hit the "acquire" button again to end your acquisition.
- The high-MI (flash) duration at rest should be set at around five frames and adjusted as needed depending on the destruction of the microbubbles. This will be the same for the post-stress images. If too many bubbles are being destroyed in the LV cavity, then the flash duration (or MI) needs to be turned down.
- When using the Philips iE33 scanner, the "iScan" button should be used only in the beginning when resting images are taken. For all systems, the frame rate should be around

---

TABLE 9-7 VASODILATOR STRESS AGENTS UTILIZED FOR REAL-TIME PERFUSION ECHOCARDIOGRAPHY PHARMACOLOGIC STRESS

Agent	Infusion Rate	Acquisition Time for Post-Stress Images
Regadenoson	400-µg bolus × 1	Immediate postinfusion
Adenosine	140 µg/kg/min for up to 6 min	2–4 min after infusion started
Dipyridamole	0.56–0.84 mg/kg over 4–6 min	3–7 min after infusion started

22 to 25 Hz; it can be slightly higher at increased heart rates. The MI should be set at around 0.18 and no higher than 0.20.

- As with other stress protocols, communication between the nurse and sonographer/physician is important to achieving the best results. The infusion rate may need to be decreased or increased to achieve adequate destruction of the microbubbles in the myocardium. This will vary from patient to patient. It is important to have adequate destruction of the bubbles in the myocardium so that a perfusion defect can be identified. The perfusion defect may be transient and observable only during the first cardiac cycle of replenishment postflash. If you see an area of the myocardium that does not replenish (perfusion defect) after approximately two to three heartbeats after the high-MI flash, then this indicates a stenosis (Table 9-8).

Analysis

- The physician will analyze the images after both stages have been acquired. During vasodilator-induced hyperemia, the normal time period of replenishment to reach the plateau intensity following a flash impulse should be less than 2 seconds.
- With vasodilator stress, wall motion abnormalities are not typically induced even when a physiologically relevant stenosis is present. Therefore, the analysis is focused mainly on perfusion. An example of a perfusion defect during Regadenoson stress is demonstrated in Figure 9-13.

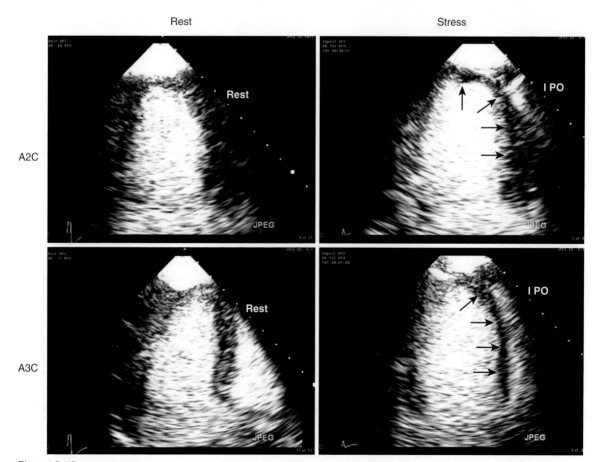

Figure 9-13. An inducible distal septal and apical perfusion defect (*arrows*) observed within the first cardiac cycle following a flash impulse. The images on the right were obtained within the first 2 minutes following a 400-μg Regadenoson bolus. IPO, immediate post; A2C, apical two-chamber view; A3C, apical three-chamber view.

TABLE 9-8   ACQUISITION PROTOCOL FOR VASODILATOR STRESS REAL-TIME PERFUSION ECHOCARDIOGRAPHY

Acquisition Philips iE33 Regadenoson Vasodilator Two-Stage Stress Echocardiogram	Acquisition Acuson Sequoia Regadenoson Vasodilator Two-Stage Stress Echocardiogram
Stage 1. Rest Images Choose protocol (MCE). Focus at the level of the MV. Set TGCs in the middle, hit iScan and then adjust your TGCs higher in the near field. You may have to adjust your overall gain if the image is too bright or adjust your flash duration. Accept your images and the protocol will automatically advance to the next stage.	**Stage 1. Rest Images** Choose protocol (MCE). Cadence turned on. Focus at the level of the MV. Triggers are turned on. Set TGCs in the middle, and adjust them higher in the near field as needed. You may have to adjust your CPS gain (overall) if the image is too bright or adjust your flash duration. Clip store your images and review/label images. Advance protocol to next stage.
Stage 2. Post-Stress Images Repeat your images following the same protocol used for the resting images. Please reference the above parameters for correct acquisition time depending on the agent that is administered.	**Stage 2. Post-Stress Images** Repeat your images following the same protocol used for the resting images. Clip store your images and review/label images. Please reference the above parameters for correct acquisition time depending on the agent that is administered.

KEY POINTS

- Vasodilator perfusion echocardiography is performed using real-time perfusion imaging or triggered approaches.
- Additional nonstandard views (apically foreshortened) may be needed to image the basal and middle portions of the LV.
- Perfusion abnormalities may be seen only transiently after the high-MI flash.
- Infusion rates and machine settings must be optimized for both rest and vasodilator images.

Reference

1. Wei K, Jayaweera AR, Firoozan S, et al. Quantification of myocardial blood flow with ultrasound-induced destruction of microbubbles administered as a constant venous infusion. *Circulation.* 1998;97:473-483.
   This is a landmark publication in the field of myocardial perfusion echocardiography demonstrating that myocardial blood flow can be quantified with MCE during a venous infusion of microbubbles.

Suggested Reading

1. Porter, TR, Xie F. Myocardial perfusion imaging with contrast ultrasound. *J Am Coll Cardiol Img.* 2010;3: 176-187.
   This state-of-the-art review covers the development and clinical application of myocardial perfusion imaging with MCE. It includes a discussion of the methods used to quantify myocardial perfusion, a review of the clinical studies that have examined the clinical utility of myocardial perfusion imaging, and an overview of the limitations.
2. Tsutsui JM, Elhendy A, Anderson JR, et al. Prognostic value of dobutamine stress myocardial contrast perfusion echocardiography. *Circulation.* 2005;112:1444-1450.
   This paper reports that myocardial perfusion imaging during dobutamine stress provides incremental prognostic information over clinical risk factors and other echocardiographic data in patients with known or suspected coronary artery disease. Patients with normal myocardial perfusion have a better outcome than patients with normal wall motion.
3. Rafter P, Phillips P, Vannan MA. Imaging technologies and techniques. *Cardiol Clin.* 2004;22:181-197.
   This review covers myocardial perfusion imaging techniques and the technologies available to perform this form of imaging.
4. Peltier M, Vancraeynest D, Pasquet A, et al. Assessment of the physiologic significance of coronary disease with dipyridamole real-time myocardial contrast echocardiography. Comparison with technetium-99m sestamibi single-photon emission computed tomography and quantitative coronary angiography. *J Am Coll Cardiol.* 2004;43:257-264.
   This study shows that real-time myocardial perfusion echocardiography with dipyridamole can define the presence and severity of coronary disease in a manner that compares favorably with quantitative SPECT.
5. Elhendy A, O'Leary EL, Xie F, et al. Comparative accuracy of real-time myocardial contrast perfusion imaging and wall motion analysis during dobutamine stress echocardiography for the diagnosis of coronary artery disease. *J Am Coll Cardiol.* 2004;44:2185-2191.
   This study sought to compare the accuracy of MCE and WMA during DSE for the diagnosis of CAD. It reported that MCE provides better sensitivity than WMA, particularly in patients with submaximal stress and in identifying patients with multivessel CAD.
6. Kirkpatrick J, Wong T, Bednarz JE, et al. Differential diagnosis of cardiac masses using contrast echocardiographic perfusion imaging. *J Am Coll Cardiol.* 2004;43:1412-1419.
   The study describes how echocardiographic contrast perfusion imaging aids in the differentiation of cardiac masses. Compared with the adjacent myocardium, malignant and vascular tumors hyperenhance, whereas stromal tumors and thrombi hypoenhance.
7. Bhatia VK, Senior R. Contrast echocardiography: evidence of clinical use. *J Am Soc Echocardiogr.* 2008; 21:409-416.
   This review provides an overview of the clinical evidence supporting the efficacy of contrast echocardiography in the assessment of myocardial structure, function, and perfusion.

8. Shimoni S, Frangrogiannis NG, Aggeli CJ, et al. Identification of hibernating myocardium with quantitative intravenous myocardial contrast echocardiography: Comparison with dobutamine echocardiography and thallium-201 scintigraphy. *Circulation.* 2003;107:538-544.

   This study demonstrates that MCE identifies myocardial hibernation in humans. Prediction of viable myocardium with MCE is best using quantification of myocardial blood flow and provides improved accuracy compared with dobutamine echocardiography and thallium-201 scintigraphy.

9. Tong KL, Kaul S, Wang XQ, et al. Myocardial contrast echocardiography versus thrombolysis in myocardial infarction score in patients presenting to the emergency department with chest pain and a nondiagnostic electrocardiogram. *J Am Coll Cardiol.* 2005;46:920-927.

   This study demonstrates that contrast echocardiography can rapidly and accurately provide short-, intermediate-, and long-term prognostic information in patients presenting to the emergency department with suspected cardiac chest pain even before serum cardiac markers are known.

10. Galiuto L, et al. The extent of microvascular damage during myocardial contrast echocardiography is superior to other known indexes of post-infarct reperfusion in predicting left ventricular remodeling. *J Am Coll Cardiol.* 2008;51:552-559.

    This study demonstrates that among patients with thrombolyis in myocardial infarction (TIMI) flow grade 3, the extent of microvascular damage, detected and quantitated by MCE, is the most powerful independent predictor of LV remodeling after ST elevation myocardial infarction as compared with persistent ST segment elevation and myocardial blush grade.

Evaluation of Coronary Blood Flow by Echo Doppler

10

Nozomi Watanabe

Background

Anatomy *(Fig. 10-1)*

The coronary arteries provide arterial blood to the myocardium. Transthoracic Doppler echocardiography allows us to detect coronary blood flow in the epicardial coronary arteries, septal branches, and perforator branches.

- The left main coronary artery originates from the left coronary sinus of the aortic root, and then bifurcates into the left anterior descending (LAD) and the left circumflex (LCx) arteries.
- The LAD runs over the anterior interventricular sulcus and extends apically, ending distal to the apex.
- The LCx is covered by the left atrial appendage in its proximal portion, and then takes position in the left atrioventricular sulcus.
- The right coronary artery (RCA) originates from the right coronary sinus of the aortic root, and goes into the right atrioventricular sulcus. The posterior descending artery (PDA) runs into the posterior interventricular sulcus.
- Commonly, Doppler echocardiography can detect:
  - the left main coronary and its bifurcation (proximal LAD and LCx),
  - middle to distal segments of the LAD,
  - the proximal segment of the RCA,
  - the PDA, and
  - the distal segment of the LCx.

Pathophysiology

- Normal coronary flow is characterized by a biphasic flow profile, consisting of small systolic and large diastolic flow (Fig. 10-2).
- The color Doppler signal is detected mainly in diastole.
- Doppler spectral tracings of coronary flow provide some useful clinical information such as coronary flow direction, flow velocity, and flow pattern.
- Coronary flow reserve (CFR) is expressed as a ratio of maximum flow to resting flow, with the normal response being an increase in flow to four times baseline (Fig. 10-3).

- CFR begins to decrease at 40% to 50% diameter stenosis for a vasodilatory stimulus.[1]
- CFR decreases to only twice baseline at approximately 75% diameter stenosis, which indicates significant myocardial stenosis.

Overview of the Transthoracic Approach in Coronary Detection

Strengths

- Noninvasive
- Portable
- Cost effective
- Physiologic assessment of coronary flow
- CFR measurement

Weaknesses

- Limited sites of coronary detection
- Low success rate in the RCA and LCx
- No histologic assessment
- Requires technical training

Anatomic Imaging and Physiologic Data Acquisition

Acquisition

Before Scanning

- A high-resolution and high-sensitivity ultrasound system is required.
- Choose a high-frequency transducer (~7 to 12 MHz) to detect the mid- to distal LAD.
- A relatively low-frequency transducer (~2 to 5 MHz) is used for the proximal LAD, RCA, and LCx.
- The Doppler velocity range is set in the range of 10 to 30 cm/s (Fig. 10-4).
- The Doppler wall filter is set to the lowest level so that low-velocity signals are recorded close to the baseline (Fig. 10-5).
- The patient is examined in the left lateral decubitus position.
- Intravenous injection of a contrast agent enhances Doppler signal intensity.

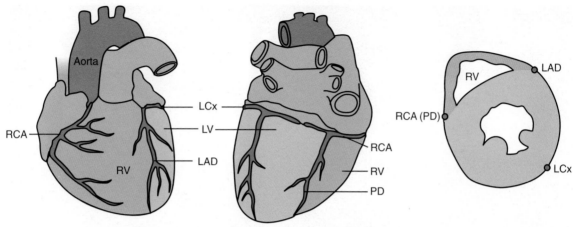

Figure 10-1. Anatomy of coronary arteries, shown in an anterior (*left*) and posterior (*center*) view of the heart and in a cross-sectional view of the papillary muscle level (*right*). The left main coronary artery bifurcates into the LAD, which runs over the anterior interventricular sulcus, and the LCx, which is related to the left atrioventricular sulcus. The LAD extends down, ending distal to the apex, often extending up into the posterior interventricular sulcus. The septal branches arise in an acute angle from the LAD, coursing close to the endocardium on the right side of the interventricular septum. The LCx is covered by the left atrial appendage in its proximal portion and then takes position in the left atrioventricular sulcus. The RCA has its origin at the right coronary aortic sinus and goes into the right atrioventricular sulcus. The posterior descending (PD) artery runs in the posterior interventricular sulcus.

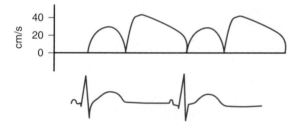

Figure 10-2. Normal coronary flow is characterized by a biphasic flow profile, which consists of low velocity systolic and diastolic flow, with higher flow velocities in diastole compared to systole.

Figure 10-3. Coronary flow reserve (CFR) expressed as a ratio of maximum flow to resting flow. With progressive coronary stenosis, baseline flow remains normal until the coronary artery is narrowed by 80% to 85% diameter stenosis. However, with a vasodilatory stimulus, CFR begins to decrease at 40% to 50% diameter stenosis compared to the normal response of a fourfold increase in flow.

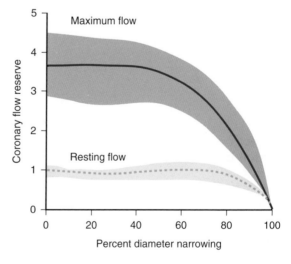

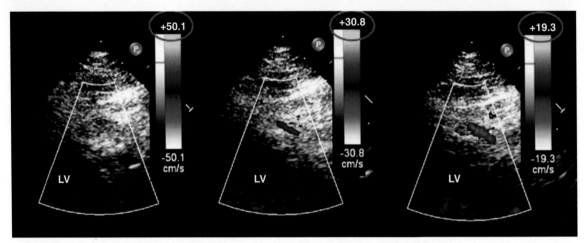

Figure 10-4. Detection of the coronary flow signal. The Doppler velocity range is set in the range of 10 to 30 cm/s because coronary flow velocities are low compared with intracardiac flow. In this example, as the color Doppler velocity scale is decreased sequentially from 50 to 30 to 19 cm/s, the color flow signal in the LAD is better visualized.

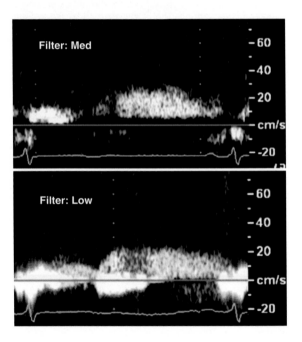

Figure 10-5. The Doppler filter should be set to "low" or "minimum" to obtain the full coronary flow spectrum. Use of a medium (med) filter results in a black band of missing signals on both sides of the baseline (*top panel*). With the filter on the low setting (*bottom panel*), the complete Doppler signal is recorded.

Detection of Coronary Flow Signal by Color Doppler

Left Main Trunk, Proximal Left Anterior Descending Artery, and Left Circumflex Artery (Use Low-Frequency Transducer)

- The basic steps for detection of coronary blood flow are shown in Figure 10-6.
- The left main trunk (LMT) and its bifurcation can be detected at the level of the left coronary sinus, in a short axis view (Fig. 10-7).
- The proximal segment of the LAD and LCx can be detected occasionally.

- The proximal RCA can be identified at the level of the right coronary sinus in a short axis or long axis view.

Middle to Distal Portion of the Left Anterior Descending Artery

- The middle portion of the LAD can be identified in short axis images of the left ventricle (LV), located in the anterior interventricular sulcus (Fig. 10-8).
- Visualization is optimized with a high-frequency transducer.
- The LAD appears in a circular cross section containing the color Doppler flow signal.

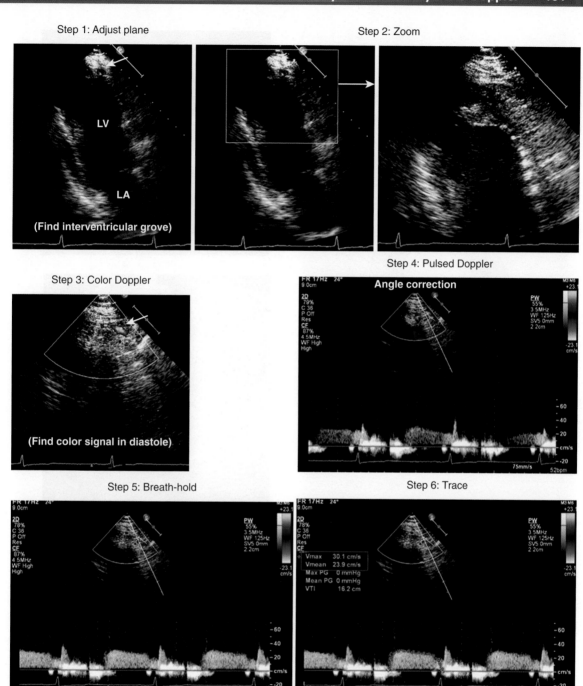

Figure 10-6. Step-by-step approach for coronary flow by color and PW Doppler.

- Rotate the transducer counterclockwise to image the LV in a long axis view along the intraventricular sulcus under the guidance of color Doppler flow mapping.
- The distal portion of the LAD can be found in the apical long axis view at the intraventricular sulcus, again as a circular cross section containing the color Doppler flow signal.

- Rotate the transducer clockwise (toward the two-chamber view position) to detect the flow signal in the long axis view.
- Coronary flow detection in the distal portion of the LAD is important because CFR should be measured distal to a stenosis.

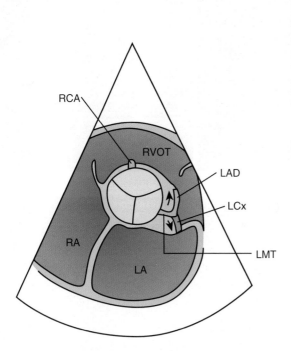

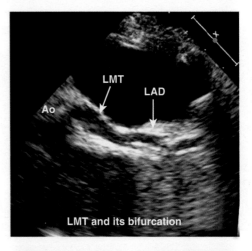

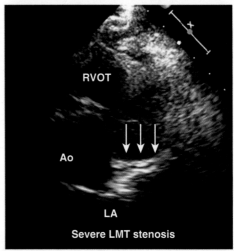

Figure 10-7. To visualize the LMT and proximal LAD, position the transducer at the level of the aortic root in the parasternal short axis view. Often these images can be acquired using a relatively low-frequency transducer. The LMT is identified as a tubular structure that originates from the left coronary sinus. By adjusting the orientation of the ultrasound beam from the distal side of the LMT, the proximal LAD can be visualized. *Right upper panel*, Tubular structure of the LMT and proximal LAD are clearly visualized in a patient with Marfan syndrome. *Right lower panel*, Severe stenosis in the left main coronary artery showing the thickened arterial wall and narrowed lumen (*white arrows*). Ao, aorta; LA, left atrium; RA, right atrium; RVOT, right ventricular outflow tract.

Right Posterior Descending Artery

- Obtain an apical two-chamber image of the LV and angle the ultrasound beam superiorly to image the posterior interventricular sulcus using a low-frequency transducer (Fig. 10-9).
- Examine this area using color Doppler flow mapping to locate the right posterior descending coronary artery.
- Contrast-enhanced Doppler technique improves the success rate.

Left Circumflex Artery

- The circumflex artery can be found in the modified four-chamber view using a low-frequency transducer (Fig. 10-10).

- The color Doppler signal is normally detected along the basal lateral wall.

KEY POINTS

- Carefully adjust the transducer position (remember the anatomy) before pushing the "Color" button.
- The color Doppler signal in the normal epicardial coronary artery is mainly seen in diastole with a red color (flow toward the transducer).
- Typically a breath-hold is needed to obtain a stable coronary Doppler signal.

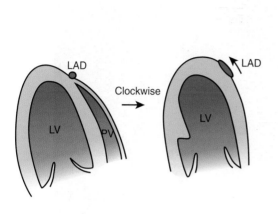

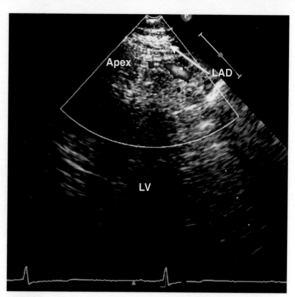

Figure 10-8. Detection of LAD flow signal by color Doppler. To visualize the distal portion of the LAD, image the LV in long axis section from the apex and search the coronary flow signal around the intraventricular sulcus. Choose a high-frequency transducer to detect the LAD signal and use color Doppler for flow detection. Once the LAD is found in cross section (*left panel*), rotate the transducer clockwise (toward the two-chamber view position) as shown to detect the flow signal in the long axis view.

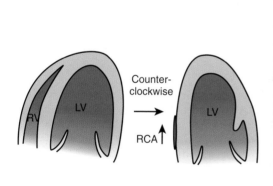

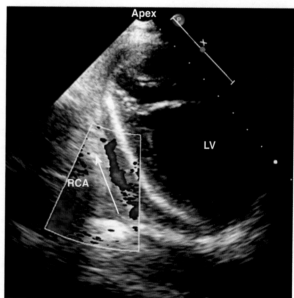

Figure 10-9. Detection of RCA flow signal by color Doppler. After obtaining the apical two-chamber view of the LV, angle the ultrasound beam superiorly to image the posterior interventricular sulcus. For detection of RCA flow, a lower frequency probe is recommended because this area is distant from the transducer compared with the location of the LAD. Carefully examine this area using color Doppler flow mapping to locate the right posterior descending coronary artery (RCA).

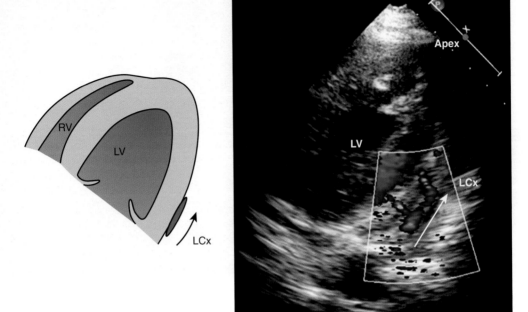

Figure 10-10. The LCx is best visualized in the modified four-chamber view. Typically, the LCx is seen as a color flow signal running along the basal lateral wall. As with the RCA, a lower frequency probe is recommended due to the distance of the artery from the transducer.

Pulsed Doppler Spectral Tracings of Coronary Flow

Analysis
Measurements in the Coronary Flow Spectrum

- Coronary flow velocity (peak velocity, mean velocity) and diastolic deceleration time are measured by tracing the pulsed wave (PW) Doppler velocity signal (Fig. 10-11).
- CFR is calculated with the diastolic flow components only.

Coronary Flow (Velocity) Reserve Measurement

- CFR can be assessed as the ratio of hyperemic to basal coronary flow velocity after drug-induced coronary vasodilatation.
- After recording baseline spectral Doppler signals in the distal portion of the targeted artery, administer the vasodilator (adenosine 140 μg/kg/min or dipyridamole 0.56 mg/kg intravenously) and then record spectral Doppler signals during hyperemic conditions.
- Measure the mean diastolic velocity and peak diastolic velocity of each flow spectrum.
- Coronary flow velocity reserve is defined as the ratio of hyperemic to basal peak diastolic coronary flow velocity, or the ratio of

hyperemic to basal mean diastolic coronary flow velocity (Fig. 10-12).
- The adverse effects of adenosine (flushing, headache, hypotension or bradycardia) diminish immediately after finishing the infusion.

Pitfalls

- The success rate in detecting a coronary flow signal in the PDA and LCx is lower compared with the LAD because of their anatomic variations and because they are located far from the transducer.
- PW Doppler recordings provide coronary flow velocity, not the absolute coronary blood flow volume.
- Coronary flow (velocity) reserve by transthoracic Doppler echocardiography is derived from changes in the velocity of coronary blood flow, which has been shown to correlate with absolute CFR.
- PW Doppler often misses the systolic component of coronary flow because of cardiac motion.
- CFR by echo Doppler is derived by tracing the diastolic flow velocity.
- Pericardial fluid may appear as a coronary flow signal at the epicardium. Pericardial fluid is seen mainly in systole and can easily be discriminated by PW Doppler recording.

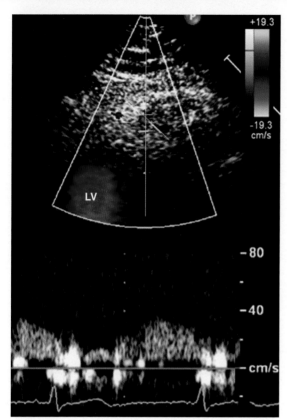

Figure 10-11. Coronary flow velocity measurements by PW Doppler. Doppler spectral tracings of coronary flow velocity can be recorded using a PW Doppler technique by positioning a sample volume (1.5–2.5 mm wide) on the color Doppler signal. Angle correction is needed for coronary blood flow because of the angle between blood flow and the Doppler beam. The coronary flow velocity provides some useful clinical information such as coronary flow direction, coronary flow velocity, and coronary flow pattern. Normal coronary flow is characterized by a biphasic flow profile with low-velocity systolic and higher-velocity diastolic flow.

KEY POINTS

- The resting coronary flow pattern is characterized by a diastolic dominant biphasic flow.
- Position a sample volume (1.5–2.5 mm wide) on the color Doppler signal of coronary flow.
- Angle correction may be needed depending on the signal direction of coronary flow.

Practical Use of the Noninvasive Measurements of Coronary Flow in the Echo Laboratory

Phasic Flow Characteristics and Coronary Stenosis

- The diastolic-to-systolic flow velocity ratio (DSVR) decreases in severe coronary stenosis.

- Cut-off points of 1.6 for peak DSVR and 1.5 for mean DSVR have high sensitivities and specificities in the detection of severe coronary stenosis[2] (Fig. 10-13).

Diagnosis of Coronary Stenosis by Coronary Flow Velocity Reserve Measurement

- A diminished coronary flow velocity reserve, defined as a mean diastolic velocity ratio less than 2.0, has a sensitivity of 91% to 92% and a specificity of 75% to 86% for the presence of significant LAD stenosis[3] (Fig. 10-14).
- Compared with thallium-201 single-photon emission computed tomography, mean CFR less than or equal to 2.0 predicted reversible perfusion defects, with a sensitivity and specificity of 92% and 90%, respectively.
- CFR improves after coronary stenting. A persistent CFR of less than 2.0 had high sensitivity (91%) and specificity (95%) in the diagnosis of in-stent restenosis after coronary intervention.[4]
- A CFR of less than 1, which may reflect coronary steal phenomenon, can discriminate high-risk patients with severe stenosis from patients with nonsevere stenosis.[5]
- Using the cut-off value of 2.0 for coronary flow velocity reserve in the RCA, sensitivity and specificity in the detection of significant stenosis are 84% to 91% and 83% to 91%, respectively.[6–8]
- Coronary flow velocity reserve of less than 2 in the LCx has a sensitivity of 92% and specificity of 96% for reversible perfusion defect detected by single-photon emission computed tomography.[9]
- Although additional coronary risk factors (pretest likelihood of disease) influence the diagnostic value of coronary flow velocity reserve, a cut-off value of less than 2.0 is still adequate in terms of the diagnosis of significant coronary stenosis. A cut-off value of less than 2.0 of CFR has a sensitivity of 90%, a specificity of 93%, a positive predictive value of 77%, and a negative predictive value of 97% for the presence of significant coronary stenosis in patients with various coronary risk factors.[10]

Detection of Total Occlusion of the Coronary Arteries by Retrograde Coronary Flow

- The retrograde blood flow velocity distal to a totally occluded coronary vessel represents collateral flow to the occluded region.

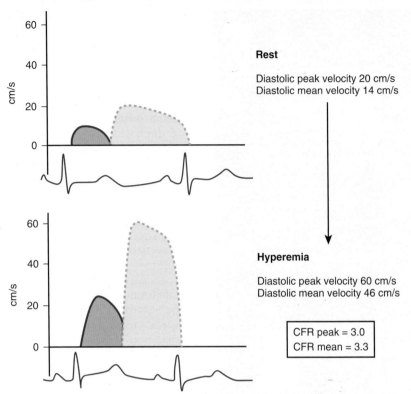

Figure 10-12. Coronary flow reserve (CFR) measurements. After recording baseline spectral Doppler signals in the distal portion of the LAD, administer the vasodilator (adenosine 140 μg/kg/min or dipyridamole 0.56 mg/kg intravenously) to record spectral Doppler signals during hyperemic conditions. Then measure the mean diastolic velocity and peak diastolic velocity of each flow spectrum. Coronary flow velocity reserve by the transthoracic Doppler technique is measured from only diastolic mean velocities, not mean velocities throughout the entire cardiac cycle, because in some cases it is difficult to obtain a complete Doppler spectral envelope throughout the entire cardiac cycle because of cardiac motion.

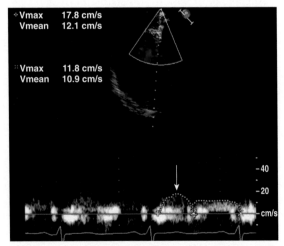

Figure 10-13. Diagnosis of severe LAD stenosis by DSVR measurement. In severe coronary stenosis, diastolic flow decreases and the DSVR decreases at rest. This example shows a resting flow signal in the distal LAD in a patient with chest pain. The DSVR (peak) was 11.8/17.8 = 0.66. Coronary angiography revealed a 90% stenosis in the proximal portion of the LAD.

- Retrograde LAD flow by transthoracic Doppler echocardiography had a sensitivity of 93% and a specificity of 100% for the detection of total LAD occlusion. Retrograde flow in the LAD or septal artery had a sensitivity of 96% and a specificity of 100% for the detection of total LAD occlusion.[11]
- Detection of reverse flow in the distal RCA and the inferior septal branches has a sensitivity of 100% and a specificity of 97.8% for identification of an occluded RCA[12] (Fig. 10-15).

Coronary Flow Measurements in Acute Coronary Syndrome

- The diagnosis of thrombolysis in myocardial infarction (TIMI) grade 3 coronary flow based on a diastolic peak distal LAD flow velocity of 25 cm/s had a sensitivity, specificity, and accuracy of 77%, 94%, and 89%, respectively[13] (Fig. 10-16).

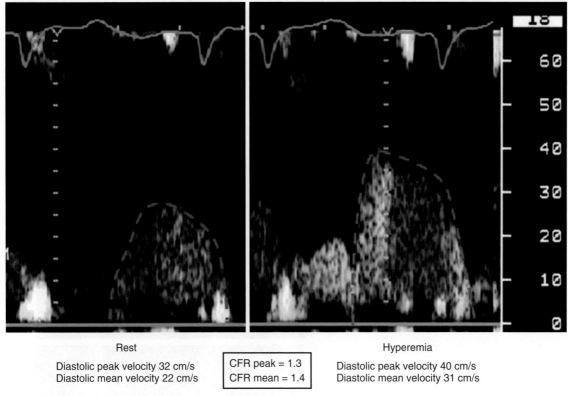

Rest

Diastolic peak velocity 32 cm/s
Diastolic mean velocity 22 cm/s

CFR peak = 1.3
CFR mean = 1.4

Hyperemia

Diastolic peak velocity 40 cm/s
Diastolic mean velocity 31 cm/s

Figure 10-14. Diagnosis of LAD stenosis by CFR measurement. CFR expressed as a ratio of maximum flow to resting flow. In this case, CFR was measured in a study requested in a patient with atypical chest pain. The CFR (mean) was 1.4, which indicates significant coronary stenosis. Subsequent coronary angiography showed greater than 75% stenosis in the middle portion of the LAD.

- The presence of signals from perforator arteries in the anterior-apical wall by transthoracic color Doppler echocardiography is an early noninvasive marker of myocardial viability.[14]
- Transthoracic detection of coronary flow pattern is useful in the direct monitoring of coronary flow augmentation during intra-aortic balloon pumping.[15]

KEY POINTS

Simple signs of coronary artery disease:
- Small diastolic flow component (at rest)
- Retrograde flow signal (at rest)
- Decreased CFR (after vasodilator infusion)

Coronary Flow in No-reflow Phenomenon

- Coronary flow velocity shows a characteristic "to-and-fro" pattern in no-reflow after coronary revascularization for acute myocardial infarction (Fig. 10-17).

- Evaluation of the coronary flow profile after revascularization is useful in predicting recovery of regional LV function.
- Optimal cut-off values to predict viable myocardium were 6.5 cm/s for average systolic velocity and 600 ms for diastolic deceleration time (sensitivity = 0.79 and specificity = 0.89, and sensitivity = 0.86 and specificity = 0.89, respectively).
- Persistence of abnormal coronary flow pattern can predict LV remodeling after myocardial infarction.[16,17]

Alternate Approaches

- The advantages and disadvantages of echocardiography evaluation of coronary blood flow are compared with other approaches in Table 10-1.
- In clinical practice, coronary angiography remains the standard approach for diagnosis in most clinical settings.
- CT and MRI angiography are particularly useful in specific clinical settings, such as evaluation of coronary anomalies.

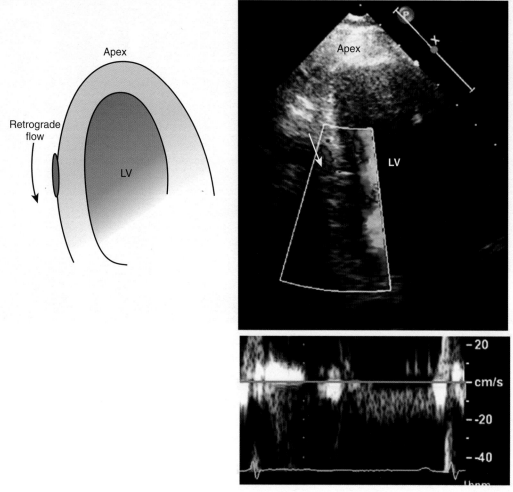

Figure 10-15. Diagnosis of total occlusion in the RCA. The retrograde blood flow velocity distal to a totally occluded coronary vessel represents collateral flow to the occluded region. This patient was referred for echo examination because of progressive chest pain. The standard two-dimensional examination showed mild hypokinesis in the inferior wall. The resting coronary flow examination found retrograde flow (*blue signal*) in the posterior descending artery (PDA), suggesting an occluded proximal vessel with retrograde flow from collateral vessels. This was confirmed on coronary angiography, which showed total occlusion in the proximal RCA with rich collateral flow from the LAD.

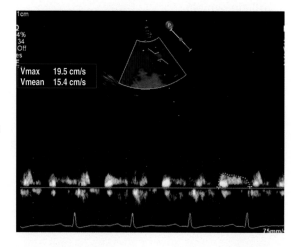

Figure 10-16. Diagnosis of severe LAD stenosis in a patient with acute coronary syndrome. Transthoracic Doppler echocardiography enables a rapid noninvasive differentiation of TIMI 3 from TIMI 2 coronary reperfusion in patients with acute myocardial infarction in the acute phase before emergent coronary intervention. This example shows the LAD flow velocity recording in a patient with acute coronary syndrome. The peak diastolic velocity is 19.5 cm/s. Coronary angiography showed a 99% LAD stenosis with TIMI 2 flow.

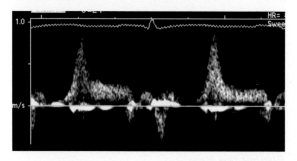

Figure 10-17. Coronary flow in no-reflow phenomenon. In no-reflow after coronary revascularization for acute myocardial infarction, the coronary flow velocity shows a characteristic "to-and-fro" pattern. This low systolic flow velocity and rapid deceleration time of the diastolic coronary blood flow spectrum immediately after primary coronary intervention reflects a greater degree of microvascular damage in the risk area.

TABLE 10-1 DIAGNOSTIC METHODS FOR EVALUATION OF CORONARY BLOOD FLOW

	Advantage	Disadvantage
Catheterization with coronary angiography	Full coverage of the coronary arteries, high resolution	Invasive Radiation exposure Needs nephrotoxic contrast agents
TTE	Noninvasive No radiation exposure Portable Cost effective Physiologic assessment of coronary circulation CFR measurement	Limited sites of coronary flow detection Low success rate in RCA and LCx (need contrast agent) Needs vasodilator infusion in measuring CFR
CT coronary angiography	Noninvasive Relatively high resolution Anatomic assessment of coronary stenosis Tissue characterization Plaque volume measurements	Radiation exposure Expensive Needs nephrotoxic contrast agents Motion artifacts Limited accuracy in the diagnosis of coronary stenosis Needs a beta-blocker before exam Not available in the heavily calcified lesion
MRI coronary angiography	Noninvasive No radiation exposure Anatomic assessment of coronary stenosis Soft tissue characterization CFR measurement	Expensive Time consuming Slower acquisition Motion artifacts Limited accuracy in the diagnosis of coronary stenosis

References

1. Gould KL, Lipscomb K. Effects of coronary stenoses on coronary flow reserve and resistance. *Am J Cardiol.* 1974; 34:48-55.
2. Higashiue S, Watanabe H, Yokoi Y, et al. Simple detection of severe coronary stenosis using transthoracic Doppler echocardiography at rest. *Am J Cardiol.* 2001;87:1064-1068.
3. Hozumi T, Yoshida K, Ogata Y, et al. Noninvasive assessment of significant left anterior descending coronary artery stenosis by coronary flow velocity reserve with transthoracic color Doppler echocardiography. *Circulation.* 1998;97: 1557-1562.
4. Pizzuto F, Voci P, Mariano E, et al. Assessment of flow velocity reserve by transthoracic Doppler echocardiography and venous adenosine infusion before and after left anterior descending coronary artery stenting. *J Am Coll Cardiol.* 2001;38:155-162.
5. Voci P, Pizzuto F, Mariano E, et al. Usefulness of coronary flow reserve measured by transthoracic coronary Doppler ultrasound to detect severe left anterior descending coronary artery stenosis. *Am J Cardiol.* 2003;92:1320-1324.
6. Ueno Y, Nakamura Y, Takashima H, et al. Noninvasive assessment of coronary flow velocity and coronary flow velocity reserve in the right coronary artery by transthoracic Doppler echocardiography: comparison with intracoronary Doppler guidewire. *J Am Soc Echocardiogr.* 2002;15:1074-1079.
7. Watanabe H, Hozumi T, Hirata K, et al. Noninvasive coronary flow velocity reserve measurement in the posterior descending coronary artery for detecting coronary stenosis in the right coronary artery using contrast-enhanced transthoracic Doppler echocardiography. *Echocardiography.* 2004;21:225-233.
8. Takeuchi M, Ogawa K, Wake R, et al. Measurement of coronary flow velocity reserve in the posterior descending coronary artery by contrast-enhanced transthoracic Doppler echocardiography. *J Am Soc Echocardiogr.* 2004;17:21-27.
9. Fujimoto K, Watanabe H, Hozumi T, et al. New noninvasive diagnosis of myocardial ischemia of the left circumflex coronary artery using coronary flow reserve measurement by transthoracic Doppler echocardiography: comparison with thallium-201 single photon emission computed tomography. *J Cardiol.* 2004; 43:109-116.

10. Matsumura Y, Hozumi T, Watanabe H, et al. Cut-off value of coronary flow velocity reserve by transthoracic Doppler echocardiography for diagnosis of significant left anterior descending artery stenosis in patients with coronary risk factors. *Am J Cardiol.* 2003;92:1389-1393.

11. Watanabe N, Akasaka T, Yamaura Y, et al. Noninvasive detection of total occlusion of the left anterior descending coronary artery with transthoracic Doppler echocardiography. *J Am Coll Cardiol.* 2001;38:1328-1332.

12. Otsuka R, Watanabe H, Hirata K, et al. A novel technique to detect total occlusion in the right coronary artery using retrograde flow by transthoracic Doppler echocardiography. *J Am Soc Echocardiogr.* 2005;18: 704-709.

13. Lee S, Otsuji Y, Minagoe S, et al. Noninvasive evaluation of coronary reperfusion by transthoracic Doppler echocardiography in patients with anterior acute myocardial infarction before coronary intervention. *Circulation.* 2003;108:2763-2768.

14. Voci P, Mariano E, Pizzuto F, et al. Coronary recanalization in anterior myocardial infarction: the open perforator hypothesis. *J Am Coll Cardiol.* 2002;40:1205-1213.

15. Takeuchi M, Nohtomi Y, Yoshitani H, et al. Enhanced coronary flow velocity during intra-aortic balloon pumping assessed by transthoracic Doppler echocardiography. *J Am Coll Cardiol.* 2004;43: 368-376.

16. Hozumi T, Kanzaki Y, Ueda Y, et al. Coronary flow velocity analysis during short term follow up after coronary reperfusion: use of transthoracic Doppler echocardiography to predict regional wall motion recovery in patients with acute myocardial infarction. *Heart.* 2003;89:1163-1168.

17. Shintani Y, Ito H, Iwakura K, et al. Usefulness of impairment of coronary microcirculation in predicting left ventricular dilation after acute myocardial infarction. *Am J Cardiol.* 2004;93:974-978.

Suggested Reading

1. Watanabe N. Echocardiographic evaluation for coronary blood flow: approaches and clinical applications. In: Otto C, ed. *The Practice of Clinical Echocardiography.* 3rd ed. Philadelphia: Saunders/Elsevier; 2007:393-402.

2. Takeuchi M. Transthoracic coronary artery imaging. In: Lang RM, Goldstein SA, Kronzon I, Khandheria BK, eds. *Dynamic Echocardiography.* Philadelphia: Saunders/ Elsevier; 2010:426-427.

3. Meimoun P, Tribouilloy C. Non-invasive assessment of coronary flow and coronary flow reserve by transthoracic Doppler echocardiography: a magic tool for the real world. *Eur J Echocardiogr.* 2008;9:449-457. Epub 2008 Feb 19.

4. Rigo F, Murer B, Ossena G, Favaretto E. Transthoracic echocardiographic imaging of coronary arteries: tips, traps, and pitfalls. *Cardiovasc Ultrasound.* 2008;6:7.

Stress Testing for Structural Heart Disease

Catherine M. Otto and David S. Owens

11

Basic Principles

- The physiologic effects of structural heart lesions may not be evident at rest (Table 11-1).
  - Flow across a stenotic valve that is adequate at rest may fail to increase appropriately with exercise or pharmacologic stress.
  - Intracardiac pressures that are normal at rest may increase significantly as cardiac output increases, with either stenotic or regurgitant valve lesions.
  - Changes in ventricular geometry with stress may result in altered valve dynamics with an increase in regurgitant severity.
  - Changes in ventricular function and loading conditions with stress may "provoke" dynamic outflow obstruction in hypertrophic cardiomyopathy (HCM).
- Exercise is the most physiologic type of stress test as it mimics normal physical activity (Table 11-2).
  - The typical hemodynamic target for an exercise stress test is 85% of the age-adjusted maximum predicted heart rate (HR) (about 220 minus patient age).
  - Systolic blood pressure (BP) normally increases by at least 20 mm Hg with exercise; a blunted BP rise suggests significant cardiovascular limitation.
  - With standard treadmill exercise protocols, exercise duration provides an estimate of functional aerobic impairment (FAI) using a nomogram based on age, gender, and degree of physical conditioning (Fig. 11-1).
  - Metabolic equivalents (METs) are a measure of oxygen (O_2) consumption, where 1 MET equals 3.5 mL O_2 per kg/min, equivalent to the resting metabolic state, 3 to 6 METs is equivalent to moderate exercise, and greater than 6 METs corresponds to strenuous exercise.
  - With treadmill exercise, echocardiographic data are recorded at baseline and immediately following exercise, after the patient transfers back to the stretcher (Fig. 11-2).
- With a supine bicycle ergometer, an incremental increase in workload is achieved either by maintaining a constant pedaling speed (mechanically braked bicycles) or by maintaining a desired workload regardless of pedaling rate (electronically braked ergometers).
- Supine bicycle exercise allows continuous recording of echocardiographic data, although the maximum workload may be lower than with upright treadmill exercise.
- Because of physiologic differences in preload between upright and supine exercise, supine ergometry typically elicits a:
  - HR increase that is 15 to 20 beats/min lower.
  - Systolic BP response that is 15 to 20 mm Hg higher.
- Pharmacologic stress testing is useful in patients who cannot exercise and for specific clinical indications.
  - A pharmacologic agent, most often intravenous dobutamine, can be used as a cardiac stressor, based on the induced increase in HR and left ventricular (LV) contractility.
  - The starting and maximum dobutamine dose is lower for stress testing in patients with structural heart disease, compared with the doses used for evaluation of ischemic heart disease.
- Continuous electrocardiographic (ECG) monitoring is needed during all stress testing.
  - HR, determined by ECG, is a primary determinant of cardiac workload.
  - Continuous ECG monitoring is a standard safety measure for detection of cardiac arrhythmias during stress testing.
  - The ECG usually is not accurate for detection of coronary disease in patients undergoing stress testing for structural heart disease because:

TABLE 11-1   PRIMARY INDICATIONS FOR STRESS TESTING WITH STRUCTURAL HEART DISEASE

Indication	Stress Type	Echo Data Acquisition	Parameters Used in Clinical Decision Making	Comments
Aortic stenosis—symptom status	ETT	Optional	Exercise duration Symptoms BP response	
Aortic stenosis—low-gradient low-output AS*	Low-dose dobutamine	Aortic jet velocity (CW Doppler) LV outflow velocity (PW Doppler) EF (2D)	Severe AS is present if: $V_{max} > 4.0$ m/s or mean $\Delta P > 40$ mm Hg with an AVA ≤ 1.0 cm^2 at any flow rate.	Contractile reserve is defined as an ↑EF or ↑transaortic SV > 20%
Mitral stenosis	ETT or supine bicycle	TR jet velocity (CW Doppler)	PA systolic pressure > 60 mm Hg with exercise	
Mitral regurgitation	ETT or supine bicycle	TR jet velocity (CW Doppler)	PA systolic pressure > 60 mm Hg with exercise	
Hypertrophic cardiomyopathy	ETT or supine bicycle	LV outflow velocity (CW Doppler)	Evidence for dynamic outflow obstruction with exercise MR severity BP response	Supine bicycle allows continuous monitoring of Doppler parameters

PA, pulmonary artery; BP, blood pressure; AS, aortic stenosis; MR, mitral regurgitation; LV, left ventricular; PW, pulsed wave; CW, continuous wave; TR, tricuspid regurgitant; AVA, aortic valve area; EF, ejection fraction; SV, stroke volume.
*Low-gradient low-output AS is defined as an AVA < 1.0 cm^2 with an LV EF < 40% and mean ΔP < 30–40 mm Hg.

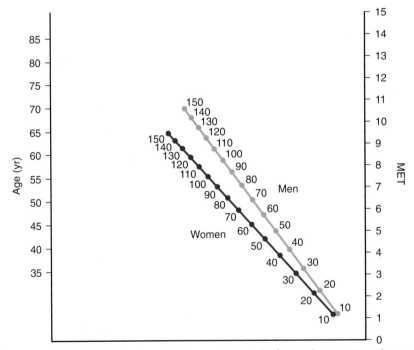

Figure 11-1. Nomogram of the percentage of predicted exercise capacity for age in asymptomatic men and women. A line drawn from the patient's age on the scale on the left to the MET value on the scale on the right crosses the percentage line at the point corresponding to the patient's percentage of predicted exercise capacity for age. The risk for death among asymptomatic and symptomatic women whose exercise capacity was less than 85% of that predicted for age is approximately twice that for women whose exercise capacity is more than 85%. *(From Gulati M, Black HR, Shaw LJ, et al. The prognostic value of a nomogram for exercise capacity in women. N Engl J Med. 2005;353:468.)*

TABLE 11-2	STRESS PROTOCOLS FOR STRUCTURAL HEART DISEASE		
	Upright Treadmill Exercise	**Supine Bicycle Ergometer**	**Dobutamine Stress**
Protocols*	• Several symptom-limited protocols available • Most common are Bruce protocol and Naughton protocol	• Stepwise increase in resistance with patient maintaining steady pedaling rate • Stepwise increase in workload, regardless of patient pedaling speed (electronic controlled mode)	• IV dobutamine infusion beginning at 5 μg/kg/min, with increases every 3 min to 10, 15, and then 20 μg/kg/min
Study end point	• Patient's exercise limit (100% maximum predicted heart rate) • Early termination for symptoms, a fall in blood pressure or significant arrhythmia	• Patient's exercise limit (100% maximum heart rate) • Early termination for symptoms or echocardiographic findings	• Symptom onset • Aortic velocity >4 m/s • End of protocol
Advantages	• Mimics daily activities and exercise induced symptoms • High workload • Provides objective measure of exercise tolerance • Documents BP response to upright exercise (a strong predictor of clinical outcome) • Allows determination of maximum HR	• Ability to record Doppler data at each stress stage • Ability to maintain a steady workload until data are collected • Increases in HR and respiratory rate limit data recording, but not to the extent seen with upright treadmill exercise	• Provides cardiac stress (increase in HR and contractility) in patients unable to exercise • In adults with low-output AS, allows evaluation of both LV function and AS severity with graded increases in stress level
Disadvantages	• Need to transfer quickly from the treadmill to the stretcher at the end of exercise • Data recording only at baseline and immediately post-exercise • Challenges in data recording due to increases in HR and respiratory rate • Need to record data quickly before HR returns towards normal	• Unfamiliar exercise modality for most patients • Lower maximum workload • BP response is less predictive of clinical outcome than with upright exercise • Patient may not achieve maximum HR	• Does not mimic normal physiology of exercise • Protocol for evaluation of low-output, low-gradient AS is not useful for diagnosis of coronary artery disease
Clinical data obtained	• Exercise capacity • Hemodynamic response to upright exercise • Provocable symptoms • Measurement of Doppler hemodynamics at rest and immediately post-stress	• Provocable symptoms • Measurement of Doppler hemodynamics at rest and each stress stage	• Measurement of Doppler hemodynamics at rest and each stress stage • Measurement of LV systolic function at rest and each exercise stage
Clinical indications	• Asymptomatic severe aortic stenosis • Moderate to severe mitral stenosis • Mitral regurgitation • Hypertrophic cardiomyopathy	• Hypertrophic cardiomyopathy • Moderate to severe mitral stenosis • Mitral regurgitation	• Low-output, low-gradient AS

*General principles of stress protocols; each center may choose a different protocol from several published options.

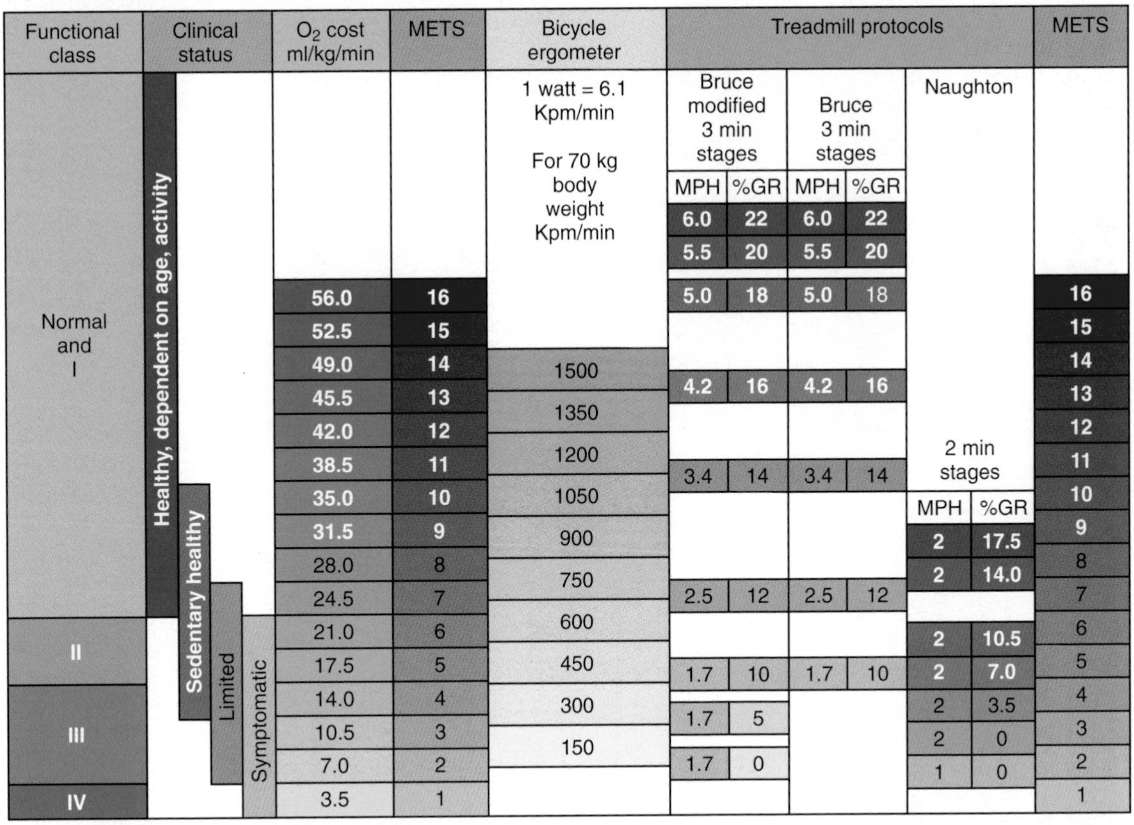

Functional class	Clinical status	O₂ cost ml/kg/min	METS	Bicycle ergometer (1 watt = 6.1 Kpm/min, For 70 kg body weight Kpm/min)	Bruce modified 3 min stages MPH	Bruce modified 3 min stages %GR	Bruce 3 min stages MPH	Bruce 3 min stages %GR	Naughton 2 min stages MPH	Naughton 2 min stages %GR	METS
					6.0	22	6.0	22			
					5.5	20	5.5	20			
Normal and I	Healthy, dependent on age, activity	56.0	16		5.0	18	5.0	18			16
		52.5	15								15
		49.0	14	1500	4.2	16	4.2	16			14
		45.5	13	1350							13
		42.0	12	1200							12
		38.5	11		3.4	14	3.4	14			11
	Sedentary healthy	35.0	10	1050							10
		31.5	9	900					2	17.5	9
		28.0	8	750					2	14.0	8
		24.5	7		2.5	12	2.5	12			7
II	Limited	21.0	6	600					2	10.5	6
		17.5	5	450	1.7	10	1.7	10	2	7.0	5
	Symptomatic	14.0	4	300	1.7	5			2	3.5	4
III		10.5	3	150					2	0	3
		7.0	2		1.7	0	1.7	0	1	0	2
IV		3.5	1								1

Figure 11-2. Relation of METs to stages in selected stress testing protocols. Functional class refers to New York Heart Association class. Kpm, kilopond-meters; MPH, miles per hour; %GR, percent grade. *(From Fletcher GF, Balady GJ, Amsterdam EA, et al. Exercise standards for testing and training: a statement for healthcare professionals from the American Heart Association. Circulation. 2001;104[14]:1694–1740.)*

- The resting ECG often is abnormal in these patients.
- The total workload may not be adequate to induce ischemia (false negative).
- ST changes may be present in the absence of ischemia in patients with LV hypertrophy due to valvular or myocardial disease (false positive).
- Stress-induced wall motion abnormalities also are not sensitive for detection of coronary disease in patients with structural heart disease because:
  - The total workload often is not adequate to induce ischemia.
  - Diffuse myocardial ischemia with stress related to LV hypertrophy may mask regional ischemic changes.
  - However, a definite stress-induced regional wall motion abnormality in the distribution of a coronary artery is likely to be specific for ischemia.
- Exercise stress testing is safe in adults with structural heart disease with appropriate patient selection and careful clinical monitoring (Box 11-1).
- Overall risk is similar to stress testing for coronary disease with very low risk for death or myocardial infarction.
- Risk is related to the severity of the underlying structural heart disease, with a higher risk for syncope when severe aortic stenosis (AS) is present; stress testing is contraindicated when symptoms are present in AS patients.
- Other major complications include arrhythmias and hypotension; the stress test should be stopped immediately if BP fails to increase appropriately or at the onset of an arrhythmia.
- ST depression on ECG is common and does not correlate well with underlying coronary disease; however, it is prudent to stop the stress test if excessive (>4 mm) ST depression is seen.
- Careful monitoring is needed for stress testing in adults with structural heart disease (Box 11-2).

BOX 11-1 Risks of Stress Testing in Adults with Structural Heart Disease

Cardiac Risks
- Bradyarrhythmias
- Tachyarrhythmias
- Acute coronary syndromes (risk is 10 per 10,000)
- Heart failure
- Hypotension, syncope, and shock
- Death (risk is 5 per 100,000 for patients with coronary disease)

Noncardiac Risks
- Musculoskeletal trauma
- Soft tissue injury

Risk for major complications is reported for populations primarily including patients with coronary artery disease (CAD). Large databases on adults with structural heart disease are not available. Risk may be higher in patients with more severe structural heart disease, particularly for exercise or dobutamine stress testing in patients with severe AS or HCM.

BOX 11-2 Recommended Set-up and Monitoring for Stress Testing in Adults with Structural Heart Disease

Stress Testing Requirements
People
- Physician, physician assistant, or nurse practitioner for supervision
- Registered nurse or other qualified health professional for patient monitoring
- Cardiac sonographer (if echocardiography performed)
Equipment
- Treadmill or bicycle ergometer
- Patient stretcher with apical cutout for echocardiographic imaging
- Echocardiographic system with permanent recording of images
- Crash cart should be immediately available
Space
- Adequate room size for equipment and for additional personnel if needed for an adverse event

Monitoring
Continuous 12-lead ECG
- HR
- Arrhythmias
- ST-segment changes
Intermittent BP
- Every 3 min, more frequent if needed
Pulse oximetry (optional)
- Recommended when chronic lung disease, sleep apnea, or congenital heart disease is present
- May be diagnostically helpful in patients with exertional symptoms

- A physician or other highly trained health professional should be present during the stress test.
- Monitoring with a continuous 12-lead ECG and intermittent BP measurements is mandatory.
- Use of pulse oximetry also may be appropriate in some patients.
- The patient should be monitored for onset of symptoms or signs of hemodynamic compromise.

KEY POINTS

- The physiologic effects of structural heart disease may be evident with stress, but not at rest.
- Important stress test parameters for clinical decision making include exercise capacity and the systemic and pulmonary arterial pressure response to exercise.
- Exercise stress testing, either upright treadmill or supine bicycle, is preferred for evaluation of structural heart disease, except for low-output, low-gradient AS, when dobutamine stress is preferred.

Asymptomatic Severe Aortic Stenosis

Indications
- Symptom onset is a definite indication for aortic valve replacement in adults with severe AS.
  - A clinical history often is adequate to elicit the onset of decreased exercise tolerance or subtle symptoms of exertional dyspnea, chest discomfort, or dizziness.
  - When the clinical history is ambiguous or when there has been an unexplained interval decline in the patient's level of physical activity, stress testing should be considered.
- The goals of stress testing in adults with severe AS and unclear symptom status are:
  - An objective measure of exercise tolerance.
  - Assessment of the hemodynamic response to exercise, specifically the increase in BP.
  - Symptom status with exercise of known intensity.
- Doppler data are not routinely recorded with exercise testing for evaluation of AS symptom status but may be helpful in selected cases.
- Exercise testing should not be performed if the patient reports definite symptoms.
  - When symptoms are present, there is a high risk for a hypotensive response to exercise, or even syncope and sudden death.

- Exercise testing provides no additional data for clinical decision making if symptoms are present.

Step-by-step Approach
Test Preparation
- Review the clinical history and ask the patient directly about possible symptoms; if symptoms are present, stress testing should not be performed.
- Examine the patient:
  - Measure and record HR and BP.
  - Document the cardiac murmur and other physical examination findings of severe AS.
  - Look for signs of heart failure (pulmonary rales, elevated jugular venous pressure). If present, stress testing should not be performed.
- Record the baseline ECG, determine cardiac rhythm, and compare with previous ECGs to ensure there are no acute changes.
- Instruct the patient about the stress test protocol, including:
  - Continue treadmill exercise until limited by symptoms, fatigue, or leg discomfort.
  - Transfer rapidly to the echo stretcher immediately after treadmill exercise if Doppler data will be recorded.
  - For bicycle stress tests, keep the pedaling speed at set limits.
- Obtain informed consent for the exercise stress test.
  - The primary risk of stress testing in adults with severe AS is provocation of symptoms, including angina or syncope.
  - If a careful history just before beginning the stress test is negative for symptoms, the risks of stress testing are low (see Box 11-1).
- Reported adverse events with stress testing in adults with asymptomatic AS include:
  - Horizontal ST depression >2 mm in up to 80% of patients, which is not predictive of coronary artery disease.
  - Provoked symptoms of angina, dizziness, or dyspnea in up to one third of patients. The test should be stopped promptly at symptom onset.
  - Exertional hypotension (a decrease in or failure of systolic BP to increase by at least 10 mm Hg) in 10% of patients.

Review the Baseline Echocardiogram
- A complete resting quantitative echo-Doppler study is needed before stress testing in adults with AS.
- The resting study should provide evaluation of:
  - Aortic valve anatomy and cause of AS.

- AS severity: velocity, mean gradient, valve area.
- Coexisting aortic regurgitation (AR).
- LV hypertrophy, dilation, and systolic function.
- Evaluation of regional LV systolic function.
- LV diastolic dysfunction.
- Mitral valve (MV) anatomy and function.
- Pulmonary pressure estimate and right heart function.
- Review the windows used to record the AS jet if Doppler data with stress will be obtained.
- If very severe AS is present (AS jet velocity >5.5 m/s), stress testing is not recommended.

Exercise Stress Test
- A standard symptom-limited treadmill or supine bicycle stress test protocol is preferred for evaluation of exercise duration and the BP response to upright exercise.
- With the upright treadmill Bruce protocol, treadmill speed and incline are increased every 3 minutes until the study end point is achieved (Fig. 11-3).
- In some cases, supine bicycle exercise may be reasonable if the goal is to measure Doppler hemodynamics at rest and with exercise.
- Stress testing in adults with severe AS should be monitored by a physician, including:
  - Continuous ECG and HR monitoring.
  - BP monitoring at least every 3 minutes, more often if needed.
  - Close patient observation for symptoms or signs of hemodynamic compromise.
- Exercise is stopped for:
  - Symptoms of chest discomfort, lightheadedness, or dyspnea.
  - A systolic BP that decreases or fails to increase by at least 10 mm Hg.
  - Any significant arrhythmia, including sustained ventricular tachycardia (absolute indication) and multifocal premature ventricular beats, new-onset atrial fibrillation, supraventricular tachycardia, heart block, or bradyarrhythmias (relative indications).
  - Excessive ST-segment depression (>4 mm) (Fig. 11-4).
  - Maximum exercise is reached based on HR (treadmill) and/or inability to exercise further due to leg fatigue or shortness of breath (bicycle ergometer).

Interpretation of Stress Test
- Adults with severe AS who have abnormal symptoms with exercise testing are then classified as having severe symptomatic AS and should be referred for consideration of valve replacement.

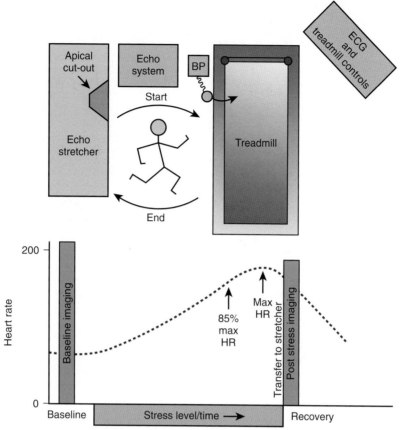

Figure 11-3. Diagram of the exercise stress protocol for patients with structural heart disease. The top part of the figure shows the room layout with the stretcher for echocardiographic imaging, the echocardiography instrument, and the treadmill with ECG monitor and treadmill controls. The physician stands between the treadmill and echocardiographic system to measure BP. The cardiac sonographer has a small wheeled stool to sit on while recording images, but can move it out of the way as needed. The patient lies on the stretcher for the baseline images, transfers to the treadmill for the stress test, and then transfers back to the stretcher as quickly as possible at the end of exercise. A removal apical cut-out in the stretcher aids in obtaining optimal apical images and Doppler data. The bottom part of the figure illustrates the increase in HR with exercise and the timing of echocardiographic data acquisition. The patient exercises to maximum tolerance (100% maximum HR), but HR declines rapidly post-exercise so that imaging needs to be completed as quickly as possible.

- Exercise duration, compared with normal standards for age and gender, is a strong predictor of clinical outcome; limited exercise tolerance suggests hemodynamically significant AS.
- In the absence of symptoms, achieving an HR at least 85% of the predicted maximum indicates that an adequate workload was achieved; a lower maximum HR suggests inadequate effort or the effects of beta-blocker therapy.
- A blunted BP response to exercise (failure to increase by at least 10 mm Hg) is consistent with flow limiting severe AS, and valve replacement should be considered.
- ST changes on ECG are a common nonspecific finding in adults with severe AS, even in the absence of associated coronary disease, most likely related to LV hypertrophy.

Doppler Echocardiographic Data
- Doppler data are not routinely recorded with exercise testing for evaluation of AS symptom status but may be helpful in selected cases.
  - Aortic valve velocity and gradient increase with exercise due to the increase in transaortic flow rate.
  - When stenosis is not severe, the valve leaflets are still somewhat flexible so that orifice area increases slightly (by about 0.2 cm^2) with the increase in flow rate.
  - When the valve leaflets are rigid so that leaflet opening does not increase with exercise, there is a greater increase in transaortic velocity and gradient compared with a flexible valve.
  - A resting mean gradient of greater than 35 mm Hg plus an increase in mean gradient by at least 20 mm Hg with exercise

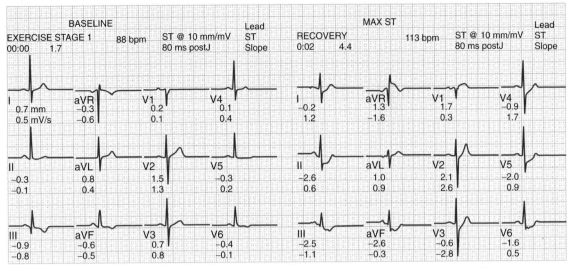

Figure 11-4. ECG tracings for a patient with severe AS undergoing exercise treadmill stress testing. ST-segment depression is seen in the inferior leads, but this finding is not specific for diagnosis of coronary disease because LV hypertrophy is present. This patient had no significant coronary disease on preoperative coronary angiography at the time of aortic valve replacement.

predicts a high rate of symptom onset over the next 1 to 2 years.

- Recording accurate Doppler data with stress testing for AS is challenging.
  - Velocity data post-exercise must be recorded as quickly as possible, before HR and flow rate decline significantly.
  - Rapid respiration with exercise limits recording of the aortic jet.
  - Echocardiographic windows post-exercise may differ from the rest windows due to changes in cardiac size and position with exercise.
  - The expected change in valve area is close to the limits of measurement variability; although these data are useful for comparing groups of patients, use in an individual patient is problematic.
- Baseline data are recorded with the patient supine in a left lateral decubitus position:
  - Left ventricular outflow tract (LVOT) diameter in mid-systole.
  - LV outflow velocity using pulsed wave (PW) Doppler from an apical approach.
  - Continuous wave (CW) Doppler aortic jet velocity.
- Immediately post-exercise, LV outflow velocity and aortic jet velocity are again recorded.
  - Aortic jet velocity often is recorded from the apical window in order to record the data as quickly after exercise as possible; if the highest jet is from a different window, this needs to be taken into account.

- LVOT diameter does not change significantly with exercise, so the baseline measurement is used for both rest and stress valve area calculations.
- Analysis of the Doppler data includes:
  - Aortic jet velocity (in m/s).
  - Mean transaortic gradient (mm Hg).
  - Aortic valve area (AVA) calculated with the continuity equation (cm^2).
  - An increase in AVA of greater than 0.2 cm^2 suggests flexible valve leaflets; an increase in mean gradient of greater than 20 mm Hg with no change in AVA suggests a fixed orifice area.

Potential Pitfalls

- Stress testing in adults with severe AS is contraindicated when symptoms are present; there is a high risk for sudden death with stress testing in this situation.
- Exercise duration may be limited by comorbid conditions, such as pulmonary or systemic diseases, rather than by severe AS.
- BP may be difficult to measure with exercise in AS patients; if the BP cannot be measured, the test should be promptly stopped because hypotension may be present.
- Stress testing is not accurate for diagnosis of coronary disease when severe AS is present.
- Recording and interpretation of Doppler data during stress testing for severe AS is challenging; clinical decision making should not rely on these data if they are discordant with other clinical data.

Alternate Approaches

- Stress testing is not needed in all patients with severe AS; if an accurate clinical history is obtained, watchful waiting and patient education about early symptoms is appropriate.
- Serum brain natriuretic peptide levels are higher in adults with symptomatic AS than in those who are asymptomatic and may be helpful in evaluation of equivocal symptoms.
- Direct imaging of valve anatomy with transesophageal echocardiography, cardiac computed tomographic (CT) imaging, or with cardiac magnetic resonance (CMR) imaging also may be helpful in clinical decision making.
- CT imaging allows quantitation of aortic valve calcification.

KEY POINTS

- Stress testing is contraindicated in adults with severe AS and definite symptoms.
- When symptom status is unclear, exercise testing may provoke symptoms or reveal exertional hypotension.
- Upright treadmill exercise is appropriate when the primary goal is to assess symptoms and BP; if Doppler data are needed, supine bicycle ergometry is reasonable.
- A higher increase in velocity and gradient with exercise are predictive of symptom onset in the near future.

Low-output, Low-gradient Aortic Stenosis

Indications

- Low-output, low-gradient AS is defined as a mean transaortic pressure gradient of less than 30 mm Hg and an aortic velocity of less than 3.5 m/s with an AVA of less than 1.0 cm^2.
- LV systolic function typically is moderately to severely reduced, with an ejection fraction (EF) of less than 50%.
  - Some patients with low-gradient, low-output AS have severe valve obstruction with LV dysfunction due to the high afterload imposed by the stenotic valve.
  - Other patients have only moderate AS with primary LV dysfunction due to cardiomyopathy or ischemic disease.
- Dobutamine stress echocardiography (DSE) is helpful for distinguishing severe AS with afterload mismatch from primary LV

dysfunction with moderate AS in the setting of a reduced LV EF.

- DSE is less helpful in patients with low-gradient AS and normal LV systolic function; these patients typically have a small hypertrophied LV with a small stroke volume.

Step-by-step Approach
Test Preparation

- Review the clinical history with attention to any potential contraindications to dobutamine infusion (e.g., significant arrhythmias, allergy history, uncontrolled hypertension).
- Examine the patient:
  - Measure and record HR and BP.
  - Document the cardiac murmur.
  - Look for signs of heart failure (pulmonary rales, elevated jugular venous pressure). If present, stress testing should be deferred until loading conditions are optimized.
- Obtain informed consent for the dobutamine stress protocol.
- Place an intravenous line for dobutamine infusion and set up appropriate monitoring.
- Review the dobutamine infusion protocol with the registered nurse before beginning the test and ensure that other pharmacologic agents are available to treat any complications or to slow the HR at the end of the protocol.

Baseline Echocardiogram

- The most recent complete transthoracic study is reviewed to determine the optimal windows for data recording and to ensure that the baseline stress test data are recorded correctly.
- Baseline data are then repeated before beginning the stress protocol, including:
  - LVOT diameter by two-dimensional (2D) imaging in the parasternal long axis view.
  - LVOT velocity with PW Doppler from the apical window.
  - Aortic jet velocity from the window that will be used during the stress protocol.
  - Biplane LV EF.
- Data are recorded with the patient optimally positioned, usually in a steep left lateral decubitus position on am echo stretcher with an apical cutout, and this position is maintained during the stress protocol.

Stress Protocol

- After baseline Doppler echo data and monitoring data are recorded, dobutamine infusion is started, typically at 5 µg/kg/min (Fig. 11-5).
- Careful patient monitoring is needed to ensure patient safety, which is critically important

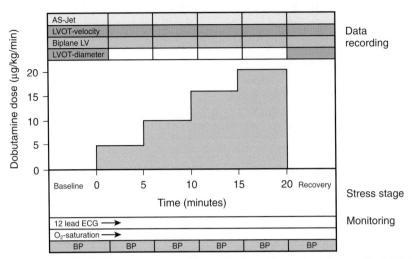

Figure 11-5. Diagram of the dobutamine stress protocol for evaluation of low-output, low-gradient AS. The dobutamine dose is increased every 3 to 5 minutes with Doppler-echo data recording (as shown in the bars at the top of the figure) and patient monitoring (as shown in the bars along the bottom). AS-jet, aortic stenosis maximum velocity recorded with CW Doppler; Biplane LV, biplane images for calculation of LV EF.

given the presence of LV dysfunction and aortic valve obstruction in these patients.
- The ECG is continuously monitored during the test, with periodic (usually every 3 minutes) 12-lead ECG recording.
- BP is measured periodically, at least every 3 minutes, with an increased frequency of monitoring as dictated by the clinical situation.
- The pulse oximetry oxygen saturation is continuously displayed.
- The patient is monitored for symptoms or any signs of distress.
- The dobutamine infusion is increased every 3 to 5 minutes by 5 µg/kg/min to a maximum dose of 20 µg/kg/min (e.g., stress stages at 5, 10, 15, and 20 µg/kg/min).
  - Dobutamine starting and maximum doses are lower compared with stress testing for coronary disease.
  - The stress test end point is not determined by HR because there usually is only a modest increase from baseline.
  - At each stage of the stress test, 2D and Doppler data are recorded, including:
    - LVOT velocity with PW Doppler from the apical window.
    - Aortic jet velocity from the window that will be used during the stress protocol.
    - Biplane LV EF.
- The stress test may be stopped before reaching the maximum dose for:
  - Significant arrhythmias.
  - Patient symptoms.

- An excessive increase (to >220 mm Hg) or decline (to <100 mm Hg) in systolic BP.
- An aortic velocity greater than 4.0 m/s.

Doppler Data Recording
- AS maximum velocity is recorded at baseline and at each stage of the dobutamine protocol.
  - Ideally, AS velocity is recorded from the acoustic window where the highest velocity jet was obtained on the baseline study; however, if this requires excessive patient repositioning, the aortic jet recorded from the apical view may be used, keeping in mind any difference from the true highest jet velocity.
  - A dedicated CW Doppler transducer is used for an optimal signal-to-noise ratio, with careful patient positioning and transducer angulation to record the highest AS jet at each stress stage.
  - The AS signal should have a smooth velocity curve with a well-defined edge and clear peak velocity.
  - The high-velocity mitral regurgitant (MR) jet should not be mistaken for the aortic signal. Compared with the AS jet, the MR jet is higher in velocity, longer in duration, and has a more rounded velocity curve.
- LVOT diameter is recorded at baseline, with the same diameter used for AVA calculations at each stress stage.

- LVOT diameter in adults is relatively constant on serial studies; any apparent change in measurement during a stress study likely is due to measurement variability.
- LVOT diameter is recorded in the parasternal long axis view using zoom mode to maximize the image quality.
- Care is needed to image the septal endocardium and the anterior mitral leaflet, both immediately adjacent to the valve, for accurate measurements.
- Shadowing by leaflet calcium is avoided by using a window where the aortic valve is not between the transducer and LVOT.
- Measurements are made in mid-systole, parallel and immediately adjacent to the aortic valve or within 1 cm of the valve closure plane if edges are not well defined closer to the valve leaflets.
- LVOT velocity is recorded with PW Doppler from an apical approach at baseline and at each step of the test protocol.
  - An apical long axis view is used, when possible, to align the Doppler beam parallel to flow. Alternately, an anteriorly angulated four-chamber view (sometimes called a five-chamber view) is used.
  - The sample volume is positioned just on the LV side of the valve, with this position verified by the presence of an aortic valve closing (but not opening) click on the Doppler recording.
  - The spectral Doppler signal should show a smooth velocity curve, with a well-defined edge and a narrow band of velocities at peak flow.
  - The zero baseline is set near (but not at) the top of the scale, with the velocity scale adjusted so the Doppler signal just fits in the velocity range.
- 2D (or three-dimensional [3D]) views of the LV in apical four-chamber and two-chamber views are recorded for measurement of LV EF at baseline and at each stage of the stress protocol.
  - Standard four-chamber and two-chamber views are recorded with image depth adjusted to maximize the image of the LV while including the entire LV, from the mitral annulus to the apex in the image.
  - Harmonic imaging is used to optimize endocardial definition; left-sided echo-contrast should be used if needed for accurate identification of endocardial borders.
  - 3D imaging of the LV may be used if available for measurement of EF.

Measurements

- AS severity is measured at baseline and each stage of the stress protocol.
- The primary measures of stenosis severity are (Fig. 11-6):
  - Aortic jet velocity in m/s.
  - Mean transaortic gradient in mm Hg, calculated with the Bernoulli equation ($4v^2$) by tracing the outer edge of the AS velocity curve, with integration of instantaneous gradients over the ejection period.
  - AVA in cm^2, calculated using the continuity equation, with LVOT diameter (baseline) and the AS and LV outflow velocity recorded at each stage of the stress protocol.
- EF and stroke volume are measured at rest and each stress stage.
  - EF is measured using the biplane apical approach with calculation of end-diastolic volume (EDV) and end-systolic volume (ESV): EF = (EDV − ESV) / EDV
  - Stroke volume (SV) is measured as the product of LVOT cross-sectional area (CSA) and the velocity time integral (VTI) in the LVOT (the same recording used for valve area calculations): $SV = CSA_{LVOT} \times VTI_{LVOT}$
  - The modal LVOT velocity (not the outer edge of the signal) is used when tracing the LVOT velocity signal for stroke volume calculation.

Test Interpretation

- The report is best formatted (Table 11-3) showing the stress stage in rows with echocardiographic measurements in columns.
- The goal of dobutamine stress testing in AS is to increase LV contractility, resulting in an increase in EF and transaortic flow rate.
  - EF typically increases by at least 20% with dobutamine infusion unless there is irreversible myocardial damage, such as scarring due to myocardial infarction or a primary cardiomyopathy.
  - Although there is only a modest increase in transaortic SV with exercise in adults with AS, the maximum transaortic flow rate increases because the systolic ejection period shortens slightly as HR increases.
- With any degree of AS, velocity and mean gradient increase with the increase in transaortic flow rate; with severe AS, the increase is greater than with less severe AS.
  - When AS is not severe, AVA increases with the increased flow rate across the valve, typically by about 0.2 cm^2, so the increase in velocity and gradient is less than expected for a fixed valve area.

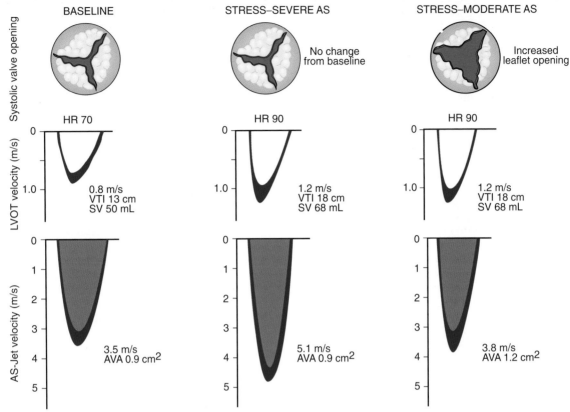

Figure 11-6. Schematic diagram of the changes in AV opening and Doppler flows with dobutamine stress echocardiography (DSE) for low-output, low-gradient AS. The baseline data show a hypothetical patient with an EF of 35% and limited AV systolic opening, an aortic jet velocity (AS-jet) of 3.5 m/s, and AVA of 0.9 cm². If true severe AS is present (*middle panel*), as EF increases from 35% to 45%, transaortic flow rate increases but aortic opening is fixed, resulting in a marked increase in aortic velocity (and pressure gradient) with no change in valve area. In a patient with the same baseline data but "pseudo-severe AS," the increase in EF and transaortic stroke volume "push" the aortic leaflets to open more so there is a smaller increase in aortic velocity in association with an increase in AVA. Current diagnostic testing relies on Doppler data with dobutamine stress testing because direct imaging of valve anatomy is not adequate for visualization of the exact systolic orifice.

Dobutamine Dose (μg/kg/min)	Aortic Velocity (m/s)	Mean Gradient (mm Hg)	AVA (cm²)	Transaortic Stroke Volume (mL)	EF (%)
Rest					
5					
10					
15					
20					
Change from rest to peak stress					

TABLE 11-3   REPORT FORMAT FOR DOBUTAMINE STRESS ECHO FOR LOW-OUTPUT, LOW-GRADIENT AS

- With a rigid valve, the degree of leaflet opening does not change from rest to stress so that the increase in velocity and gradient corresponds to the expected values for that valve area.
- Severe AS on dobutamine stress testing is defined as an aortic velocity greater than 4.0 m/s at any flow rate with an AVA less than 1.0 cm² (Fig. 11-7).
- These patients are likely to benefit from AV replacement.
- Lack of contractile reserve is defined as an increase from rest to stress in EF or SV less than 20% (Fig. 11-8).

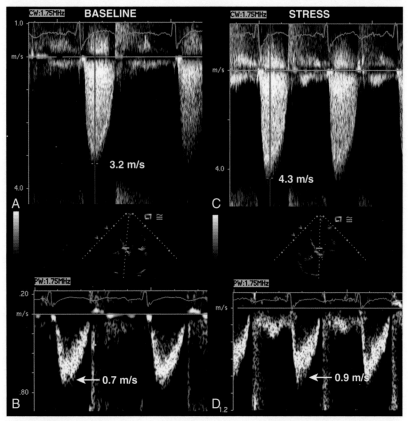

Figure 11-7. DSE for evaluation of low-output, low-gradient AS in an 84-year-old man with calcific valve disease shows (**A**) a resting aortic velocity of 3.2 m/s and mean gradient of 26 mm Hg, and (**B**) LV outflow velocity of 0.7 m/s and valve area of 0.8 cm². With dobutamine infusion at a maximum dose of 15 μg/kg/min, HR increased from 74 to 95 beats/min from rest to stress and blood pressure fell slightly from 132/74 mm Hg at rest to 116/58 mm Hg at peak stress. Doppler data recorded at peak dose showed (**C**) an aortic velocity of 4.3 m/s and mean gradient of 47 mm Hg, and (**D**) LV outflow velocity of 0.9 m/s and valve area of 0.8 cm². These findings are consistent with true severe AS.

- If there is lack of contractile reserve and AS measures are equivocal for severe AS, clinical management is controversial; outcomes are poor with either medical therapy or valve replacement.
- If there is lack of contractile reserve with hemodynamics suggesting severe AS or with severe valve calcification, valve replacement is likely to be beneficial, although surgical risk is high.

Potential Pitfalls
- Recording accurate stress Doppler data in AS patients is challenging, in part due to the increase in HR; study quality depends on the experience of each laboratory and cardiac sonographer.
- Aortic velocity may be underestimated during stress testing because optimal patient positioning is more difficult.
- The changes in AVA with stress testing are close to the limits of measurement variability,

which makes interpretation problematic in an individual patient.
- The known variability in recording and measuring each of the variables used in these calculations may lead to erroneous test results.
- There is little clinical outcome data to support the use of dobutamine stress testing in adults with low-output, low-gradient AS; many other factors need to be considered in clinical decision making. Patients should not be denied the potential benefit of valve replacement solely based on a stress test result.
- Dobutamine stress testing is not accurate for diagnosis of coronary artery disease when moderate to severe AS is present.

Alternate Approaches
- In adults with AS and LV dysfunction, careful evaluation for other causes of myocardial dysfunction is needed, including evaluation of coronary anatomy and myocardial viability.

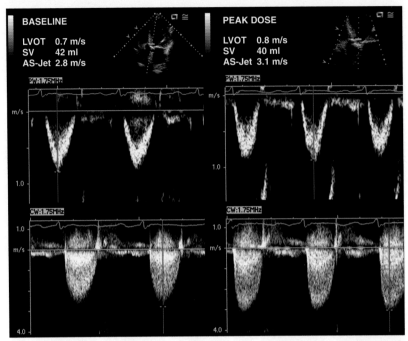

Figure 11-8. DSE in a patient with lack of contractile reserve. This 83-year-old man with heart failure symptoms, an EF of 22%, and a calcified AV underwent DSE for evaluation of low-gradient, low-output AS. The baseline (*left*) and peak dose (*right*) Doppler recordings of LVOT flow (*top*) and aortic velocity (*bottom*) are shown. The following data were obtained:

Stress Stage	Heart Rate	Stroke Volume (mL)	Cardiac Output (L/min)	Ejection Fraction (%)	Aortic Velocity (m/s)	Mean Gradient (mm Hg)	Aortic Valve Area (cm²)
Rest	76	42	3.2	22	2.8	18	0.8
Peak dose	110	40	4.4	14	3.1	27	0.8

In this patient, the slight increase in cardiac output was mediated by an increase in HR with no change in stroke volume and a fall in EF. The failure of stroke volume and EF to increase by at least 20% indicates contractile reserve with primary myocardial dysfunction. In this situation, evaluation of AS severity is problematic. This patient had a very calcified valve, and it is likely that severe AS is present even though the aortic velocity did not increase to over 4.0 m/s. The fall in EF likely was due to concurrent coronary disease (known to be present in this patient) with inducible ischemia.

- Direct visualization of valve anatomy to identify the number of leaflets and degree of valve calcification may be helpful using TEE, CT, or CMR imaging.
- However, the degree of leaflet opening can be misleading because leaflet opening is reduced in parallel with the degree of LV dysfunction, even with normal valve leaflets (e.g., reduced leaflet motion with a severe cardiomyopathy or the lack of leaflet motion when an LV assist device is present).
- When severe LV dysfunction is present, another approach is careful medical therapy for heart failure with a repeat resting echocardiogram after optimization of therapy.

KEY POINTS

- Low-output, low-gradient AS is defined as a mean transaortic pressure gradient of less than 30 mm Hg and aortic velocity of less than 3.5 m/s with a valve area less than 1.0 cm², typically in association with an EF of less than 50%.
- Dobutamine stress testing is helpful in low-output, low-gradient AS to distinguish true severe AS from moderate AS with primary ventricular dysfunction.
- Severe AS is defined as an aortic velocity greater than 4 m/s with a valve area less than 1.0 cm², at any flow rate.
- Lack of contractile reserve is defined as a failure of transaortic stroke volume or EF to increase by at least 20%; evaluation of AS severity in these patients is problematic.

Mitral Stenosis

Indications
- Recommendations for percutaneous balloon mitral commissurotomy (BMC) for patients with moderate to severe mitral stenosis (mitral valve area [MVA] = 1.5 cm^2) include:
  - Symptoms.
  - Pulmonary artery systolic pressure (PAP) greater than 50 mm Hg at rest or greater than 60 mm Hg with exercise.
  - New-onset atrial fibrillation (may be considered in these patients).
- Thus, exercise testing is helpful in:
  - Asymptomatic patients with MVA less than or equal to 1.5 cm^2 and PAP less than 50 mm Hg at rest.
  - Patients with symptoms greater than expected given resting echocardiographic data.
- The goals of stress testing are:
  - An objective measure of exercise tolerance.
  - Assessment of the HR and BP response to exercise.
  - Measurement of PAP with exercise; an exercise PAP greater than 60 mm Hg is an indication for intervention.
  - Measurement of transmitral pressure gradient with stress.
- MVA typically does not change with exercise because the rheumatic orifice has a fixed size due to commissural fusion. The transmitral gradient increases in parallel with the increase in flow rate.

Step-by-step Approach
Test Preparation
- Review the patient history, current medications, allergies, and indications for the stress test.
- Review the baseline echocardiographic study with particular attention to:
  - MV anatomy and area by 2D planimetry.
  - Pressure half-time MVA.
  - Tricuspid regurgitant (TR) jet velocity—used for estimation of PAP.
  - Inferior vena cava (IVC) diameter and respiratory variation.
  - Presence and severity of coexisting MR.
- Review the optimal window and patient position for recording TR velocity; ensure signal strength is adequate for PAP calculations.
  - The TR signal should be denser than background noise and clearly identifiable.
  - The TR signal should show a smooth velocity curve with a well-defined maximum velocity.

- Ideally, the TR signal is dense around the outer edge ("envelope"), indicating that the Doppler beam is intersecting the TR vena contracta.
- Interrogation from multiple windows is needed to ensure a parallel intercept angle with flow, with the highest velocity used in PAP calculations.
- Ensure each member of the medical team understands the primary goals of the stress test (measurement of PAP with stress).
- Obtain informed consent from the patient for the stress test.

Stress Protocol
- Either upright treadmill or supine bicycle stress testing can be used for mitral stenosis patients.
- Advantages and disadvantages of upright versus supine exercise are shown in Table 11-2.
- A maximal stress test is performed with either stress type, stopping only when patients reach their exercise limit. HR should increase to at least 85% of maximum predicted HR to ensure an adequate workload.
- As with all stress testing, monitoring by a physician or other qualified health professional includes a continuous 12-lead ECG, intermittent BP, and assessment of any symptoms.

Echocardiographic and Doppler Data
- The primary goal of stress testing in patients with mitral stenosis is measurement of PAP with exercise, so this measurement is the first priority in data recording (Fig. 11-9).
  - Using the baseline complete transthoracic study as a guide, the highest TR velocity is recorded at baseline.
  - Patient position is noted and the best acoustic window is marked to ensure reproducible data recording with stress.
  - If atrial fibrillation or another irregular rhythm is present, enough beats should be recorded to calculate a representative average peak velocity.
  - The TR signal should have a well-defined edge, smooth velocity curve, and clear maximum velocity.
  - TR velocity is recorded immediately post-exercise (treadmill) or at each stress stage (supine bicycle).
- IVC diameter and respiratory variation are recorded at baseline to estimate right atrial (RA) pressure.

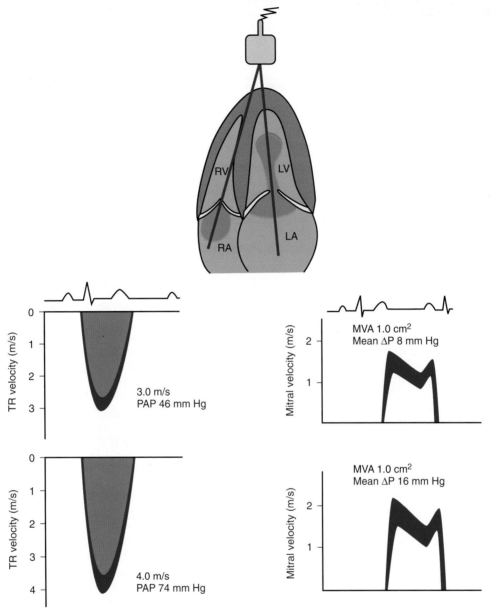

Figure 11-9. Schematic diagram showing the Doppler data recording in stress testing for evaluation of mitral stenosis. The figure at the top shows the apical transducer location for recording of the TR jet with CW Doppler in systole and the transmitral flow curve with either pulsed wave (PW) or CW Doppler in diastole. The bottom part of the figure shows that the TR velocity and transmitral gradient (ΔP) increase to levels consistent with severe valve obstruction with no change in mitral valve area (MVA) and a marked increase in PAP. The exercise data now meet criteria for percutaneous balloon mitral commissurotomy.

- Transmitral flow is recorded with CW Doppler for measurement of mean diastolic gradient and pressure half-time valve area.

Measurements
- PAP is calculated from the TR velocity at baseline, at each stress stage, and at maximum workload using the standard formula: PAP = $4(V_{TR})^2$ + RA pressure.

- RA pressure is estimated from the IVC appearance (Table 11-4).
- Typically the baseline RA pressure is used for all calculations because of the difficulty of imaging the IVC and estimating RA pressure during exercise, due to the high heart and respiratory rates.
- Mean diastolic transmitral gradient is calculated by tracing the Doppler curve to

TABLE 11-4   ESTIMATION OF RIGHT ATRIAL PRESSURE

IVC Diameter (1–2 cm from RA junction)	Change with Respiration or "Sniff"	Estimated RA Pressure
Small (<1.2 cm)	Spontaneous collapse	Intravascular volume depletion
Normal (<1.7 cm)	Decrease by ≥50%	0–5 mm Hg
Dilated (>1.7 cm)	Decrease by ≥50%	6–10 mm Hg
Dilated (>1.7 cm)	Decrease by <50%	10–15 mm Hg
Dilated (>1.7 cm)	No change	15–20 mm Hg
Dilated with dilated hepatic veins	No change	>20 mm Hg

From Otto CM, *Textbook of Clinical Echocardiography*. 4th ed. Philadelphia: Elsevier; 2009: Table 6-7.

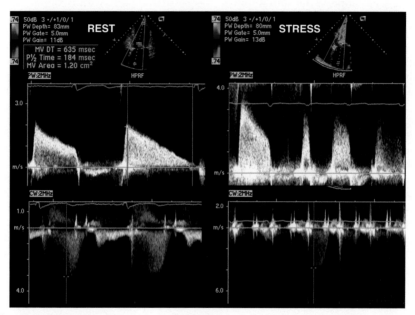

Figure 11-10. Treadmill stress echocardiography was requested in this 32-year-old woman with rheumatic mitral valve (MV) disease and mixed moderate stenosis and moderate regurgitation now with symptoms of dyspnea on exertion. At rest (*left*), MVA is 1.2 cm² with a mean transmitral gradient of 8 mm Hg (*top*). Pulmonary pressure is 48 mm Hg, based on the TR jet velocity of 3.1 m/s (*bottom*) and an estimated RA pressure of 10 mm Hg. She exercised for 4 minutes and 15 seconds on a Bruce protocol treadmill (moderately reduced exercise capacity), reaching 85% of her maximum predicted heart rate. The immediate post-stress Doppler data show a mean transmitral gradient of 18 mm Hg, although there is wide beat-to-beat variation with atrial fibrillation. The TR jet velocity was difficult to record due to rapid respiration, but a velocity of 3.8 m/s was obtained, consistent with an exercise PA systolic pressure of 67 mm Hg.

average the instantaneous gradients over the filling period.

- Mitral pressure half-time is measured from the early diastolic slope of transmitral flow, when possible.

Data Analysis

- Exercise duration and the HR response to exercise are compared with expected standards for age and gender.

- An increase in TR jet velocity indicating a PAP greater than 60 mm Hg is consistent with hemodynamically significant MV disease (Fig. 11-10).
- An exercise transmitral mean gradient greater than 15 mm Hg is consistent with severe valve obstruction.
- An increase in PAP to greater than 60 mm Hg without a high transmitral gradient suggests that underlying lung disease may be the cause of pulmonary hypertension.

Potential Pitfalls
- Recording data after treadmill stress testing is challenging due to:
  - Time needed for transfer from the treadmill to the stretcher.
  - Increased respiratory rate and excursion interfering with recording of the Doppler signal.
  - Data recording is less problematic with supine bicycle testing, but recording a weak TR jet signal still may be challenging.
- Measurement of mitral stenosis severity by Doppler is difficult because diastole becomes shorter as HR increases so that it is difficult to identify the diastolic slope of the mitral inflow curve for pressure half-time calculations, particularly if atrial contraction obscures the late diastole segment of the velocity slope.
- Doppler allows estimation of PAP; methods to estimate pulmonary vascular resistance are less well validated.

Alternate Approaches
- TEE provides better assessment of MR severity, especially if transthoracic image quality is suboptimal or if there is significant valve calcification, allowing identification of the patient with combined mild-moderate mitral stenosis and mild-moderate MR.
- Cardiac catheterization allows direct measurement of PAP and calculation of pulmonary vascular resistance.

- 3D echocardiography provides useful images of valve anatomy, including the symmetry of the valve orifice and commissural fusion, which may be helpful in clinical decision making.

Mitral Regurgitation

Indications
- Stress testing is helpful in patients with MR who have:
  - Symptoms greater than expected based on resting echocardiographic findings.
  - Unclear symptom status.
  - Unexplained episodes of pulmonary edema, particularly with ischemic MR.
  - For evaluation of the change in EF with exercise when LV resting function is abnormal.
- MR severity may increase with exercise due to increased leaflet prolapse in patients with myxomatous MV disease (Fig. 11-11).
- Myocardial ischemia also may result in an increase in MR with exercise in patients with coronary artery disease. Multivariate predictors of cardiac death in patients with ischemic MR include:
  - An exercise increase in effective regurgitant orifice area (EROA) ≥ 13 mm^2.
  - An EROA greater than 20 mm^2 at rest.
- With rheumatic MV disease, regurgitant severity may increase with exercise even when only mild regurgitation is present at rest.

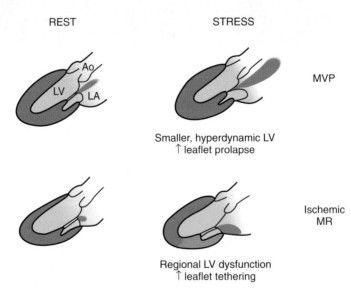

REST   STRESS

MVP

Smaller, hyperdynamic LV
↑ leaflet prolapse

Ischemic
MR

Regional LV dysfunction
↑ leaflet tethering

Figure 11-11. Examples of mechanisms for increased MR with exercise. When mitral valve prolapse (MVP) is present, the increased contractility and smaller size of the LV may result in increased mitral leaflet prolapse with an increase in MR severity. This example shows posterior leaflet prolapse with an anteriorly directed MR jet. With ischemic MR, stress results in myocardial ischemia. This increases the degree of mitral leaflet tethering with an increase in the posteriorly directed MR jet. In both cases, the increased LA pressure due to the MR in turn leads to an increase in pulmonary systolic pressure and a higher tricuspid regurgitant jet. Ao, aorta.

- The goals of stress testing are:
  - An objective measure of exercise tolerance.
  - Assessment of the HR and BP response to exercise.
  - Measurement of PAP with exercise; an exercise PAP greater than 60 mm Hg is an indication for intervention.
  - Evaluation of the change in EF with exercise; a normal increase predicts preservation of ventricular function after MV surgery.
- Quantitative measurement of MR severity at peak exercise is challenging, so the primary focus of the study is measurement of PAP.
- Evaluation of LV mechanics with stress—for example, with speckle tracking measures of myocardial deformation—is an area of interest, but currently there are few data to guide clinical practice (see Chapter 7).

Step-by-step Approach
Test Preparation
- Review the patient history, current medications, allergies, and indications for the stress test.
- Review the baseline echocardiographic study with particular attention to:
  - MV anatomy and mechanism of MR.
  - Quantitative measures of MR severity (vena contracta width, regurgitant volume, and regurgitant orifice area).
  - The TR velocity signal used for estimation of pulmonary systolic pressure.
  - IVC diameter and respiratory variation.
  - LV regional and global systolic function, including quantitative measurement of EF.
- Review the optimal window and patient position for recording TR velocity; ensure signal strength is adequate for PAP calculations.
  - The TR signal should be denser than background noise and clearly identifiable.
  - The TR signal should show a smooth velocity curve with a well-defined maximum velocity.
  - Ideally, the TR signal is dense around the outer edge ("envelope"), indicating the Doppler beam is intersecting the TR vena contracta.
  - Interrogation from multiple windows is needed to ensure a parallel intercept angle with flow, with the highest velocity used in PAP calculations.
- Ensure that each member of the medical team understands the primary goals of the stress test (measurement of PAP with stress).
- Obtain informed consent from the patient.

Stress Protocol
- Either upright treadmill or supine bicycle stress testing can be used for MR patients (see Table 11-2).
- A maximal stress test is performed with either stress type, stopping only when patients reach their exercise limit. HR should increase to at least 85% of maximum predicted HR to ensure an adequate workload.
- As with all stress testing, monitoring by a physician or other qualified health professional includes a continuous 12-lead ECG, intermittent BP, and assessment of any symptoms.

Echocardiographic and Doppler Data
- The primary goal of stress testing in patients with MR is measurement of PAP with exercise, so this measurement is the first priority in data recording.
  - Using the baseline complete transthoracic study as a guide, the highest TR velocity is recorded at baseline (Fig. 11-12).
  - Patient position is noted and the best acoustic window is marked to ensure reproducible data recording with stress.
  - If atrial fibrillation or another irregular rhythm is present, enough beats should be recorded to calculate a representative average peak velocity.
  - The TR signal should have a well-defined edge, smooth velocity curve, and clear maximum velocity.
  - TR velocity is recorded immediately post-exercise (treadmill) or at each stress stage (supine bicycle).
- IVC diameter and respiratory variation are recorded at baseline to estimate RA pressure.
- A secondary goal is evaluation of global and regional LV function at rest and with exercise.
  - Apical four- and two-chamber views for calculation of EF are recorded.
  - Standard views for evaluation of regional LV function are recorded, including long axis and short axis views, in addition to apical four- and two-chamber views.
  - 3D echocardiography may be used to evaluate LV function if available.
- If imaging time allows, MR severity can be recorded at baseline and each stress stage including:
  - Color Doppler imaging of vena contracta width in the parasternal view.
  - CW Doppler recording of the MR signal.
  - Color Doppler visualization of the proximal isovelocity surface area.
  - All these measurements can be challenging at the high HR associated with exercise.

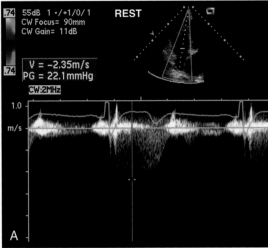

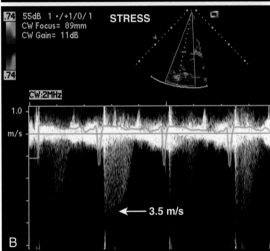

Figure 11-12. Treadmill stress echocardiography in a 46-year-old woman with mitral valve prolapse, moderate MR at rest, and exertional dyspnea shows (**A**) a resting TR jet velocity of 2.4 m/s, consistent with a right ventricular (RV) to RA pressure difference of 23 mm Hg and a pulmonary systolic pressure of 33 mm Hg (with RA pressure of 10 mm Hg). She exercised for 11 minutes and 38 seconds on the Bruce treadmill protocol, achieving 13 METs, which is an above average functional capacity. HR increased from 75 to 164 beats/min (94% maximum predicted), with an increase in BP from 100/64 to 150/54 mm Hg. Immediately post-exercise she transferred back to the echo stretcher in a left lateral decubitus position. **B,** The TR jet velocity of 3.5 m/s indicates an RV to RA pressure difference of 49 mm Hg and a PA systolic pressure of 59 mm Hg. Notice how the higher HR and respiratory variation in the angle between the Doppler beam and TR jet are challenges in recording the velocity signal at peak stress.

Measurements
- PAP is calculated from the TR velocity at baseline, at each stress stage, and at maximum workload using the standard formula: PAP = $4(V_{TR})^2$ + RA pressure.
- RA pressure is estimated from the IVC appearance (see Table 11-4).
- Typically the baseline RA pressure is used for all calculations because of the difficulty of imaging the IVC and estimating RA pressure during exercise, due to the high heart and respiratory rates.
- EF is measured using the apical biplane approach or by 3D echocardiography.
- Mitral regurgitant severity is measured qualitatively as mild, moderate, or severe based on the vena contracta width and CW Doppler signal; if quantitative measures are needed (and are feasible) standard quantitative approaches are used.

Data Analysis
- Exercise duration and the HR response to exercise are compared with expected standards for age and gender.
- An increase in TR jet velocity indicating a PAP greater than 60 mm Hg is consistent with hemodynamically significant MR.
- If MR severity can be quantitated at rest and with stress, an increase in MR severity supports MR as the cause of pulmonary hypertension and patient symptoms.

Potential Pitfalls
- Recording data after treadmill stress testing is challenging due to :
  - Time needed for transfer from the treadmill to the stretcher.
  - Increased respiratory rate and excursion interfering with recording of Doppler signals.
  - Data recording is less problematic with supine bicycle testing, but recording a weak TR jet signal still may be challenging.
- Measurement of MR severity with exercise is difficult because of the increased respiratory and HRs and the inherent measurement variability of these approaches.
- Doppler allows estimation of PAP; methods to estimate pulmonary vascular resistance are less well validated.

Alternate Approaches
- TEE provides better assessment of MV anatomy and regurgitant severity, especially if transthoracic image quality is suboptimal.
- Cardiac catheterization allows direct measurement of PAP and calculation of

pulmonary vascular resistance; LV angiography can be used to assess MR severity.

- CMR allows quantitation of MR severity when echocardiographic data are suboptimal or inconsistent with other clinical data.
- 3D echocardiography provides useful images of valve anatomy that may be helpful in clinical decision making.

Hypertrophic Cardiomyopathy

Background

- HCM is an inherited disease of the myocardium due to mutations in genes encoding sarcomeric proteins. The diagnosis typically is based on clinical features of the disease, although genetic testing is increasingly part of the diagnostic approach.
- HCM is characterized by LV hypertrophy (septal thickness at least 15 mm in diastole) with a nondilated chamber, in the absence of another disease that produces LV hypertrophy (such as hypertension).
- Dynamic LV outflow obstruction is a common finding in HCM patients but is not necessary for the diagnosis.
  - Obstruction is dynamic in that it occurs predominantly in mid- to late systole. A hypertrophied basal septum may redirect intracardiac flow, causing systolic anterior motion (SAM) of the MV and progressive subaortic obstruction during LV ejection.
  - Obstruction is also dynamic in that the severity of obstruction may vary with physical activity and other changes in physiologic status (such as hypovolemia).
- Although LVOT obstruction is present at rest in only about 30% of patients with HCM, an additional 33% have LV outflow obstruction with exercise, often called "latent" obstruction (Fig. 11-13).

- Exercise-induced LV outflow obstruction is a major determinant of symptoms, including dyspnea, angina, presyncope, or syncope.
- Dynamic LV outflow obstruction with a peak gradient over 30 mm Hg at rest or 50 mm Hg with exercise is generally accepted as an indication for therapy in symptomatic patients.
- HCM patients with continued dynamic LV outflow obstruction and symptoms despite medical therapy are often considered for septal reduction procedures.

Indications

- An objective measure of exercise capacity in patients with HCM before starting medical therapy or for monitoring the efficacy of therapy.
- Evaluation for latent LVOT obstruction in symptomatic HCM patients.
- Assessment of BP response to exercise in patients younger than 50 years as part of risk stratification for sudden cardiac death.
- Exercise stress testing should not be performed in HCM patients with symptoms and severe resting LVOT obstruction (peak gradient >90 mm Hg).

Step-by-step Approach
Test Preparation

- Review the patient history, current medications, allergies, and indications for the stress test.
- All cardiac medications should be held for 24 to 72 hours before the stress test, if possible.
- Review the baseline echocardiographic study with particular attention to:
  - The degree and pattern of LV hypertrophy.
  - The presence and severity of LVOT obstruction.
  - The presence and severity of MR.
- Ensure each member of the medical team understands the primary goals of the stress test (measurement of LV outflow obstruction with stress).
- Obtain informed consent from the patient.

Baseline Echocardiographic and Doppler Data

- 2D and M-mode imaging is recorded to document:
  - The degree and pattern of LV hypertrophy.
  - The presence and timing of SAM of the MV.
  - Mitral leaflet anatomy and motion.

REST

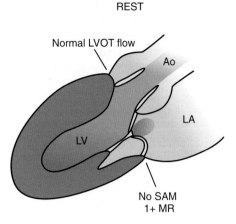

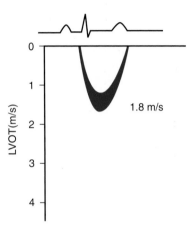

STRESS

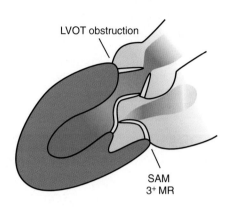

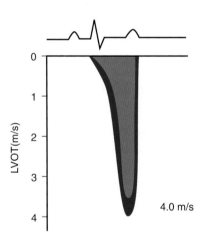

Figure 11-13. Exercise stress testing for HCM may show provocable LVOT dynamic obstruction. Typically, imaging at rest (*top left*) shows the presence of HCM without obstruction to LV outflow and with mild MR. The Doppler flow in the LVOT (*bottom left*) may be slightly higher than normal, but the shape of the curve is relatively normal. With exercise (*top right*), the ventricle is smaller and more hyperdynamic, with increased systolic anterior motion (SAM) of the MV in association with dynamic subaortic obstruction, documented with color Doppler showing an increase in velocity at this site. The SAM also may be associated with increased MR. The CW Doppler velocity recording of LVOT flow now shows the typical late-peaking high-velocity signal of dynamic subaortic obstruction.

- LVOT velocity is recorded with PW and CW Doppler (Fig. 11-14).
  - Typically a steep left lateral decubitus position on a stretcher with an apical cut-out provides the best window for Doppler data recording.
  - Patient position is noted and the best acoustic window is marked to ensure reproducible data recording with stress.
  - Either the long axis plane or an anteriorly angulated four-chamber view (the "five-chamber" view) is used, whichever provides the optimal Doppler signal.
  - LV outflow velocity is recorded with PW Doppler starting with the sample volume in the mid-LV cavity, with repeated recordings as the sample volume is moved toward the aortic valve to identify the presence and location of LV outflow obstruction.
- CW Doppler is used to record the maximum LV outflow velocity.
  - The Doppler scale is set so the signal fills but fits within the displayed velocity range.
  - Wall filters are increased to optimize the high-velocity signal-to-noise ratio.
- MR
  - The CW Doppler waveform for MR (if present) is also recorded.

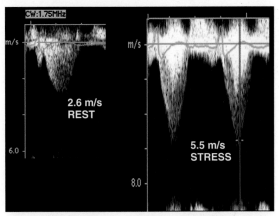

Figure 11-14. Supine bicycle stress testing in a 45-year-old man with HCM showed an LVOT velocity that peaked in mid-systole at 2.6 m/s during rest (*left*), consistent with no significant obstruction. Peak stress Doppler data documented provocable obstruction with a late-peaking LV outflow signal with a maximum velocity of 5.5 m/s. The velocity scale on the baseline and peak Doppler recordings have matched in this example.

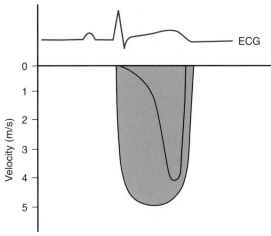

Figure 11-15. Schematic illustration of the differences between the CW Doppler velocity signal for subaortic dynamic outflow obstruction (*in red*) and MR (*in blue*). These signals often are both present and overlap each other and may be difficult to separate. The MR signal starts earlier and ends later in systole, has a high velocity throughout the ejection period, and is higher in velocity than LV outflow. Dynamic subaortic obstruction starts later in systole and typically is low in early systole, with a peak near end-ejection.

- The timing, shape, and velocity of the MR waveform must be distinguished from velocities due to LV outflow obstruction.
- MR severity may increase with stress if LV outflow obstruction due to SAM results in inadequate mitral leaflet coaptation.
- Color Doppler is used to evaluate MR in parasternal and apical long axis views. Vena contracta is recorded as a quantitative measure of regurgitant severity.

Stress Protocol
- Either upright treadmill or supine bicycle stress testing can be used for patients with HCM (see Table 11-2).
- A maximal stress test is performed with either stress type, stopping only when patients reach their exercise limit. HR should increase to at least 85% of maximum predicted HR to ensure an adequate workload.
- As with all stress testing, monitoring by a physician or other qualified health professional includes a continuous 12-lead ECG, intermittent BP, and assessment of any symptoms.

Stress Echocardiographic and Doppler Data
- The primary goal of stress testing in patients with HCM is measurement of LV outflow obstruction with exercise, so this measurement is the first priority in data recording.

- Using the baseline complete transthoracic study as a guide, LVOT velocity is recorded at baseline using both PW and CW Doppler.
- CW and PW Doppler LV outflow velocities are again recorded immediately post-exercise (treadmill) or at each stress stage (supine bicycle).
- After recording LV outflow velocity, the degree of mitral SAM and MR severity are recorded.
  - Mitral SAM is evaluated in apical and parasternal long axis views.
  - MR is evaluated with color Doppler in apical and parasternal long axis views; measurement of vena contracta is recommended at each stress stage.
  - The MR CW Doppler signal from the apical view is recorded at each stage.
- It may be challenging to distinguish the CW Doppler MR velocity from the signal due to LV outflow obstruction (Fig. 11-15).
  - The timing of the LV outflow and MR signals is one distinguishing feature:
    - Both are high-velocity systolic signals directed away from the apex that are adjacent to each other (mitral SAM causes the MR jet to originate anteriorly) and thus are often included in the wide beam of a CW Doppler transducer.
    - The duration of the MR waveform is slightly longer than LV outflow

obstruction because MR starts in the isovolumic contraction period (before aortic valve opening) and continues after aortic valve closure, during isovolumic relaxation.

- In contrast, LV outflow starts slightly later and ends slightly earlier, with flow only when the aortic valve is open.
- The maximum velocity of the signals also is different for MR and LV outflow obstruction (Fig. 11-16):
  - The MR velocity is always higher than the LVOT velocity because MR velocity reflects the LV to left atrial (LA) systolic pressure difference, whereas LV outflow velocity reflects the LV to aortic systolic pressure difference.
  - However, if signals overlap, it can be challenging to identify separate maximum velocities for each signal.
- The shape of the velocity curves may be helpful in identification of signal origin:
  - Dynamic LV outflow obstruction increases gradually during early systole, with an abrupt increase in velocity in mid- to late systole as obstruction worsens in conjunction with SAM of the MV.
  - The late-peaking velocity curve of HCM is distinctive, but this velocity curve may become more rounded with exercise if obstruction occurs earlier in systole.
  - The MR velocity curve shows a sharp increase in velocity in early systole, with the slope reflecting the rate of rise in LV pressure (*dP/dt*), and a high velocity throughout mid-systole followed by an abrupt decline in velocity at end-systole.
  - Jet shape can be misleading since the timing of the obstruction affects both the MR and LVOT waveforms, but because the change in gradient is a smaller percent of the total LV to LA (versus LV to aortic) pressure difference, the effect on the MR jet is usually less pronounced.
- In general, if an LV outflow gradient of greater than 100 mm Hg is suspected, a separate MR signal with a gradient even greater than the LV outflow gradient should be documented.

Measurements
- The severity of LV outflow obstruction is reported as the maximum (or peak instantaneous) subaortic velocity at rest and at maximum stress, as measured by CW Doppler.

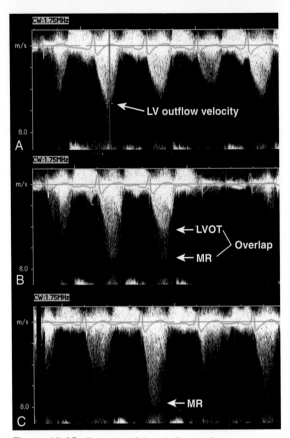

Figure 11-16. Example of the challenges in differentiating subaortic obstruction, e.g., the LVOT velocity from the MR velocity curve. There is marked respiratory variation in the flow signal at peak stress, most likely related to a changing intercept angle between the Doppler beam (which the sonographer holds still) and the direction of the high-velocity jet. The highest velocity signals represent the most parallel orientation to flow and are the beats that are measured. These recordings from the same transducer position with a similar 2D color Doppler image show (**A**) the late-peaking LV outflow velocity at about 5 m/s with the onset of flow late in the QRS signal, (**B**) overlap between the LVOT and higher velocity MR signal, and (**C**) the high-velocity MR signal that starts early in the QRS, shows a rapid increase in velocity in early systole, and has a peak close to 8 m/s, consistent with a systolic BP of 120 mm Hg and a 100 mm Hg gradient between the LV and aorta, resulting in an LV systolic pressure of about 220 mm Hg. Given a typical LA pressure of 10 to 15 mm Hg, the MR velocity is expected to be at least 7.4 m/s.

- The presence and severity of SAM is noted at rest and each exercise stage.
- MR severity is measured qualitatively as mild, moderate, or severe based on the vena contracta width and CW Doppler signal.

Data Analysis
- Exercise capacity, maximum HR, and the rise in BP with exercise are key elements in interpretation of the stress study.

- Exercise capacity is compared with expected normal standards for age and gender.
- A maximum HR at least 85% of maximum predicted indicates an adequate workload.
- Failure of systolic BP to increase by at least 20 mm Hg, or an initial rise followed by a fall in systolic BP at peak exercise, is considered a risk factor for sudden cardiac death.
- Gradients elicited with exercise are categorized as:
  - Moderate-severe obstruction (≥50 mm Hg)
  - Mild obstruction (30–49 mm Hg)
  - Nonobstructed (<30 mm Hg)
- Any increase in MR severity is documented.
- A mid-cavity increase in velocity due to a hyperdynamic ventricle with cavity obliteration at end-systole is distinguished from subaortic LV outflow obstruction, using PW and color Doppler to document the anatomic site where the velocity increases.
- A mid-systolic decrease in PW Doppler velocity ("lobster claw" appearance) either at the LV mid-cavity or outflow tract level indicates an abrupt increase in afterload due to dynamic obstruction (Fig. 11-17).

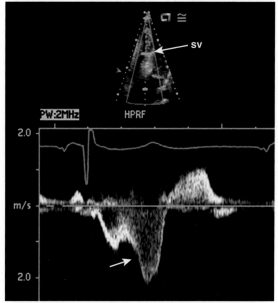

Figure 11-17. PW Doppler recording of flow in the LVOT from an apical position with the Doppler sample volume (SV) positioned at the mitral leaflet level. The high-pulse repetition frequency (HPRF) Doppler curve shows the initial normal velocity and shape of the curve in early systole as LV ejection commences but then shows an abrupt decline of velocity in mid-systole followed by a higher velocity late-peaking signal (*arrow*) once LV obstruction occurs due to SAM of the MV.

Potential Pitfalls
- Recording data after treadmill stress testing is challenging due to:
  - Time needed for transfer from the treadmill to the stretcher.
  - Increased respiratory rate and excursion interfering with recording of the Doppler signal.
- Data recording is less problematic with supine bicycle testing, but there is a lower maximum workload, and clinical symptoms may not be reproduced.
- The LVOT gradient may be overestimated if systolic BP decreases immediately post-exercise due to changes in peripheral vascular tone.
- Exercise-induced LVOT gradients must be interpreted in the context of both mitral leaflet motion and exercise duration; gradients may be due to significant obstruction or to an appropriate increase in cardiac output.
- Measurement of MR severity with exercise is challenging.
  - When there is overlap in the MR and LV outflow Doppler data, it can be difficult to separate these two velocity waveforms, resulting in overestimation of the severity of LV outflow obstruction.
- Mitral SAM typically results in a posteriorly directed jet; if the jet is central or anteriorly directed, other causes of MR should be considered.

Alternate Approaches
- Patients with HCM who are symptomatic and have LVOT obstruction at rest may not need stress testing prior to considering medical or procedural therapies.
- Cardiopulmonary exercise testing (CPET) is helpful to distinguish cardiac from respiratory causes of exercise limitation with measurement of peak oxygen uptake (VO₂).
- CPET also may help separate increased wall thickness due to an athletic heart versus HCM. Indicators of physiologic hypertrophy include a peak VO₂ greater than 50 mg/kg/min or 20% greater than predicted maximum VO₂, an oxygen pulse greater than 20 mL/beat, or an anaerobic threshold greater than 55% of predicted maximum VO₂.
- CMR is useful for assessment of the presence, degree, and pattern of LV hypertrophy and may show myocardial scarring.

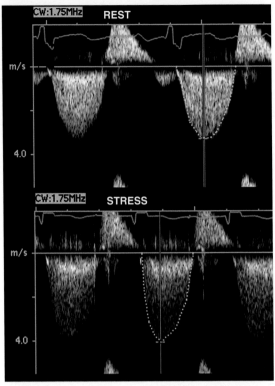

Figure 11-18. Stress echocardiography for evaluation of a bioprosthetic pulmonic valve in a 23-year-old woman with congenital heart disease (operated truncus arteriosus) shows a resting transpulmonic velocity of 3.3 m/s with a mean systolic gradient of 24 mm Hg. Severe pulmonic regurgitation also is present, as seen by the dense retrograde diastolic flow with a steep deceleration slope that reaches the baseline before end-diastole. She exercised for 6 minutes on a Bruce protocol treadmill (7 METs with an exercise capacity 35% less than predicted). The immediate post-stress Doppler recording shows a pulmonic velocity of 4.0 m/s and a mean gradient of 39 mm Hg, consistent with severe stenosis.

Stress Testing for Other Types of Structural Heart Disease

- Stress testing may be useful in selected patients with aortic regurgitation (AR).
  - Stress testing provides an objective measure of exercise tolerance and the BP and HR response to exercise.
  - The exercise change in EF is a predictor of both symptom onset and postoperative recovery of LV function.
    - Symptom onset is more likely in those with an exercise EF below 50% (symptoms occur in 9% per year) compared to those with an exercise EF over 57% (0% per year).
    - An increase in EF with exercise is associated with long-term recovery of LV function after valve replacement for severe AR.
  - However, stress testing is not widely used for evaluation of AR because resting parameters of regurgitation severity, LV size and function, and clinical symptoms are the primary factors in clinical decision making.
- Exercise testing is useful in adults with congenital heart disease (Fig. 11-18).
  - CPET typically is preferred as it allows separation of symptoms due to a cardiac versus respiratory limitation, conditions that often coexist in these patients.
  - Echocardiographic and Doppler data recording in patients with congenital heart disease is individualized based on the specific anatomy and physiology and the clinical question being addressed by the stress test.
  - A pulse oximeter with periodic recording of oxygen saturation should be used if standard stress testing, rather than CPET, is performed.
- Exercise stress testing may be helpful in patients with suspected prosthetic valve dysfunction or patient-prosthesis mismatch (Fig. 11-19).
  - Exercise capacity is normal with a normally functioning bileaflet mechanical valve, even when there is a high localized gradient at rest.

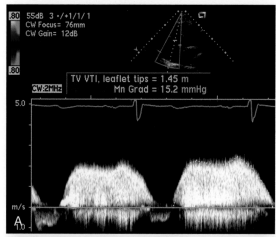

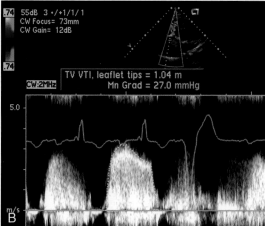

Figure 11-19. This 35-year-old man had undergone MV repair for MR and tricuspid valve replacement with a bioprosthetic valve 6 years ago. He presented with increasing dyspnea, and stress echocardiography was requested to evaluate for exercise-induced MR. However, the resting Doppler data showed a gradient across the bioprosthetic (31 mm) valve of 15 mm Hg with a flat deceleration slope, suggesting prosthetic valve stenosis. His exercise duration was limited, and the test was stopped for an asymptomatic eight-beat run of ventricular tachycardia. The immediate post-stress Doppler flow across the prosthetic valve showed a mean gradient of 27 mm Hg, confirming severe prosthetic valve stenosis.

- Exercise capacity is reduced, in association with a marked increase in prosthetic valve gradient, when patient-prosthesis mismatch is present.
- An exercise increase in gradient over 20 mm Hg for an aortic prosthesis or over 12 mm Hg for a mitral prosthesis is consistent with severe patient-prosthesis mismatch.

Suggested Reading
General
1. Pellikka PA, Nagueh SF, Elhendy AA, et al. American Society of Echocardiography recommendations for performance, interpretation, and application of stress echocardiography. *J Am Soc Echocardiogr.* 2007; 20:1021-1041.
   General guidelines for performing stress echocardiography.
2. Picano E, Pibarot P, Lancellotti P, et al. The emerging role of exercise testing and stress echocardiography in valvular heart disease. *J Am Coll Cardiol.* 2009;54:2251-2260.
   Concise review of the clinical applications of stress echocardiography in adults with valvular heart disease.

Asymptomatic Severe Aortic Stenosis
3. Ennezat PV, Maréchaux S, Iung B, et al. Exercise testing and exercise stress echocardiography in asymptomatic aortic valve stenosis. *Heart.* 2009;95:877-884.
4. Das P, Rimington H, Chambers J. Exercise testing to stratify risk in aortic stenosis. *Eur Heart J.* 2005; 26:1309-1313.
5. Lancellotti P, Lebois F, Simon M, Tombeux C, Chauvel C, Pierard LA. Prognostic importance of quantitative exercise Doppler echocardiography in asymptomatic valvular aortic stenosis. *Circulation.* 2005;112:I377-I382.
6. Maréchaux S, Hachicha Z, Bellouin A, et al. Usefulness of exercise-stress echocardiography for risk stratification of true asymptomatic patients with aortic valve stenosis. *Eur Heart J.* 2010;31:1390-1397.

Low-gradient, Low-output Aortic Stenosis
7. Baumgartner H, Hung J, Bermejo J, et al. Echocardiographic assessment of valve stenosis: EAE/ASE recommendations for clinical practice. *J Am Soc Echocardiogr.* 2009;22:1-23.
8. Grayburn PA. Assessment of low-gradient aortic stenosis with dobutamine. *Circulation.* 2006;113:604-606.
9. Monin JL, Quéré JP, Monchi M, et al. Low-gradient aortic stenosis: operative risk stratification and predictors for long-term outcome: a multicenter study using dobutamine stress hemodynamics. *Circulation.* 2003;108:319-324.
10. Blais C, Burwash IG, Mundigler G, et al. Projected valve area at normal flow rate improves the assessment of stenosis severity in patients with low-flow, low-gradient aortic stenosis: the multicenter TOPAS (Truly or Pseudo-Severe Aortic Stenosis) study. *Circulation.* 2006;113:711-721.

Mitral Valve Disease
11. Reis G, Motta MS, Barbosa MM, et al. Dobutamine stress echocardiography for noninvasive assessment and risk stratification of patients with rheumatic mitral stenosis. *J Am Coll Cardiol.* 2004;43:393-401.
12. Supino PG, Borer JS, Schuleri K, et al. Prognostic value of exercise tolerance testing in asymptomatic chronic nonischemic mitral regurgitation. *Am J Cardiol.* 2007;100:1274-1281.
13. Tischler MD, Battle RW, Saha M, et al. Observations suggesting a high incidence of exercise-induced severe mitral regurgitation in patients with mild rheumatic mitral valve disease at rest. *J Am Coll Cardiol.* 1995;25:128-133.
14. Lancellotti P, Cosyns B, Zacharakis D, et al. Importance of left ventricular longitudinal function and functional reserve in patients with degenerative mitral regurgitation: assessment by two-dimensional speckle tracking. *J Am Soc Echocardiogr.* 2008;21:1331-1336.

15. Lancellotti P, Troisfontaines P, Toussaint AC, Pierard LA. Prognostic importance of exercise-induced changes in mitral regurgitation in patients with chronic ischemic left ventricular dysfunction. *Circulation*. 2003; 108:1713-1717.

Hypertrophic Cardiomyopathy

16. Fletcher GF, Balady GJ, Amsterdam EA, et al. Exercise standards for testing and training: a statement for healthcare professionals from the American Heart Association. *Circulation*. 2001;104:1694-1740.
17. Maron MS, Olivotto I, Zenovich AG, et al. Hypertrophic cardiomyopathy is predominantly a disease of left ventricular outflow tract obstruction. *Circulation*. 2006;114:2232-2239.
18. Shah JS, Esteban MT, Thaman R, et al. Prevalence of exercise-induced left ventricular outflow tract obstruction in symptomatic patients with non-obstructive hypertrophic cardiomyopathy. *Heart*. 2008;94:1288-1294.
19. Maron BJ, Maron MS, Wigle ED, Braunwald E. The 50-year history, controversy, and clinical implications of left ventricular outflow tract obstruction in hypertrophic cardiomyopathy from idiopathic hypertrophic subaortic stenosis to hypertrophic cardiomyopathy. *J Am Coll Cardiol*. 2009;54:191-200.

Other

20. Li M, Dumesnil JG, Mathieu P, Pibarot P. Impact of valve prosthesis-patient mismatch on pulmonary arterial pressure after mitral valve replacement. *J Am Coll Cardiol*. 2005;45:1034-1040.
21. Borer JS, Hochreiter C, Herrold EM, et al. Prediction of indications for valve replacement among asymptomatic or minimally symptomatic patients with chronic aortic regurgitation and normal left ventricular performance. *Circulation*. 1998;97:525-534.
22. Wahi S, Haluska B, Pasquet A, et al. Exercise echocardiography predicts development of left ventricular dysfunction in medically and surgically treated patients with asymptomatic severe aortic regurgitation. *Heart*. 2000;84:606-614.

Multimodality Cardiac Imaging—When Is Echo Not Enough?

Nuno Cortez Dias, Ana G. Almeida, and Fausto J. Pinto

Basic Concepts

- The field of cardiovascular imaging has undergone tremendous improvements over the past decade, with the advent of advanced echo modalities (deformation, contrast, and three-dimensional imaging), advances in nuclear cardiology (single-photon emission computed tomography [SPECT], positron emission tomography [PET], and computed tomography hybrid systems) and the emergence of the new technologies of cardiac computed tomography (CCT) and cardiac magnetic resonance (CMR) and molecular imaging.
- Echocardiography maintains a central position in modern cardiac diagnosis and management, being the first choice of imaging method to assess cardiac anatomy and function. It provides portable, widely available, safe, and inexpensive imaging.
- For the majority of patients, a transthoracic echocardiogram alone is sufficient, providing all the imaging information required for making clinical decisions.
- In many clinical scenarios, the standard echo examination is not enough and clinicians need to identify when and how to combine it with other imaging tests to answer clinical questions (Tables 12-1 and 12-2).
- However, it is important not only to obtain the most complete and valid clinical information, but also to ensure that patients do not get inappropriate, unnecessary, and nondiagnostic imaging tests.
- It is critical to match rapid technological developments with a rigorous scientific evaluation to demonstrate the impact of multimodality tools on clinical decision making and patient outcome.

Cardiac Computed Tomography
- Advances in multidetector computed tomography with the introduction of multi-slice spiral computed tomography (MSCT) and dual-source CT have radically changed the role of CT in cardiac imaging.
- Electrocardiographic (ECG) gating is another important innovation that has allowed the correlation of anatomic information with the cardiac cycle phase.
  - Retrospective ECG gating is a technique in which CT data are continuously acquired and the ECG signal is used during postprocessing analysis to correlate the information with the corresponding phases of cardiac contraction.
  - Prospective ECG gating refers to the synchronization data acquisition with the electrocardiogram (ECG). Acquisition is done only in late diastole (when cardiac motion is lowest), reducing the exposure to radiation (to as low as 1.2 mSv).
- Single-source MSCT (64-, 256-, or 320-slice systems) performs spiral data acquisition that is processed to generate a three-dimensional (3D) dataset. Images are usually presented as cross-sectional slices of the heart in any desired plane or as 3D reconstructions.
  - CCT has excellent spatial resolution (maximal isotropic resolution of 0.5–0.8 mm^3) and very good image quality.
  - CCT offers excellent morphologic depiction of the heart anatomy, myocardium, heart valves, coronary arteries, and bypasses.
  - CCT allows accurate 3D anatomic evaluation of associated extracardiac structures, including the great arteries, proximal branch pulmonary arteries, and pulmonary venous and systemic connections.
  - CCT detects and quantifies calcification of cardiac structures, including the coronary arteries (the calcium score is used to stratify the risk for coronary atherosclerosis) and the pericardium (relevant in the diagnosis of constrictive pericarditis).
  - CCT provides fast data acquisition: the entire heart can be scanned in three to five

TABLE 12-1   STRENGTHS AND LIMITATIONS OF THE MOST COMMONLY USED CARDIAC IMAGING MODALITIES

Echocardiography	CCT	CMR	Nuclear Imaging Modalities (SPECT and PET)
Main Advantages			
• First-line diagnostic imaging test • Provides anatomic and functional information with the highest temporal resolution • Widely available • Low cost • Safe (no need for ionizing radiation) • Portability (bedside exam) • Can be performed in hemodynamically unstable patients	• Provides excellent anatomic evaluation with high spatial resolution • Limited functional assessment (i.e., ventricular function) • Evaluates extracardiac associated abnormalities (providing the best visualization of the lung tissue) • Detects and quantifies vascular calcifications • Detects pericardial calcification	• Provides both anatomic and functional information • Highly reproducible • Superior tissue characterization • Evaluates extracardiac-associated vascular abnormalities	• Evaluate physiologic functions of the heart: myocardial perfusion, metabolism, contractility and neural innervation
Main Limitations			
• Limited windows, narrow field of view • Poor acoustic window in case of obesity or obstructive lung disease • Operator dependent • Limited tissue characterization	• Use of radiation (limiting serial studies) • Use of iodinated contrast • Functional evaluation requires ECG gating (higher radiation dose, suboptimal temporal resolution) • Difficulties in case of tachycardia or unstable heart rhythm • Need for breath-hold • Cannot be performed in hemodynamically unstable patients	• Expensive • Long acquisition time • Associated pulmonary abnormalities are less well characterized • Calcifications are less well visualized • Use of breath-hold sequences • Difficulties in case of unstable heart rhythm • Difficulties in case of claustrophobia • Cannot be performed in hemodynamically unstable patients • Use of gadolinium is contraindicated in patients with advanced kidney disease • Contraindicated in patients with pacemakers, defibrillators, vascular clips, cochlear implants, and neurostimulators	• Use of radiation (limiting serial studies) • Very limited anatomic evaluation (low spatial resolution) • Low temporal resolution • Difficulties in case of unstable heart rhythm • Cannot be performed in hemodynamically unstable patients • Long testing time

gantry rotations, representing only one breath-hold period.

• Dual-source multidetector scanners have a maximum of 2×64 rows, providing 2×128 slices.
  • Dual-source CT shortens the time of acquisition.
  • With retrospective ECG gating, dual-source CT provides better temporal resolution (75–83 ms) than single-source CT (165 ms)

but is still clearly inferior to both two-dimensional echocardiography (2DE) and CMR.

• Dual-source CT reduces heart motion artifacts, particularly in patients with tachycardia and irregular heart rhythms.

• Computed tomography coronary angiography (CTCA) has received a great deal of attention in recent years since technologic developments made possible the simultaneous

TABLE 12-2 COMPARISON OF CARDIAC IMAGING MODALITIES

	Echocardiography	CCT		CMR	Nuclear Scintigraphy
		Ungated	ECG-gated		
Availability	+++	+++	++	++	+++
Portability	++++	−	−	−	−
Cost	+	++	++	+++	++
Exposure to radiation	−	+++	++++	−	++++
Spatial resolution	<1 mm	<1 mm	<1 mm	1–2 mm	5–10 mm
Temporal resolution	20 ms	−	60 ms	30 ms	Variable
Cardiac morphology	++++	++	++++	++++	−
Extracardiac vasculature	++	++++	++++	++++	−
Ventricular function quantification	+++	−	+++	++++	+++
Regional function	++++	−	++	++++	+
Diastolic function	+++	−	−	++	−
Tissue characterization	+	+	+	++	+
Flow quantification	+	−	−	++++	−
Valve regurgitation	+++	−	+	++++	−
Valve stenosis	++++	−	++	++	−
First-pass perfusion	++	+	++	++++	++++
Stress imaging	+++	−	−	+++	++++
Myocardial viability	+++	+	+	++++	++++
Coronary artery imaging	++	+	++++	++	−

Symbols indicate relative value of each modality ranging from none (−) to extremely useful (++++)
Adapted from Prakash A, Powell AJ, Geva T. Multimodality noninvasive imaging for assessment of congenital heart disease. *Circ Cardiovasc Imaging*. 2010;3:112-125.

TABLE 12-3   CURRENT AND EMERGING CLINICAL APPLICATIONS OF THE MOST COMMONLY USED CARDIAC IMAGING MODALITIES

CCT	CMR	Nuclear Imaging Modalities (SPECT and PET)
Current Clinical Applications • Exclusion of CAD in the setting of medium to high-risk but asymptomatic patients or in patients with atypical symptoms • Assessment of bypass graft patency • Evaluation of anomalous coronary arteries • Characterization of aortic valve apparatus for TAVI planning • Pericardial disease • Extracardiac vascular abnormalities (including aorto-pulmonary collaterals)	• LV and RV volumes, systolic function, and mass • Myocardial viability • Myocardial perfusion • CHD, including shunt calculation • Evaluation and follow-up of valvular disease • Pericardial disease • Aortic disease • Cardiac masses • Nonischemic cardiomyopathies (dilated or hypertrophic), myocarditis, sarcoidosis, arrhythmogenic RV cardiomyopathy	• Myocardial perfusion • Myocardial viability • LV volume and systolic function
Emerging Applications • Coronary angiography	• Coronary angiography • Interventional magnetic resonance	• Plaque imaging • Neurocardiac imaging

TAVI, transcatheter valve implantation; CHD, congenital heart disease.

visualization of the coronary lumen and vessel wall (Table 12-3).
- Contrast-enhanced CT is an emerging technology that examines myocardial perfusion. Using first-pass imaging (adenosine-augmented), it may detect perfusion defects. With a second scan a few minutes later, delayed enhancement may be analyzed for detection of myocardial infarction and scars.
- Recent advances include 320-slice scanners and true volumetric scanners.

CT: Limitations and Disadvantages
- Relevant radiation exposure: between 7 and 21 mSv (equivalent to 100–600 X-rays) depending on the CCT modality and use of radiation-reducing algorithms. This limits use of CCT for longitudinal follow-up.
- Use of iodinated contrast agents: adverse reactions include nephropathy and potentially life-threatening allergic reactions.
- Need for breath-holding: respiratory motion causes artifacts and degradation of image quality. However, the breath-holding duration is nowadays very short (<15 s) due to faster gantry rotation times and more efficient detectors.
- Difficulties in case of tachycardia or unstable heart rhythm: to achieve the best image quality with ECG gating, the heart rate should be less than 65 beats/min. Thus, beta-blockers are usually given to patients with heart rates over 75 beats/min.

- Since data are acquired from several heartbeats, artifacts may be produced at the transition zone between gantry rotations.
- Retrospective ECG gating uses low-pitch acquisition, resulting in longer exposure time and higher radiation dose. Since acquisition takes longer, more respiratory artifacts may be produced.
- Prospective ECG gating dramatically reduces the radiation exposure, but it does not provide information on left ventricular (LV) function, and may be impossible to apply in patients with tachycardia or unstable heart rhythm.

Cardiovascular Magnetic Resonance
- CMR is a rapidly emerging noninvasive imaging modality that consists of several techniques that can be performed separately or in various combinations during a patient examination.
- Several pulse sequences may be used for CMR. A pulse sequence is a combination of transmitted radiofrequency pulses and magnetic gradients in the presence of a strong magnetic field, from which a series of received radiofrequency echoes are obtained and processed into an image.
- The radiofrequency signal emitted by hydrogen nuclei as it returns to baseline energy state has an amplitude (which depends on tissue properties) and a phase (which depends on the velocity and direction of flow of the water molecules).

- The most frequently used pulse sequences for CMR are:
  - Spin echo and turbo spin echo sequences (T1, T2, with or without fat saturation) produce images with high tissue contrast and spatial resolution without the need for contrast agents. Flowing blood appears black, and more stationary tissues are displayed in shades of gray.
  - Gradient echo sequence provides high temporal resolution (50 ms), allowing cine display. Flowing blood appears bright, and stationary tissue is displayed in gray. Flow turbulence generates signal void, allowing the detection of regurgitation.
  - Steady-state in free precession (SSFP) pulse sequence: contrast is produced based on the ratio between T1 and T2, providing better signal-to-noise ratio and contrast between blood and myocardium. Similarly to conventional gradient echo sequences, flowing blood appears bright and flow turbulence produces signal void.
  - Phase-contrast pulse sequence (or velocity mapping) is based on the accumulated phase of moving protons. Each pixel is displayed as a velocity rather than a signal magnitude. That allows flow calculations in vessels and cardiac valves by integration over time of the product of mean velocity with cross-sectional area.
- SSFP is currently the most widely used technique for CMR cine imaging. It provides high-quality information regarding heart anatomy, chamber volume, valve anatomy, and motion.
- SSFP produces 2D images in any desired plane having multiple phases (frames) throughout the cardiac cycle with high spatial resolution (in-plane resolution of 1.4 × 1.8 mm) and reasonably high temporal resolution (25–50 ms).
- Gadolinium-based magnetic contrast agents are large molecules that shorten T1 relaxation time (leading to an increase in signal intensity on T1-weighted images). After intravenous injection, they initially transit through the heart and vessels. Then, contrast agents rapidly diffuse from intravascular to interstitial space, being unable to enter cells provided that the tissue cell membranes are intact. Finally, if wash-in and wash-out kinetics are normal, contrast concentration in the tissue will decrease in minutes.
- Several CMR techniques are based on the evaluation of the dynamics of paramagnetic contrast agents in the heart:

- CMR-angiography is used for visualization of arteries and veins throughout the body.
- First-pass contrast CMR visualizes the initial transit of contrast media in the heart and is useful to evaluate myocardial perfusion.
- Delayed contrast enhancement CMR (DE-CMR) detects myocardial retention of contrast, which might result from abnormal vascular permeability (i.e., myocarditis), passive diffusion into the intracellular space due to the loss of membrane integrity (i.e., myocardial infarction), and increase of the interstitial space due to accumulation of collagen or reduction of the capillary density (i.e., myocardial fibrosis and scars).
- CMR can be combined with pharmacological stress for the detection of ischemia and assessment of myocardial viability. The excellent imaging quality provides accurate depiction of the regional contractility, which can be assessed qualitatively or precisely quantified in terms of regional shortening and thickening.
- Tagging is a technique for quantitative analysis of myocardial contraction. Late diastolic selective saturation pre-pulses are used to superimpose a grid across the field of view. Myocardial tissue with initial saturated magnetization remains hypointense throughout the cardiac cycle. Subsequent tracking of tag line deformation through time allows direct assessment of myocardial strain and torsion.
- Recently available single-shot fast planar sequences and parallel imaging techniques significantly reduced the acquisition time for CMR imaging.
- CMR is independent of chest anatomy, body habitus, and acoustic window quality.
- CMR does not expose patients to ionizing radiation and does not require the injection of potentially nephrotoxic contrast medium. Therefore, it can be repeated as often as necessary for follow-up.
- Real time CMR imaging has been introduced recently, allowing the acquisition of the image in one cardiac cycle. However, it still faces problems related to lower spatial resolution.
- Recent advances in CMR technique made coronary artery imaging possible, although CMR-angiography still remains a research tool.

CMR: Limitations and Disadvantages
- Need for breath-holding sequences (10–20 s each) during acquisition: because respiratory movement has a major impact on image quality.

- Long acquisition time (10 to 20 min): conventional CMR imaging techniques require 10 to 12 breath-hold periods to obtain the complete data set. That may lead to patient restlessness and inaccuracy caused by slice misregistration between breath-holds.
- CMR may be unviable for patients with congestive heart failure and high-grade dyspnea, who often cannot withstand the long examination time in the supine position and repeated breath-holding.
- Difficulties in case of tachycardia or unstable heart rhythm: the ECG is used to synchronize the data, and the final image is averaged from data acquired across several cardiac cycles. ECG gating may be difficult if the heart rhythm is not regular but real-time sequences are already available for these patients.
- Metallic implants such as prosthetic valves, coronary stents, sternal wires, and hip and knee prostheses may produce local image artifacts (but pose no hazard at field strengths of 1.5 and probably 3 T).
- CMR is contraindicated in patients with neurostimulators, cochlear implants, metal fragments retained in the eye, and certain vascular clips.
- Gadolinium is contraindicated in patients with advanced kidney disease due to the risk of nephrogenic systemic fibrosis.
- CMR is contraindicated in patients with pacemakers or implanted cardioverter-defibrillators.

Nuclear Cardiology Imaging Modalities

- Nuclear cardiology imaging modalities differ from other imaging techniques since instead of providing anatomic information they evaluate physiological functions of the heart.
- Depending on the tracer used, nuclear techniques may assess myocardial perfusion, metabolism, contractility, or neural innervation.
- The integrated biological risk-benefit balance should be taken into account whenever SPECT or PET are considered since exposure to high levels of radiation occurs.

Radionuclide Ventriculography
- Red blood cells are labeled with technetium-99m (^{99m}Tc) pertechnate and reinjected into the patient.

- Equilibrium radionuclide ventriculography is a technique in which planar images in anterior and left anterior oblique projections are acquired once the radiotracer has equilibrated within the blood pool.
  - Used to quantify LV volumes and function—counts within the LV blood pool are directly proportional to the volume of blood.
- First-pass radionuclide ventriculography is a technique in which planar images are acquired immediately after the injection of radiotracer as a bolus, while the radiotracer passes through the heart.
  - Used to measure right ventricular (RV) volumes and function.

Single-photon Emission Computed Tomography
- Nuclear imaging modality in which gamma rays emitted by radionuclides (tracers) are directly detected using a rotating gamma camera.
- 2D data are acquired from multiple projections to reconstruct a three-dimensional (3D) dataset. The information is typically presented as cross-sectional slices of the heart but can be freely reformatted as required.
- SPECT combined with a cardiac stress test is used to assess myocardial perfusion and viability. Thallium-201 (^{201}Th)- or ^{99m}Tc-labeled sestamibi and tetrofosmin are the available tracers for that purpose.
- ECG triggering of SPECT acquisition allows the assessment of the tracer distribution throughout the cardiac cycle and provides additional quantitative information about wall motion, wall thickening, and LV volumes.
- Recent advances include phase analysis of gated SPECT, which enables the evaluation of LV regional mechanical activation and promises to be useful in the assessment of LV dyssynchrony.

SPECT: Limitations and Disadvantages
- Use of radioactive material: the effective dose of a single nuclear stress imaging ranges from 10 to 27 mSv, which is equivalent to exposure to 500 chest X-rays (sestamibi-SPECT) or 1200 chest X-rays (thallium-SPECT).
- Low spatial resolution, which precludes the assessment of cardiac anatomy.
- Low temporal resolution: with ECG-gated SPECT, 16 frames at most are assessed by the cardiac cycle.
- Inability to measure absolute myocardial blood flow.
- Difficulty to distinguish between true perfusion defects and fixed defects caused by

soft tissue attenuation, particularly in women (photoelectric absorption in the breast) and obese patients. Several methods of nonuniform attenuation correction are available, including the use of parametric maps obtained from low-dose CT. Wall motion analysis by ECG-gated SPECT also aids in the distinction.

- Difficulty in performing ECG gating in the case of irregular heart rhythms.
- Long image acquisition: a complete stress and rest study may take half a day or may require acquisitions on two separate days.

Positron Emission Tomography

- Nuclear imaging technique that detects pairs of gamma rays emitted indirectly by positron-emitting radionuclides (tracers), which are introduced into the heart on biologically active molecules.
- The high-energy photons released from the annihilation of positrons provide more radiation-event localization information and thus confer spatial resolution superior to SPECT.
- Computer analysis of PET datasets provides 3D reconstruction of the tracer concentration.
- The major clinical applications of PET are:
  - Assessment of myocardial perfusion at rest and during stress, using as tracers nitrogen-13 (^{13}N)-ammonia, rubidium-82 (^{82}Rb), or oxygen-15 (^{15}O)-water.
  - Assessment of myocardial metabolism and viability using the glucose analogue fluorine-18-fluorodeoxyglucose (^{18}F-FDG) (and less commonly carbon-11 acetate).
- Promising applications of PET imaging but still restricted to research purposes are:
  - Evaluation of endothelial dysfunction, by detecting low coronary flow reserve in the absence of epicardial coronary disease. The assessment of endothelial dysfunction promises to improve the long-term risk stratification by identifying early asymptomatic coronary artery disease (CAD).
  - Identification of vulnerable plaque: preliminary studies have suggested that iodine-125 (^{125}I) labeling of low-density lipoproteins and ^{99}mTc-annexine V, which localizes the apoptotic cells, may depict the unstable atheromatous plaque.
  - Assessment of ischemic memory: after a transitory ischemic event, the perfusion is restored but the myocardial metabolism remains abnormal during some days. Instead of obtaining energy through fatty acid metabolism, myocardial cells use glucose. This phenomenon can be demonstrated with labeled fatty acid scintigraphy or ^{18}F-FDG SPECT.

- Major advantages of PET are:
  - Higher spatial resolution than SPECT.
  - Ability to provide absolute quantification of myocardial perfusion.
  - Less affected by soft tissue attenuation than SPECT (leading to better accuracy for the assessment of obese individuals and women with large breasts).
  - Ability to label naturally occurring elements in the body, such as carbon, water, or nitrogen.
- ECG gating may be applied to PET, providing additional information regarding ventricular function.

PET: Limitations and Disadvantages

- Use of radioactive material.
- Low spatial resolution, which precludes the assessment of cardiac anatomy.
- Soft tissue attenuation: the use of external germanium-68 (^{68}Ge) or X-ray sources provides efficient attenuation correction.
- Not widely available and more expensive than other imaging modalities.

Hybrid Imaging

- Hybrid imaging combines the high-resolution 3D anatomic depiction of the coronary arteries by CT-angiography with the functional evaluation of myocardial perfusion by SPECT or PET.
- Integration of CTCA data with SPECT/PET information can be achieved with hybrid scanners (which combine SPECT or PET devices with high-end CT scanners) or with software fusion of datasets obtained from separate stand-alone scanners.
- The process of integration of imaging systems has also progressed to CMR.
- Hybrid imaging promises to offer a full comprehensive noninvasive assessment of CAD, yielding complementary information both on coronary stenosis anatomy and hemodynamic significance of relevant lesions.
- The clinical impact on treatment strategy and patient outcome of hybrid imaging remains to be determined in large-scale prospective studies.

Hybrid Imaging: Limitations and Disadvantages

- Higher exposure to radiation.
- Not widely available and cost-effectiveness concerns.

Assessment of Ventricular Anatomy, Systolic Function, and Mass

- Echocardiography is the first choice of imaging test in the assessment of ventricular anatomy, systolic function, and mass. However, echocardiography has three relevant limitations:
  - Image quality depends on the thoracic acoustic window.
  - Volume estimation depends on geometric assumptions.
  - High inter- and intraobserver variability.
- If the acoustic window is insufficient to provide a high degree of diagnostic certainty, ventricular opacification with echocardiographic contrast agents may be useful, improving the endocardial visualization.
- Quantification of the ventricular volumes by 2DE depends on geometric assumptions, which do not apply to the RV (due to its unique geometry) and are often incorrect even for the LV (especially when the ventricular shape deviates from assumed geometric models, as in ischemic or dilated cardiomyopathy).
- Evaluation of the ventricular geometry and systolic function using three-dimensional echocardiography (3DE) uses direct volumetric quantification, not relying on

geometric modeling and preventing errors caused by foreshortened views (Fig. 12-1).
- Specific software designed for quantification of LV volumes (disk summation) and for volumetric analysis of the RV is currently available for 3DE.
- 3DE improves the accuracy of the ventricular quantification and reduces the unacceptable high level of variability of the 2DE evaluation.
- Disadvantages of 3DE include worse image quality, lower spatial resolution (because of lower line density than 2DE), suboptimal temporal resolution, and time-consuming analysis. Hopefully, further advances in transducer and computer software technology will progressively solve these problems.
- The major limitation of 3DE relies on its dependence on adequate acoustic windows.
- 3DE may be combined with ventricular opacification with contrast to improve the accuracy of the quantitative analysis and to expand 3DE use in patients with suboptimal endocardial visualization.

Left Ventricular Anatomy, Systolic Function, and Mass

- The accurate and reproducible assessment of LV volumes, function, and mass is crucial for the determination of appropriate therapeutic procedures, monitoring disease progression, timing of surgery, and prognostic stratification in patients with cardiac disease.
- Echocardiography is the primary modality used in routine clinical practice. 2DE techniques allow reasonably accurate measurements of LV mass, volume, and ejection fraction (EF).
- LV quantification by echocardiography is based on geometric assumptions, assuming an idealized cardiac shape that may not represent the patient being studied.
- Error due to geometric modeling is particularly significant in the case of remodeled ventricles, as in patients with dilated cardiomyopathy, wall motion abnormalities, and ventricular aneurysms.
- Echocardiography is significantly operator and acoustic window dependent, which contributes to high inter- and intraoperator variability and low interstudy reproducibility.

When to Consider Additional Imaging

- The assessment of LV anatomy and systolic function is crucial in every cardiac imaging examination, but it is especially relevant in the evaluation of patients with heart failure symptoms.

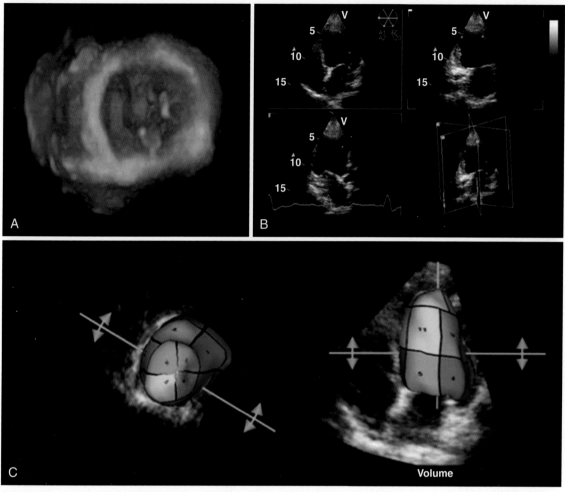

Figure 12-1. 3DE in a patient with ischemic dilated cardiomyopathy before successful cardiac resynchronization therapy. **A,** Real-time 3DE. **B,** Triplane apical views of the left ventricle. **C,** 3D reconstruction of the LV, for assessment of ventricular volumes, ejection fraction, and dyssynchrony.

- High-quality imaging is crucial to confirm the clinical diagnosis of heart failure and to assess deterioration or response to treatment during follow-up.
- Imaging evaluation aims to quantify chamber dimensions and global systolic function, detect wall motion abnormalities, search for LV hypertrophy and diastolic dysfunction, look for valvular dysfunction, and assess pulmonary hemodynamic parameters.
- If the echocardiographic image quality is good, with full visualization of endocardial and pericardial borders in all segments, standard 2DE may provide adequate evaluation of LV anatomy and accurate estimation of LV volumes, EF, and mass.
- 3DE improves the accuracy of the evaluation of LV volumes and mass by eliminating the need for geometric modeling. Thus, it may be particularly useful whenever an abnormal LV geometry is suspected, such as in patients with dilated cardiomyopathy, wall motion abnormalities, ventricular aneurysms, or abnormally shaped ventricles secondary to congenital heart disease (CHD).
- However, 3DE still requires adequate acoustic access and depends on the ability to include the entire LV cavity within the 3D pyramidal scan volume. That is frequently impossible to achieve in patients with markedly dilated LV cavities.
- If the acoustic window is insufficient to provide a high degree of diagnostic certainty in the assessment of heart failure patients, evaluation should proceed to another imaging modality, such as contrast echocardiography, CMR, CCT, or nuclear imaging.

- The most appropriate added imaging modality depends on the suspected cause for heart failure: ischemic or nonischemic myocardial dysfunction, valvular abnormality, or pericardial disease.
- In a research environment, when assessing the effects of drugs on LV volumes, function, or mass, 2DE requires large sample sizes due to its high interstudy variability. Thus, more reproducible imaging modalities such as CMR are usually used in clinical trials, resulting in significant savings.

Cardiac Magnetic Resonance

- CMR is the most precise technique for quantification of LV geometry, volumes, EF, and mass, so it is considered the gold standard for noninvasive volume measurements of LV.
- CMR has the highest reproducibility and lowest interstudy variability, which is essential for longitudinal follow-up studies of patients and especially in research. The excellent interstudy reproducibility minimizes the sample size for studies of the effects of drugs on cardiac function or mass, reducing time and cost for clinical trials.
- LV (and RV) volume and mass assessment is optimally performed with multislice 2D SSFP cine imaging covering the entirety of the ventricular chamber (Fig. 12-2).
- From contiguous LV short axis slices, each one 5 to 10 mm thick, LV volumes and mass are determined by planimetry of the blood-endocardium border (end-diastole and end-systole) and epicardial border (end-diastole) for each slice and summed for the entire ventricle (Fig. 12-3).
- Semi-automated analysis of LV mass, volume, and systolic function with intensity-based thresholding and long axis valve plane tracking is currently available, saving time.
- Besides quantifying regional and global LV systolic function, CMR may provide functional hemodynamic information by the assessment of LV stroke volume and concomitant valvular disease.
- CMR may be particularly useful in the work-up of patients with heart failure, providing detailed visualization of all areas of the heart, accurate quantification of LV and RV volumes and function, superior tissue characterization, assessment of cardiac dyssynchrony, and comprehensive assessment of valvular and hemodynamic function.
- Tissue characterization by CMR may help in the distinction between ischemic cardiomyopathy, dilated cardiomyopathy, and less common diseases, such as sarcoidosis and myocarditis. For that purpose, delayed enhancement should complement standard CMR evaluation, directly visualizing myocardial inflammation and fibrosis:
  - Ischemic pattern: characterized by the presence of myocardial scar, visualized as an area of delayed hyperenhancement invariably involving the subendocardial regions in the distribution territory of a coronary artery.
  - Nonischemic patter: characterized by patchy or linear midwall striae or scars (delayed hyperenhancement) with "noncoronary" distribution.

Cardiac Computed Tomography

- CCT using retrospective gating provides reasonably accurate assessment of LV geometry, volumes, EF, and mass. CCT is more accurate than echocardiography, nuclear imaging, or contrast ventriculography as long as a minimum temporal resolution is guaranteed.
- Performance for assessment of LV function is limited by the relatively modest temporal resolution of CCT.
- New prospective gating protocols that reduce radiation exposure do not provide information on LV function.
- The major advantage of CCT in the assessment of LV anatomy and systolic function is the shorter examination time than for CMR (<15 s), which makes it more feasible in patients with heart failure symptoms.
- The two major limitations of CCT are (1) exposure to ionizing radiation, which limits its usefulness and precludes its use in follow-up studies, and (2) use of contrast media, which may transiently change the ventricular performance due to preload and negative inotropic effect.
- Given the predominant disadvantages of contrast medium application and radiation exposure, the assessment of LV function and morphology alone is not an indication for CCT, as these parameters can be assessed by echocardiography and CMR without radiation exposure and with higher temporal resolution.
- CCT assessment of LV volumes and mass should be considered a part of an examination required for other purposes, such as evaluation of coronary anatomy. Thus, CCT may be of value for patients with heart failure and distorted ventricles to elucidate the etiology, because information in terms of LV volumes, function, and mass is complemented by data

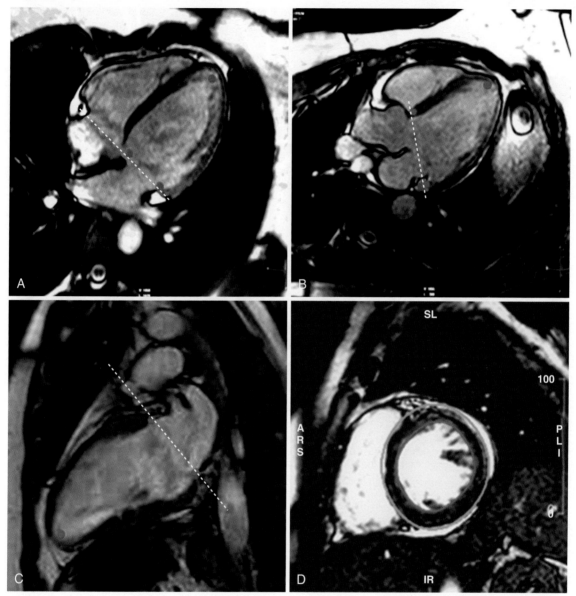

Figure 12-2. Mitral valve (*red dots* and *white dashed line*) annulus and apex (red dot) andmarks to obtain the basal LV slices in LV volumes and mass evaluation by CMR. **A–C,** Four-, three-, and two-chamber steady state in free precession (SSFP) images at end-diastole. **D,** A single representative short axis SSFP image of the mid-ventricle with the endocardial and epicardial borders traced.

concerning coronary anatomy without additional imaging time or contrast.
- CCT may be considered as an alternative for patients with contraindications to CMR.

Nuclear Cardiology
- Radionuclide ventriculography and ECG-gated nuclear imaging techniques allow calculations of the LV end-systolic and end-diastolic volumes and thus EF.
- Measurements do not rely on geometric assumptions, being derived from end-systolic and end-diastolic count densities.
- 3D tomographic techniques (PET and ^{99m}Tc-SPECT) provide better accuracy than radionuclide ventriculography (planar acquisitions).
- Errors may occur in the case of small or large hearts, including patients with ischemic dilated cardiomyopathy due to the difficulty in assigning ventricular borders to areas with low counts, such as scars or areas of infarction.

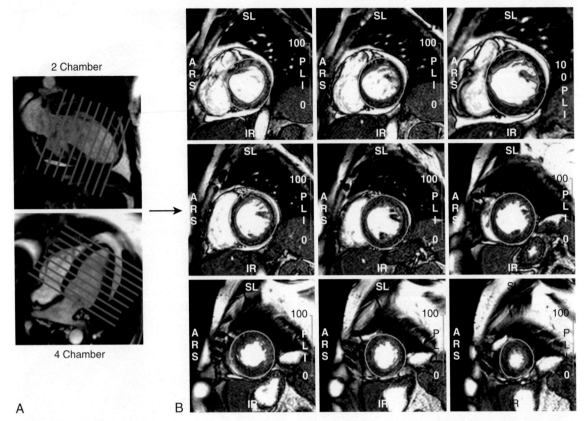

Figure 12-3. Quantification of LV volumes and mass by CMR. **A,** Two- and four-chamber SSFP images at end-diastole with lines representing the imaging locations of serial short axis images. **B,** LV volumes and mass are determined using disk summation from a short axis SSFP stack of images. The endocardial borders are traced, and the difference between end-diastolic and end-systolic area is multiplied by the sum of the slice thickness and interslice gap to calculate stroke volume.

- Spatial and temporal resolution of nuclear imaging modalities is insufficient to assess LV mass or geometry.
- The use of ionizing radiation limits the utility of nuclear techniques for longitudinal studies.

Right Ventricular Anatomy and Systolic Function

- Assessment of RV geometry and function using cardiovascular imaging techniques is considerably more challenging than the evaluation of LV function.
- These challenges are attributed to the complex geometry of the RV, which makes geometric modulation unviable.
- The RV is also difficult to visualize by echocardiography because of its crescentric shape around the LV and proximity to the sternum.
- Several 2DE approaches for quantification of RV volumes have been proposed, but none has shown to be reliable because:

- Geometric models used for calculations are inappropriate, due to the complex shape of the chamber, which is irregular, asymmetric, crescentric, and truncated.
- The RV has a unique geometry that makes it difficult to obtain orthogonal long axis views rotated around a common axis (required for biplane Simpson's and area-length techniques).
- RV chamber orientation varies considerably between patients.
- Prominent endocardial trabeculae compromise the accurate identification of the endocardial boundaries in 2D images.
- The complex geometry of the RV makes it ideally suited for 3D analytical models. Progressive development of 3DE has made it possible to evaluate the RV in the clinical setting and promises to overcome some limitations of 2DE.
- For RV quantification by 3DE, it has been shown that the disk summation technique

offers no significant advantage in comparison with 2D methods. Conversely, recently developed software specific for volumetric analysis of the RV from 3DE datasets without using geometric assumptions does improve accuracy.

- Echocardiographic contrast agents and intravenous saline contrast can facilitate RV endocardial border definition, improving the accuracy and reproducibility of echocardiographic structure and function.
- However, 3DE strongly depends on adequate acoustic windows and relies heavily on the scanning abilities of the sonographer.
- Methods for quantitatively assessing RV function with 3DE have not been widely applied in clinical practice, and the expertise in their use is currently limited to a few centers.
- Despite extensive research and promising results, quantification by 3DE cannot be recommended as a standard for routine clinical practice.

When to Consider Additional Imaging

- Careful and comprehensive evaluation of RV systolic function is indispensable in multiple clinical settings, especially in patients with suspected cardiomyopathy, arrhythmogenic RV dysplasia, inferior wall myocardial infarction, valvular heart disease, pulmonary hypertension, and CHD.
- Patients with pulmonary hypertension require accurate serial evaluation of RV function to assess the progression of the disease and to determine the effects of treatment. In fact, the severity of pulmonary hypertension as determined by the pulmonary artery pressure does not reliably predict survival, whereas indices of RV performance are strong predictors of outcome.
- Patients with repaired tetralogy of Fallot, who commonly have a significant degree of pulmonary regurgitation, and individuals who have undergone valvuloplasty for congenital pulmonary stenosis have a high risk for long-term RV dysfunction, which negatively impacts their prognosis. Longitudinal assessment of RV function can guide the timing of reintervention.
- Since RV volume measurements are not interchangeable between imaging modalities, serial evaluations should preferably be performed using the same modality.
- In most clinical settings, the assessment of RV systolic function is performed qualitatively with 2DE techniques and relies on the interpretative ability of the operator.

- When precise RV assessment is required, other nonechocardiographic imaging modalities need to be considered.

Cardiac Magnetic Resonance

- CMR is considered the reference method to assess anatomy, geometry, as well as regional and global RV systolic function (Figs. 12-4 and 12-5).
- Even CMR may face problems since it provides suboptimal discrimination of the endocardial boundary, due to the presence of heavy trabeculation.
- Among the available imaging modalities, the volumetric analysis of CMR images yields the most accurate and reproducible measurements.
- So, 2DE is the first-choice technique when screening for RV dilation or dysfunction. In most patients, echocardiography provides sufficient information to complete the diagnostic evaluation. However, if accurate serial evaluation of the RV volumes is required (namely in patients with RV compromise due to CHD or pulmonary hypertension) or exhaustive tissue characterization of the RV myocardium is pretended (namely in patients with clinical suspicion of arrhythmogenic RV cardiomyopathy), CMR should be the preferred imaging modality.

Cardiac Computed Tomography

- MSCT provides the best spatial resolution to differentiate RV trabeculae from the myocardium and blood pool, allowing the best discrimination of the inward displacement of the endocardial boundary and the most reproducible assessment of RV parameters, as long as a minimum frame rate is guaranteed.
- CCT has a relatively low temporal resolution compared with CMR and echocardiography, a limited number of phases of the cardiac cycle being analyzed. Even so, retrospective gated CT has been shown to be accurate in the quantification of RV volumes, mass, and EF in adults.
- Because of its use of ionizing radiation, CCT may cause unwanted biological effects, particularly in the case of children or repeated examinations in adults.
- The large volume of contrast medium administered at a high flow rate during acquisition may negatively affect the RV volumetric parameters due to preload and negative inotropic effect.
- The accuracy of MSCT in assessing RV anatomy and EF in patients with depressed

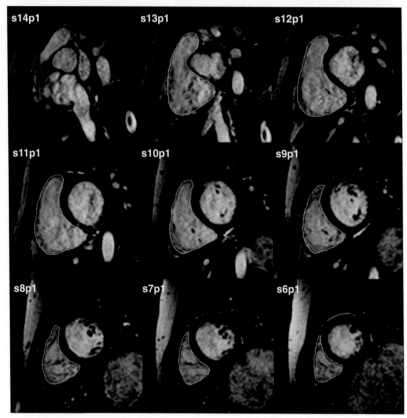

Figure 12-4. RV volumes are obtained using slice summation from a stack of short axis images where endocardial borders are manually or automatically traced.

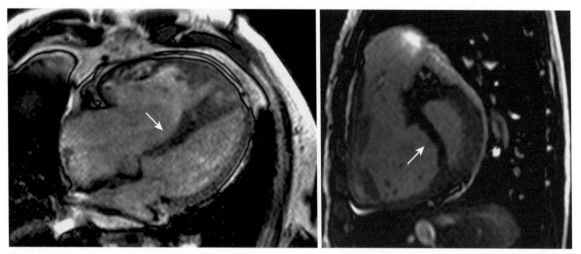

Figure 12-5. SSFP systolic images from a patient with severe pulmonary arterial hypertension (systolic pulmonary artery pressure 145 mm Hg), depicting a dilated and hypertrophied RV and a systolic septal bowing to the left due to RV pressure overload (*arrows*).

RV contractility, CHD, or valvular dysfunction needs to be further determined in large scale studies.

- CCT is not the preferred modality for RV assessment, but it can be useful when precise systolic function quantification is required in patients with contraindications to CMR.

Cardiac Nuclear Imaging

- Nuclear imaging techniques are able to accurately and reproducibly derive RV EF from radiotracer count densities.
- Because global RV systolic function is derived from end-systolic and end-diastolic count densities, it is independent of the geometric assumptions.
- Nuclear techniques that have been used to assess RV function include first-pass radionuclide angiography, equilibrium radionuclide angiography, and SPECT equilibrium radionuclide angiography.
- First-pass radionuclide ventriculography is the preferred nuclear imaging approach to calculate RV EF. It involves the injection of a bolus of radionuclide tracer into a peripheral vein followed by imaging with a gamma camera with high count rate capabilities. Data are summed over a span of several cardiac cycles, and RV EF is derived from end-systolic and end-diastolic frames.
- Its success is largely dependent on the quality of the injected bolus, and its accuracy may be affected in patients with severe RV dysfunction or significant tricuspid regurgitation.
- SPECT equilibrium ventriculography is accomplished by blood pool labeling with ^{99m}Tc followed by tomographic ECG-gated data acquisition. Because of its 3D nature, it enables precise identification and isolation of RV counts, allowing accurate quantification of RV volumes.
- SPECT and PET can also provide information on RV perfusion and metabolism, which were found abnormal in some patients with pulmonary hypertension. The clinical usefulness of this information is currently under investigation.

Myocardial Tissue Characterization

- Myocardial tissue characterization is an important issue in some heart failure patients.
- CMR is the better established imaging modality for tissue characterization, assessing tissue properties in T1- and T2-weighted sequences as well as detecting delayed hyperenhancement.
- Delayed contrast enhancement of the myocardium can also be assessed by CCT, but it has not been fully validated and requires exposition to substantial ionizing radiation.
- Late enhancement is analyzed in inversion recovery images acquired 5 to 20 min after the intravenous injection of paramagnetic contrast agent.
- The presence of delayed hyperenhancement reflects abnormal wash-in/wash-out dynamics of the contrast within myocardial tissue, which may be caused by:
  - Abnormal vascular permeability, as in acute myocarditis or the acute phase of cardiac sarcoidosis.
  - Passive diffusion of contrast into the intracellular space due to the loss of membrane integrity, as within necrotic areas of acute myocardial infarction. Some acute infarcts have a central dark zone in the area of hyperenhancement, representing microvascular obstruction.
  - Increase of the interstitial space due to accumulation of collagen or reduction of the capillary density, as occurs with myocardial fibrosis in the chronic stage of myocardial infarction (ventricular scar) or the setting of cardiac sarcoidosis and myocarditis.
- The pattern of distribution of delayed hyperenhancement provides relevant clues regarding the etiology of LV dysfunction since fibrosis due to CAD invariably involves the subendocardial areas.
- Thus, tissue characterization may direct or confirm the diagnosis of cardiac sarcoidosis, cardiac amyloidosis, siderotic cardiomyopathy, arrhythmogenic right ventricular cardiomyopathy, and myocarditis (Fig. 12-6).

Arrhythmogenic Right Ventricular Cardiomyopathy

- Primary myocardial disorder characterized by localized or diffuse atrophy of predominantly RV myocardium, with subsequent replacement with fatty and fibrous tissue.
- CMR is the best imaging modality to detect the characteristic abnormalities in RV anatomy: presence of fatty infiltration (T1-weighted images) and hyperenhancement in regions of fibro-fatty replacement, RV dilatation, and detection of areas with wall thinning, regional dyskinesia, focal bulging, or aneurysms.

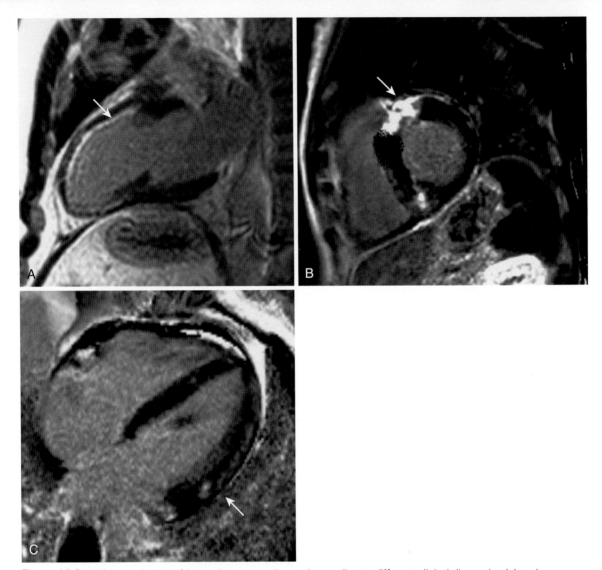

Figure 12-6. Different patterns of late enhancement (*arrows*) according to different clinical diagnosis, delayed hyperenhancement of the subendocardium along the anterior wall and apex in a patient with a subendocardial myocardial infarction (**A**), hypertrophy and scarring of the basal septum in a patient with hypertrophic cardiomyopathy (**B**), and focal patchy mid-myocardial fibrosis in a patient with myocarditis (**C**).

Myocarditis

- The clinical diagnosis of myocarditis is often difficult and may mimic myocardial infarction.
- Acute myocardial inflammation appears as regions of bright signal on T2-weighted sequences that also have hyperenhancement on images acquired 1 to 2 min after gadolinium injection.
- Delayed hyperenhancement may be preferentially located in the subepicardial region of the lateral wall.
- Persistence of late enhancement after the acute phase suggests chronic fibrosis.

Cardiac Amyloidosis

- Cardiac amyloidosis is typically characterized by global subendocardial delayed hyperenhancement, reflecting the preferential endocardial deposition of amyloid.

Cardiac Sarcoidosis

- Active cardiac sarcoidosis appears in CMR as regions of bright signal on T2-weighted sequences that also have delayed hyperenhancement.
- Myocardial fibrosis in sarcoidosis appears as a hyperenhanced midwall or transmural area with a "noncoronary" distribution.

Siderotic Cardiomyopathy

- Secondary myocardial disorder due to tissue accumulation of iron, with oxidative cellular damage and organ dysfunction.
- Since ferrihydrite (the main form of ferritin) is ferromagnetic, myocardial relaxation parameter T2* measured by CMR can be used to directly quantify the myocardial iron loading.

Hypertrophic Cardiomyopathy

- CMR should be performed when the diagnosis of hypertrophic cardiomyopathy is not clear after echocardiographic evaluation.
- CMR demonstrates the distribution of hypertrophy more precisely than 2DE. It is especially useful for detecting localized hypertrophy occurring in the inferolateral wall or in the apical region.
- CMR provides superior evaluation of RV involvement, assesses the dynamic obstruction in the outflow tract or at mid-cavity level, and quantifies concomitant mitral valve regurgitation (MR).
- The extent of patchy midwall delayed hyperenhancement reflects fibrosis and has been linked to the risk for sudden death or heart failure.

KEY POINTS

- Standard echocardiographic evaluation is adequate for clinical decision making in most patients with heart failure.
- 3DE is useful when LV geometry is abnormal because it provides more accurate LV volume data compared with 2D imaging.
- CMR is the most precise method for measurement of LV geometry, volume, EF, and mass and should be considered when more accurate data are needed for clinical decision making.
- CCT can be used to measure LV volumes and should be considered when CCT is performed for other indications.
- Radionuclide ventriculography provides LV volumes and EF data that do not rely on geometric assumptions.
- RV volumes and EF are best evaluated by CMR.
- Myocardial tissue characterization is helpful in some heart failure patients and is best evaluated by CMR.

Assessment of Left Ventricular Synchrony

- Cardiac resynchronization therapy (CRT) is one of the most important advances in the treatment of heart failure patients. It consists of multisite pacing in order to improve the electrical and mechanical coordination of the LV.
- CRT has been shown to improve survival, quality of life, exercise capacity, LV EF, and functional class in patients with moderate to severe heart failure resistant to optimal medical treatment, a low LV EF (35% or less), and a wide QRS (at least 120 ms).
- Around one third of patients who meet the criteria for CRT fail to respond symptomatically.
- Response to CRT is influenced by the presence and severity of dyssynchrony, scar burden, lead placement, pacing A-V and V-V intervals, and disease progression.
- QRS duration as a measure of delayed electrical activation inadequately identifies mechanical dyssynchrony. It is conceivable that the direct evaluation of mechanical dyssynchrony may eventually better identify patients who are more likely to benefit from CRT.
- Echocardiography is the most widely used cardiac imaging modality and the one with the best temporal resolution, making it an attractive tool for assessing LV synchrony.
- Many echocardiographic techniques have emerged to quantify dyssynchrony, including M-mode septal to posterior wall motion delay, pulsed wave (PW) Doppler measures of LV ejection in relation to RV ejection, diastolic filling time as a ratio of cycle length, tissue Doppler imaging techniques to assess intraventricular opposing wall delay or dispersion of time to peak velocities, and speckle tracking techniques to assess time differences for peak radial strain (Fig. 12-7). (See Chapter 8.)
- These sophisticated echocardiographic techniques have substantial intra- and interobserver variability owing to technical issues including available acoustic windows, operator experience, echocardiographic settings, and angle of incidence effects.
- Results of recent clinical trials have challenged the applicability of contemporary echocardiographic techniques in evaluating dyssynchrony since no single echocardiographic measure of dyssynchrony was able to predict clinical benefit from cardiac resynchronization. Thus, current guidelines do not include these approaches for patient selection.
- Several centers are currently using the dyssynchrony information as an adjunct for clinical decision making in patients who are

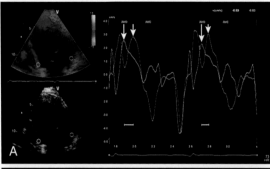

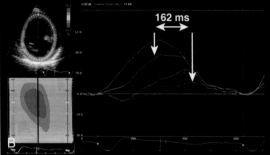

Figure 12-7. Quantification of intraventricular dyssynchrony by echocardiography in a responder prior to resynchronization therapy. **A,** Tissue Doppler imaging assessment of opposing wall delay in apical four-chamber view. Myocardial longitudinal velocity curves demonstrate a significant septal-to-lateral peak systolic delay (76 ms). **B,** Speckle tracking-derived evaluation of radial strain in short axis view. Myocardial radial strain curves show a significant delay between the anteroseptal (*red*) and posterior (*purple*) walls (*vertical arrows*). The difference in time to peak radial strain is 162 ms, indicating significant intraventricular dyssynchrony.

borderline candidates for CRT (borderline QRS duration, functional class, or EF).

- Recent clinical trials have also demonstrated that CRT is not beneficial for patients with a narrow QRS and echocardiographic evidence of dyssynchrony as assessed by current tools. Thus, CRT cannot be recommended for heart failure patients with narrow QRS.
- Accordingly, the application of dyssynchrony information for patient selection is not clear, and its evaluation remains investigational.
- Thus, alternative methods to detect delayed mechanical activation are currently the subject of extensive research, namely CMR and nuclear imaging modalities.

Real-time Three-dimensional Echocardiography

- Real-time 3DE is emerging as an alternative approach to tissue Doppler imaging for the detection and quantification of LV dyssynchrony.
- Regional wall motion excursion can be quantified after segmentation of the LV chamber with contour tracing. Most studies have used the standard deviation of the regional ejection times (interval between the R wave and minimum systolic LV volume) as an index of dyssynchrony.
- The advantage of 3DE is that it allows a segmental analysis of dyssynchrony in a comprehensive view of the heart.
- Disadvantages include lower spatial resolution than 2DE, lower temporal resolution with frame rates at 20 to 30 frames per second and high dependence on the acoustic window.
- Patients with severe LV dysfunction frequently have 3DE regional volume curves with low-amplitude and high-noise signal, resulting in inaccurate identification of regional ejection times.
- It may be impossible to evaluate some patients with severe LV dilation by 3DE since the LV cavity often is larger than the 3D pyramidal scan volume.

Cardiac Magnetic Resonance

- CMR allows for high-resolution and highly reproducible 3D wall motion tracking, providing highly reproducible and operator-independent estimates of myocardial velocity, strain, displacement, torsion, and twist.
- Several techniques have been investigated to assess LV dyssynchrony, but they remain mainly as investigational tools:
  - Velocity-encoded magnetic resonance imaging (MRI) quantifies myocardial velocities from sample volumes placed at different parts of the ventricular wall, without the need for tracking tissue tags. Similarly to tissue Doppler imaging, LV dyssynchrony is detected based on the delay in peak systolic velocity of basal parts of the septum and lateral wall.
  - Harmonic phase analysis of standard CMR tagging.
  - Strain-encoded CMR of sinusoidal tagging, which allows instantaneous real-time quantitative circumferential and longitudinal strain assessment (Figs. 12-8 and 12-9).
  - Displacement encoding with stimulated echoes CMR, which encodes deformation in the phase of each image pixel.
- Combining CMR tagging data with scar quantification by DE-CMR further improves predictive accuracy:

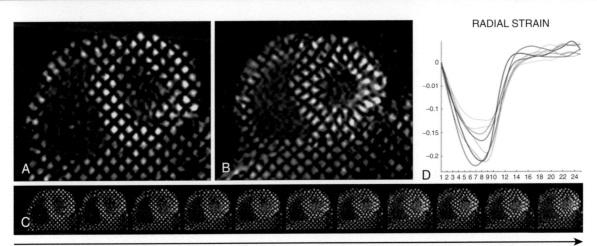

Sequence of tagging images from end-diastole to end-systole (every third cardiac phase shown)

Figure 12-8. Evaluation of mechanical dyssynchrony with CMR tagging. End-diastolic (**A**) and end-systolic (**B**) images from a short axis mid-ventricular grid-tagging sequence (**C**), depicting the grid deformation along the systole. (**D**) Radial strain curves showing synchronous negative strain for each segment along the circumference of the LV.

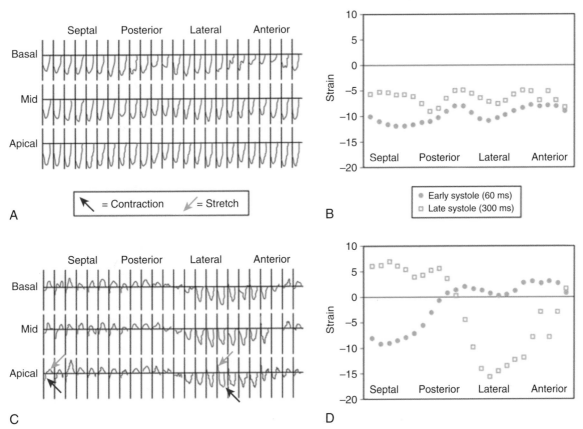

Figure 12-9. CMR tagging-derived circumferential strain maps for a normal subject and a patient with cardiomyopathy and dyssynchrony. **A**, In the normal subject, the progression of the strain versus time is uniform, and (**B**) there is synchronous negative strain for each segment along the circumference of the LV. **C**, In the patient with dyssynchrony and cardiomyopathy, the strain versus time maps show variable timing of contraction (*blue arrows*, negative strain) and stretch (*red arrows*, positive strain) in septal versus lateral segments. **D**, In this subject, some segments have positive strain (stretch) and others have negative strain (contraction) during systole. *(From Bilchick KC, Dimaano V, Wu KC, et al. Cardiac magnetic resonance assessment of dyssynchrony and myocardial scar predicts function class improvement following cardiac resynchronization therapy. JACC Cardiovasc Imaging. 2008;1[5]:561-568.)*

- Scar burden, transmurality, and posterolateral scar location are strong negative predictors of response to CRT in patients with ischemic cardiomyopathy.
- Transmural scar tissue in the posterolateral wall, where the LV lead is usually positioned, often leads to ineffective pacing.
- Contrast-enhanced CMR (as well as CCT) can be used to characterize the cardiac venous anatomy. That is of great value in planning the implant procedure, allowing more directed lead implantation.
- CMR is an attractive pre-CRT imaging modality since it may simultaneously identify the latest activated viable region, assesses the feasibility of lead implantation in cardiac veins nearby, and evaluates the scar extent and distribution.
- A clinical trial comparing empiric lead placement with lead placement guided by identification of the site of greatest LV delay would be of outstanding clinical value.

Nuclear Cardiology Imaging Modalities

- LV synchrony can be assessed with ECG-gated equilibrium ventriculography and ECG-gated SPECT.
- To assess dyssynchrony with ECG-gated SPECT, the following processing steps are required:
  - Images are reconstructed and reoriented to the gated short axis, and subsequent 3D sampling is performed during the cardiac cycle.
  - For each myocardial segment, a time-activity curve (8–16 frames/cardiac cycle) is generated by approximation of first Fourier harmonic function, wherein amplitude provides end-systolic wall thickness and phase reflects the onset of mechanical contraction.
  - Phase analysis assesses the sequence of mechanical activation of the entire LV and is displayed as polar maps or histogram format (Fig. 12-10).
- Dyssynchrony can be quantified by several parameters:
  - Intraventricular dyssynchrony: measured by the standard deviation of phase angle within the LV.
  - Interventricular dyssynchrony: estimated by the difference between mean phase angles of the RV and LV.
- Preliminary clinical studies suggest that nuclear imaging techniques may have a role in the evaluation of heart failure patients with wide QRS who are considered for CRT. In a small patient population, CRT responders were identified with a sensitivity and specificity of 74%.
- The major advantages of nuclear imaging techniques, particularly ECG-gated SPECT myocardial perfusion imaging (MPI), in the assessment of LV dyssynchrony include:
  - More automated and reproducible analysis (as opposed to tissue Doppler imaging).
  - Integration of information on LV volumes and EF together with location and degree of myocardial ischemia, viability, and scar (important determinants of the success of CRT).
  - The latest activated viable region (theoretically preferable LV lead location) can be identified.
- The major limitation of ECG-gated SPECT MPI is the low temporal resolution (in the range of 20–40 frames per second), which may reduce its ability to recognize less severe situations of dyssynchrony.
- Large prospective trials are required to fully elucidate the role of nuclear imaging techniques in the prediction of response to CRT.

Coronary Artery Disease

- The imaging assessment of patients suspected to have CAD aims to provide:
  - Detailed characterization of anatomic sequelae of CAD, including regional contractile abnormalities due to infarction or ongoing ischemia, myocardial wall thinning secondary to fibrosis, ventricular aneurysms, and cardiac chamber dilation.
  - Assessment of the coronary artery anatomic course, lumen size, and atherosclerotic plaques.
  - Detection of myocardial perfusion defects.
  - Assessment of myocardial viability.
  - Assessment of LV global systolic function.
- Resting echocardiographic examination is the first-line imaging modality to detect the anatomic sequelae of CAD. However, standard echo neither directly evaluates the coronary anatomy and function nor excludes the presence of coronary disease.
- Resting echocardiography provides valuable information that may guide the choice of imaging technique and assist in its interpretation:
  - If there is adequate image quality, allowing full visualization of the endocardial border

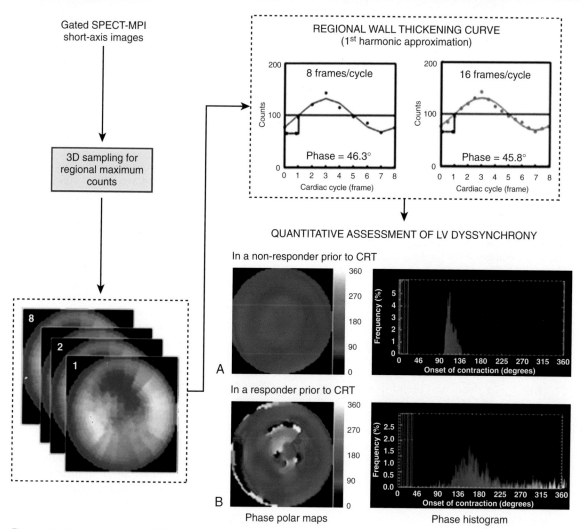

Figure 12-10. Assessment of LV synchrony by ECG-gated SPECT-MPI phase analysis in a nonresponder (**A**) and a responder (**B**) to CRT. Both patients had New York Heart Association functional class III, depressed LV EF, and prolonged QRS duration. In the responder, LV dyssynchrony was evident as a significant phase delay (bright region at the anterior and apical walls) in the phase polar map and as high bandwidth and phase standard deviation in the phase histogram. *(From Chen J, Bax JJ, Henneman MM, et al. Is nuclear imaging a viable alternative technique to assess dyssynchrony? Europace. 2008;10(suppl 3):iii101-iii105.)*

and wall thickening in all myocardial segments, dobutamine stress echocardiography (DSE) may be the test of choice to assess myocardial ischemia and viability.

- If the acoustic window is insufficient to provide a high degree of diagnostic certainty despite contrast enhancement, another imaging approach should be used.
- If extensive regional contractile abnormalities are present at rest, DE-CMR may be preferable to assess viability, since it performs better in patients with severe LV dysfunction than stress tests (either DSE or dobutamine-CMR).

Coronary Anatomy

- In patients with excellent acoustic windows, it may be possible to visualize the origin and proximal coronary arteries with 2DE. That is especially the case in children, in whom 2DE is often used to screen the coronary involvement of Kawasaki disease. (See Chapter 10.)
- However, transthoracic echocardiography is insufficient to delineate the anatomic course or lumen size of coronary arteries and does not visualize atherosclerotic plaques.
- Catheterization with coronary angiography is the gold standard imaging modality to assess coronary artery anatomy:

- Provides excellent visualization of the coronary artery lumen, with an image spatial resolution of 0.25 mm and a temporal resolution of 6 ms.
- Allows diagnosis and, if necessary, treatment in the same session.
- Is an invasive procedure and has very rare but potentially serious complications.
- Requires exposure to ionizing radiation (in average, 3 mSv).
- Does not assess the coronary vascular wall properties, which can be done by complementing with intracoronary ultrasound imaging.
- An alternative noninvasive diagnostic modality for coronary artery visualization with similar diagnostic accuracy would be desirable.
- Noninvasive coronary artery imaging is very challenging:
  - High spatial resolution is needed to assess such small and tortuous vessels.
  - High temporal resolution is required since the coronary arteries undergo substantial motion throughout the cardiac cycle with superimposed respiratory movements.
  - High tissue detail and blood-tissue contrast are required to delineate the lumen size throughout the coronary system, to identify calcified and noncalcified coronary plaques, and to distinguish epicardial coronary arteries from surrounding epicardial fat and the parallel running veins.
- The only noninvasive modality that currently provides adequate depiction of coronary arteries is CCT.

Computed Tomography Coronary Angiography

- CT is able to obtain a quantitative measure of coronary calcium and provides information related to coronary tree anatomy, including anatomic course, lumen size, and artery wall status. Furthermore, CT has the potential to detect not only calcified but also noncalcified atherosclerotic plaques.
- The Agatston coronary calcium score is used in standard clinical practice to quantify the extent and density of calcification of the coronary tree:
  - It is the product of the area of each calcified lesion with the maximum CT attenuation within the lesion. The sum of these values in all the identified lesions provides the total calcium score.
  - The following categories are considered: minimal (score 1–10), mild (score 11–100), moderate (score 101–400), and severe calcification (score >400).

- The coronary calcium score has elevated sensitivity but low specificity for detection of CAD: the vast majority of stenotic segments are calcified, but the presence of calcified plaques does not necessarily imply the presence of significant stenosis.
- Absence of severe calcification does not exclude the possibility of flow-limiting CAD, since noncalcified lesions may be present.
- The coronary calcium score is mainly useful to evaluate the long-term risk of coronary events in patients with intermediate likelihood of disease: the presence of significant plaque burden suggests the need for aggressive preventive approaches.
- Recent studies suggest that the coronary calcium score is useful for prognostic stratification of asymptomatic type 2 diabetic patients, performing better than the Framingham Risk Score. Clinical trials are being conducted to determine its cost effectiveness and usefulness to target low-density lipoprotein cholesterol goals.
- MSCT and dual-scan MSCT improved the spatial and temporal resolution and made possible the use of CCT for noninvasive coronary angiography. In fact, CCT is the noninvasive modality that better visualizes the coronary anatomy (Fig. 12-11).
- ECG gating should be used when coronary artery visualization is required, to improve coronary delineation and image quality.
- Recent studies have demonstrated that MSCT is able not only to visualize the vessel lumen but also the wall, detecting and characterizing the atherosclerotic plaque (Fig. 12-12).
  - CCT easily identifies calcified plaques, but also has moderate accuracy to detect noncalcified (lipid-rich) and mixed plaques.
  - Intracoronary ultrasound imaging studies have suggested that plaques at higher risk of rupture may not be associated with a significant degree of stenosis but tend to have higher lipid content.
  - In patients with chest pain, the extent of noncalcified atherosclerosis as assessed by MSCT was found to be correlated with mortality. Prospective clinical studies are required to clarify the prognostic value of CCT in this context.
  - Plaque characterization promises to help in the detection of vulnerable plaques. Currently, however, it is not possible or recommended in routine clinical practice.
- Single- and multicenter studies demonstrated that CTCA has a high negative predictive

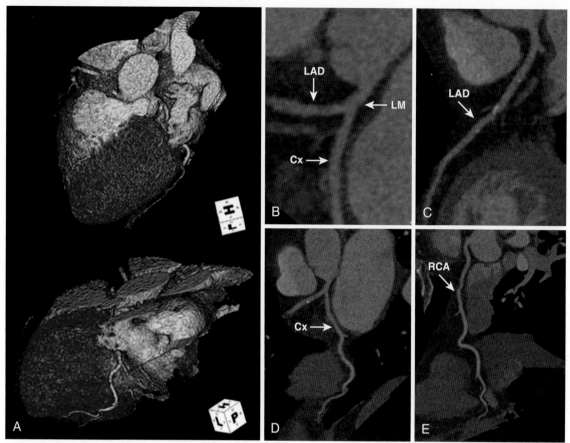

Figure 12-11. 3D-rendered image of the heart (**A**) and multiplanar reconstruction of the coronary arteries (**B–E**). Nonstenotic atheromatous plaques are identified in the proximal and medium segments of the left anterior descending coronary artery (LAD).

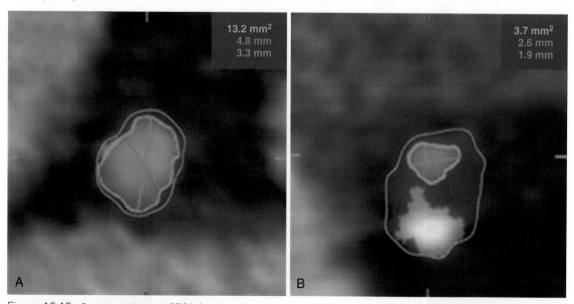

Figure 12-12. Contrast-enhanced CTCA for detection of plaque, minimal lumen area of the plaque, and percent atheroma volume showing a normal coronary arterial segment with measurements of luminal diameter (**A**). In an adjacent stenotic segment of the vessel, the narrowed lumen is seen in green with the plaque components coded in color, with yellow for calcification, red for fibro-fatty components, and blue for fatty components as determined by Hounsfield units (**B**). *(From Akram K, Rinehart S, Voros S. Coronary arterial atherosclerotic plaque imaging by contrast-enhanced computed tomography: fantasy or reality? J Nucl Cardiol. 2008;15(6):818-829.)*

value (ruling out significant disease) but a low positive predictive value (plaque calcification frequently precludes accurate visualization of the lumen, leading to overestimation of luminal stenosis).
- Thus, from a clinical perspective, the most important advantage of MSCT is the possibility to convincingly rule out significant CAD.
- Current clinical applications of CTCA include:
  - Noninvasive exclusion of CAD in patients at an intermediate risk who have undergone one or more inconclusive stress tests, including patients with atypical angina pectoris and ambiguous results of previous stress tests.
  - Evaluation of the origin and course of anomalous coronary arteries: provides better characterization than CMR, but special efforts to reduce the radiation exposure should be undertaken since these patients are often young.
  - Assessment of the patency of coronary grafts and detection of stenosis within the bypass or at the connection with the primitive coronary tree (Fig. 12-13).
- CTCA is not recommended in high-risk patients (such as individuals with typical angina or positive stress test results), in whom prognosis is more related to functional parameters such as ischemia and LV

dysfunction than to anatomic plaque measurement.
- CTCA is not appropriate as a screening examination in asymptomatic individuals or in patients at low risk because of its associated radiation exposure, contrast administration, and risk for false-positive results.

Magnetic Resonance Coronary Angiography

- Advances in CMR technique with use of parallel imaging acquisition, fat suppression (T2 preparation), ECG gating algorithms, and diaphragmatic monitoring with navigator echoes improved the spatial and temporal resolution and made possible the visualization of coronary arteries.
- The anatomic evaluation of the entire coronary tree and lumen size are still very difficult, partially because the spatial resolution of CMR is still worse than that of CCT (0.8–1.1 mm vs. 0.4–0.5 mm).
- CMR coronary angiography is not ready for reliable determination of the location and extent of CAD in the routine clinical practice.
- However, CMR coronary angiography has proven clinically valuable to assess the proximal portions of the coronary system and coronary grafts:
  - Evaluation of the origin and course of the proximal coronary artery, to detect

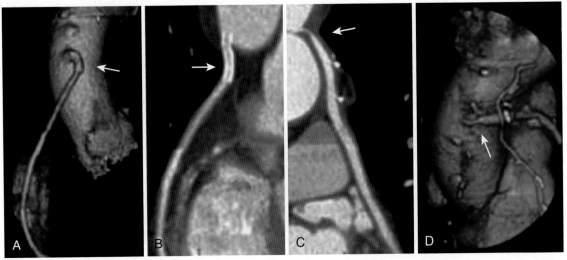

Figure 12-13. **A, B,** 3D rendering and multiplanar reconstruction of a coronary artery bypass graft to the right coronary artery after stent implantation in the proximal part. **C, D,** Stenosis of a proximal coronary artery bypass graft to the right coronary artery in another patient. A left mammary artery bypass to the left anterior artery is crossing the coronary artery bypass graft. *(From Lehmkuhl L, Grothoff M, Nitzsche S, et al. Contrast-enhanced multislice computed tomography of the heart. Eur Cardiol. 2009;5:8-11.)*

anomalous coronary artery origins and coronary fistulas (Fig. 12-14).

- Detection and follow-up of coronary aneurysms caused by Kawasaki disease.
- Assessment of the patency of coronary artery bypass grafts, although difficulty remains for visualization of the connection with the native coronary circulation, where stenoses are often located.
- Further technological advances, with acquisitions by whole heart sequences, higher field magnets, higher multiple receiver channel coils, and new intravascular paramagnetic agents, promise to improve the quality of coronary CMR images.

Myocardial Perfusion and Ischemia

- Currently, there are many noninvasive techniques to assess myocardial perfusion and ischemia, including stress echocardiography, SPECT-MPI, PET, CMR, and CCT.
- All of them use either exercise or pharmacologic stress to produce heterogeneity of blood flow between myocardial regions supplied by normal arteries and those perfused by stenotic vessels, in order to induce ischemia (Table 12-4).
- Pharmacologic stress can be produced by infusion of vasodilators (dipyridamole or adenosine) or inotropic agents (dobutamine stress). Despite acting by different

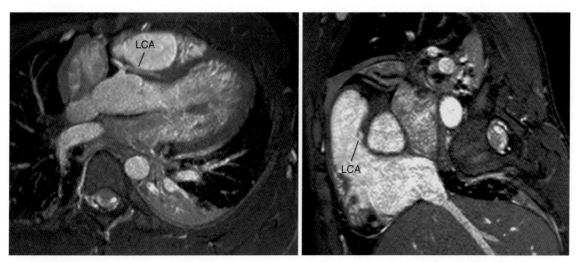

Figure 12-14. MRI with real-time navigator technique demonstrates anomalous origin of the left main coronary artery (LCA) from the right sinus of Valsalva with course between the aorta and pulmonary artery. Patient is a 13-year-old boy. *(From Vick G III. The gold standard for noninvasive imaging in coronary heart disease: magnetic resonance imaging.* Curr Opin Cardiol. *2009;24:567-579.)*

TABLE 12-4   SUMMARY OF STRESS TEST PROTOCOLS

	Exercise	Adenosine	Dipyridamole	Dobutamine
Mechanism of action	Secondary coronary vasodilatation	Primary coronary vasodilatation via A2 adenosine receptor stimulation	Primary coronary vasodilatation	Mainly secondary coronary vasodilatation
Half-life	—	10 s	40 min	2 min
Side effects	Tachyarrhythmia Hypotension	Bronchospasm Heart block	Bronchospasm Heart block	Tachyarrhythmia Hypotension
Contraindications	Limited mobility Severe three-vessel disease Severe LV outflow tract obstruction ACS/PE/acute illness <24 h prior	Severe asthma Second or third degree heart block without pacemaker ACS/PE/acute illness <24 h prior	Severe asthma Second or third degree heart block without pacemaker ACS/PE/acute illness <24 h prior	Severe three-vessel disease ACS/PE/acute illness <24 h prior

Adapted from Stirrup J, Maenhout A, Wechalekar K, et al. Radionuclide imaging in ischaemic heart failure. *Br Med Bull.* 2009;92: 43-59.

mechanisms, at appropriate doses all have similar ischemic potency.

- Dobutamine increases contractility and myocardial oxygen demand, resulting in ischemia of regions supplied by stenotic arteries.
- Dipyridamole inhibits adenosine uptake, inducing adenosine accumulation. The stimulation of adenosine receptors induces potent vasodilatation, which is less pronounced in those areas supplied by stenotic coronary arteries. Thus, flow is diverted away (coronary steal), and the blood flow misdistribution produces ischemia.
- Standard stress echocardiography detects stress-induced myocardial ischemia but is unable to directly assess myocardial perfusion. This reduces its sensitivity since regional wall motion abnormalities do not become apparent until disease becomes moderate to severe.
  - Major advantages of stress echocardiography are higher specificity, wider availability, ability for bedside examinations, lower cost, radiation-free nature, and higher temporal/spatial resolution.
- Myocardial contrast echocardiography is a technique that uses microbubbles to assess myocardial perfusion.
  - Microbubbles remain within the intravascular space. Thus, steady state myocardial contrast intensity reflects the capillary blood volume.
  - The delivery of high-energy ultrasound destroys microbubbles within myocardium capillaries. The subsequent rate of contrast replenishment reflects myocardial blood flow at the tissue level.
  - Combination of myocardial contrast echocardiography with pharmacologic stress provides incremental value for the assessment of CAD.
- Stress echocardiography has several limitations that justify the permanent search for alternatives: high dependence on operator skills, high inter- and intraobserver variability, and dependence on the acoustic window quality.
- The imaging stress test most widely used to assess myocardial perfusion is stress SPECT-MPI, but the use of CMR and PET continues to increase (Fig. 12-15).

Single-photon Emission Computed Tomography

- SPECT MPI performed at rest and during stress is a robust, well-validated, and widely available technique to assess regional myocardial perfusion.
- SPECT is based on the detection of heterogeneous uptake of the radiotracers during stress, caused by the inability to increase myocardial perfusion within the territory of stenotic arteries (Fig. 12-16).
- The major advantages of SPECT in comparison with stress echocardiography are:
  - Higher feasibility and lower operator dependency.
  - Higher sensitivity ($\approx$86%), especially for single-vessel disease involving the left circumflex.
  - Higher accuracy in the presence of extensive resting wall motion abnormalities.
  - Most cost-effective technique in patients with intermediate risk for coronary events.
- SPECT is unable to provide absolute quantification of blood flow; only relative differences in perfusion are assessed from one region of the myocardium to the region with highest myocardial counts.
  - The extent of CAD may be underestimated in patients with three-vessel and/or left main CAD, particularly if balanced ischemia occurs during stress.
- The three available perfusion tracers (^{201}Th- or ^{99m}Tc-labeled sestamibi and tetrofosmin) provide similar accuracy in the identification of CAD.
- Although SPECT is very sensitive for detection of CAD (absence of reversible perfusion defects has a negative predictive value of 95%), it is moderately specific (~74%).
- The specificity of SPECT-MPI is diminished when artifacts caused by soft tissue attenuation are interpreted as perfusion defects.
- Dedicated hardware and software enable image reconstruction for different types of attenuation, reducing artifacts originated from the diaphragm, breast tissue, or adipose tissue in obese patients.
- ECG-gated SPECT, only possible with the use of ^{99m}Tc-labeled tracers, besides assessing myocardial perfusion evaluates regional and global LV contractility and wall thickening.
- Use of ECG gating, with the simultaneous evaluation of perfusion and myocardial function, improves the differentiation of scars from attenuation artifacts and provides important prognostic information.
- The extent and severity of inducible perfusion defects has not only diagnostic value, but also identifies patients who are likely to benefit from revascularization

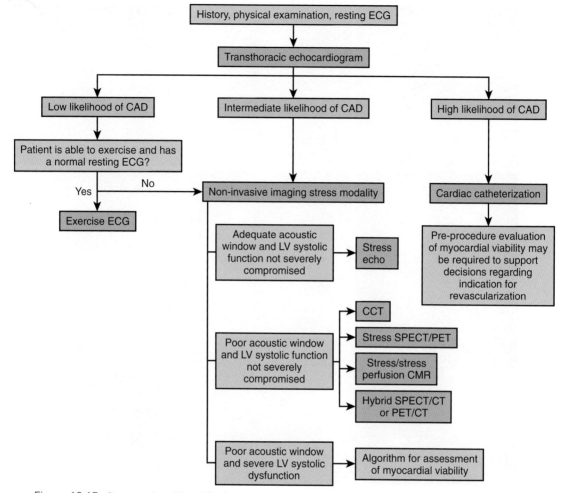

Figure 12-15. Suggested multimodality imaging approach to evaluation of the patient with suspected CAD.

procedures and provides prognostic stratification (correlates with the risk for coronary events and sudden death).

- The absence of perfusion defects indicates a very low likelihood of flow-limiting coronary stenosis and is associated with a low risk (<1%) for future coronary events.
- The prognostic accuracy of gated SPECT derives from the simultaneous assessment of the most important prognostic factors:
  - Extension of necrotic myocardial tissue.
  - Extension and severity of inducible ischemia, the best predictor of nonfatal myocardial infarction.
  - LV volumes and systolic function: the post-stress EF is the best predictor of cardiac death.

Positron Emission Tomography

- PET is the gold standard for assessment of myocardial perfusion, as it is the only

technique that allows absolute quantification of coronary blood flow at rest and coronary reserve during hyperemia.

- Quantification of myocardial blood flow improves accuracy in patients with multivessel disease and balanced myocardial ischemia, in whom the absence of a normal reference segment may produce false-negative results by SPECT-MPI (Fig. 12-17).
- The most commonly used tracers for assessment of myocardial perfusion with PET are ^{13}N-ammonia, ^{82}Rb, and ^{15}O-water.
- These tracers have a high-energy emission, so are particularly indicated in obese subjects, and have a short half-life, guaranteeing that the tissues are exposed to radiation for a short time.
- ^{13}N-ammonia is the preferred tracer for myocardial perfusion provided that a cyclotron is available because it allows the acquisition of high-quality images due to the high

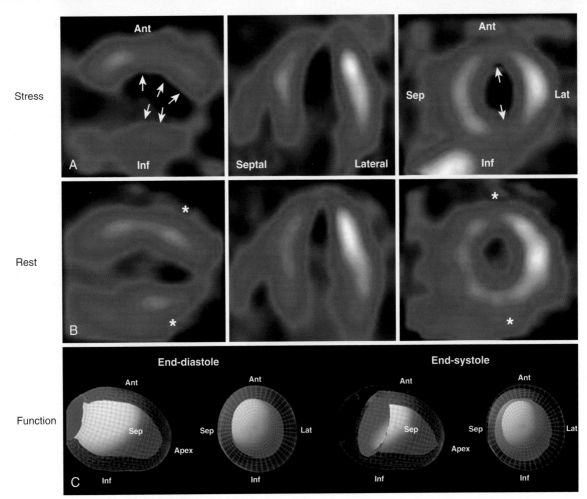

Figure 12-16. Exercise and rest ^{99m}Tc tetrofosmin SPECT images in a patient with three-vessel coronary artery disease and severe LV systolic dysfunction. **A,** On images obtained after stress, uptake is absent at the apex and is severely reduced at the inferior and anterior walls (*arrows*). **B,** At rest, there is significant improvement in the mid-apical parts of the anterior and inferior walls (*asterisk*). However, there is no change at the apex. **C,** ECG gating of the resting tomograms showing the endocardial border at end-systole and end-diastole. There is akinesis of the apical parts of the anterior and inferior walls. As the latter two regions are ischemic, viable, and akinetic, they fulfill the criteria for myocardial hibernation and are likely to recover function after revascularization. In contrast, there is akinesis of the apex, which, combined with the lack of viability and ischemia, suggests myocardial infarction.

single-pass extraction, prolonged retention in the myocardium, and rapid blood-pool clearance.
- ^{82}Rb has the advantage of being readily produced without the need for a cyclotron.
- With ECG gating, PET can additionally assess regional and global LV systolic function.
- PET offers many advantages, including higher spatial and contrast resolution, improved image quality, accurate attenuation correction, higher diagnostic accuracy, and excellent risk stratification.
- However, the cost and availability of PET tracers are important limitations, hampering their widespread use in clinical practice.

Cardiac Magnetic Resonance
- The presence and extent of myocardial ischemia can be evaluated with dobutamine stress CMR and first-pass stress perfusion CMR.
- The major advantages of CMR in the assessment of myocardial ischemia are:
  - Higher resolution.
  - No radiation.
  - No attenuation related to breast tissue, diaphragmatic elevation, or obesity.

Dobutamine Stress Cardiac Magnetic Resonance
- Dobutamine CMR is based on the detection of stress-induced wall motion abnormalities,

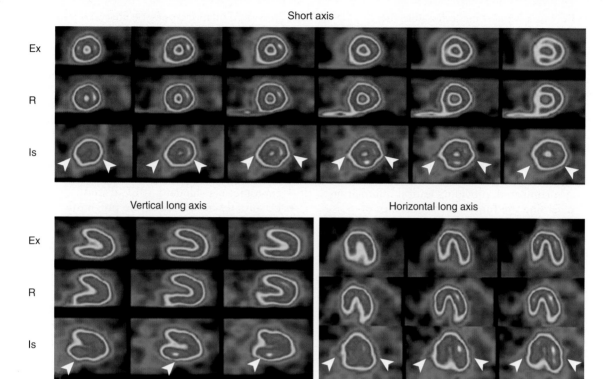

Figure 12-17. Exercise (Ex) and rest (R) ^{99m}Tc sestamibi and exercise ^{18}F-FDG ischemia images (Is) in a patient with three-vessel CAD. The perfusion images show no focal defects since balanced ischemia was present. However, the ^{18}F-FDG images show intense abnormally increased global uptake in all three vascular territories (*arrows*). *(From Jain D, He ZX. Direct imaging of myocardial ischemia: a potential new paradigm in nuclear cardiovascular imaging. J Nucl Cardiol. 2008;15[5]:617-630.)*

without direct assessment of myocardial perfusion
- Dobutamine is the preferential pharmacologic stressor for CMR studies.
- Similar to echocardiography, CMR allows visualization of regional wall motion and systolic wall thickening but is characterized by superior endocardial border definition.
- Regional function is qualitatively assessed as normal, hypokinetic, akinetic, or dyskinetic.
- Several methods for quantification of wall thickening and myocardial deformation have been investigated. Small clinical studies suggest that the quantification of myocardial strain by tagging analysis may not only reduce the observer variability, but also increase the sensitivity of stress CMR.
- The diagnostic performance of dobutamine-CMR is comparable with stress echocardiography in patients with good acoustic windows and is clearly superior in those patients with poor acoustic windows. Thus, CMR is an excellent option when stress echocardiography is inconclusive or not feasible.

Stress Perfusion Cardiac Magnetic Resonance

- Myocardial perfusion is analyzed at rest and during infusion of adenosine by measuring the first-pass signal changes in the myocardium after fast intravenous injection of paramagnetic contrast.
- Myocardial concentration of the contrast agent at rest and during stress directly reflects blood flow. Thus, as for PET, regional myocardial perfusion and perfusion reserve can be measured.
- Myocardial areas supplied by coronary vessels with high-grade stenosis receive less contrast than adjacent normally perfused regions and will appear relatively hypointense.
- The excellent spatial resolution of CMR allows the detection of perfusion defects limited to the subendocardium (impossible for all the other imaging modalities) and the evaluation of ischemia transmurality.
- In routine clinical practice, myocardial perfusion is qualitatively scored or semiquantitatively analyzed (using the upslope method).

- Recent advances made possible the quantification of myocardial perfusion using the deconvolution methodology.
  That promises to improve the diagnostic accuracy and to allow the identification of myocardium dependent on collateral perfusion.
- Further advances in perfusion analysis software will hopefully make it less time consuming and clinically applicable.
- In stress perfusion CMR, regional wall motion and thickening at rest and during stress are also compared, providing critical information regarding the functional significance of perfusion defects.
- Late gadolinium enhancement images are also acquired, yielding additional information about infarction/scar and the differentiation of peri-infarct ischemia (Fig. 12-18).

First-pass Perfusion Cardiac Computed Tomography

- Myocardial perfusion assessment with MSCT may be done dynamically or as first-pass perfusion.

- MSCT 3D datasets may be analyzed with precise volumetric quantification of myocardial perfusion.
- CCT may provide a comprehensive assessment with anatomic evaluation of the coronary tree (by CTCA), assessment of myocardial perfusion (with first-pass perfusion CCT), and detection of delayed hyperenhancement (to evaluate for infarction and necrosis).
- The total radiation dose required to acquire the complete dataset is comparable with the exposure in a standard SPECT study.
- Despite recent advances, the prognostic value and diagnostic accuracy of CCT for assessing myocardial perfusion remain unclear.

Hybrid Imaging: SPECT/CT and PET/CT

- Hybrid nuclear and CT scanners and software fusion of datasets obtained from stand-alone scanners allow image fusion of CTCA and nuclear imaging.
- The major advantage of hybrid imaging is the integration of information regarding

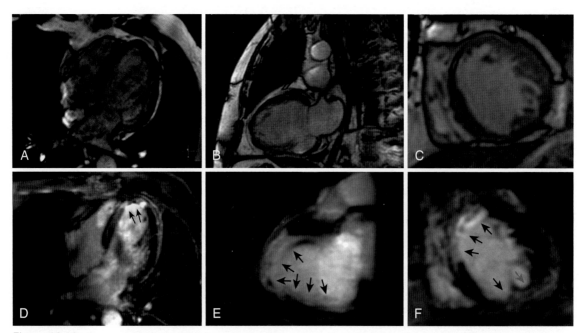

Figure 12-18. Assessment of myocardial scarring in a responder with ischemic cardiomyopathy (three-vessel CAD) prior to cardiac resynchronization therapy. **A–C,** SSFP cine-CMR demonstrating severe LV systolic dysfunction, with akinesis and severe thinning at the apex, mid-apical anterior and septal walls, and mid-basal segments of the inferior wall. **D–F,** DE-CMR demonstrating transmural myocardial scarring in those areas (*black arrows*) and nontransmural hyperenhancement in the basal posterior wall (*red arrow*). The absence of transmural scar tissue in the mid-posterolateral wall, where the LV lead is usually positioned, suggests that effective pacing is possible.

coronary calcium and coronary anatomy obtained by CT, with functional information in terms of cardiac perfusion and/or metabolism obtained with SPECT or PET (Figs. 12-19 and 12-20).

- The potential of such comprehensive noninvasive evaluation appears great, since the visualization of coronary stenosis complemented by the simultaneous assessment of its hemodynamic significance can theoretically improve the specificity without compromising test sensitivity.
- With multimodality imaging, maximum diagnostic and prognostic information can be potentially obtained, including subclinical coronary atherosclerosis that would not be detected with nuclear imaging alone.
- These new multimodality imaging systems carry enormous potential for rapid and efficient diagnosis, but their clinical impact and cost effectiveness still have to be evaluated in large clinical trials.

Myocardial Viability

- Systolic LV dysfunction due to CAD is the complex result of necrosis and scarring, but also of functional and morphologic adaptive abnormalities of the viable myocardium.
- Although the viable myocardium encompasses normally contracting and hypocontractile tissue, that term usually refers to the downregulation of contractile function in surviving myocardium in response to periodic or sustained reduction in coronary blood flow.
- The main goal of myocardial viability assessment is to detect dysfunctional myocardium that can potentially improve contractile function if normal blood supply is restored with coronary revascularization (either surgical or percutaneous) (Table 12-5).
  - In patients with extensive areas of viable myocardium, revascularization may improve symptoms, ventricular function, and survival (fivefold lower annual mortality rate when compared with medical treatment alone).
  - For patients with nonviable myocardium, revascularization seems to have no survival benefit over medical therapy.

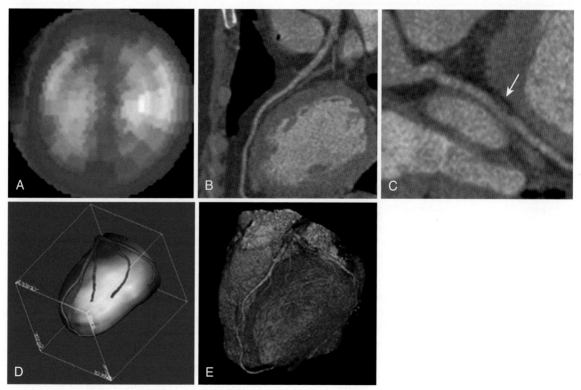

Figure 12-19. Image fusion of a myocardial perfusion SPECT bull's-eye plot and CTCA. **A,** Stress perfusion polar map with questionable anterior and inferior reduction in counts. **B,** Normal LAD from CTCA. **C,** Thirty percent soft plaque in left circumflex coronary artery (*white arrow*). **D,** Fused MPI and CTCA showing normal perfusion in the questionable area. **E,** CTCA 3D surface projection. *(From Garcia EV, Faber TL, Cooke CD, et al. The increasing role of quantification in clinical nuclear cardiology: the Emory approach. J Nucl Cardiol. 2007;14[4]:420-432.)*

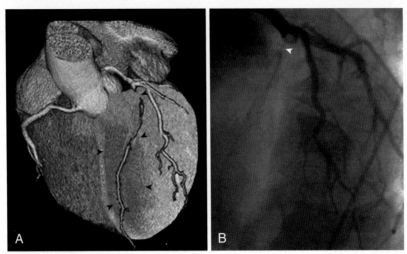

Figure 12-20. Image fusion of a low-dose gated adenosine stress SPECT-MPI with 13 MBq ^{99m}Tc-tetrofosmin and CTCA using prospective ECG triggering. **A,** Fused SPECT-CT demonstrated a perfusion defect at stress in the anterior myocardium (*arrowheads*), corresponding to the total occlusion (*white arrow*) in the proximal LAD. **B,** The invasive coronary angiography confirmed an occlusion of the LAD. *(From Herzog BA, Husmann L, Landmesser U, et al. Low-dose computed tomography coronary angiography and myocardial perfusion imaging: cardiac hybrid imaging below 3mSv. Eur Heart J. 30[6]:644.)*

TABLE 12-5	**CRITERIA INDICATING LOW PROBABILITY OF IMPROVEMENT WITH REVASCULARIZATION IN PATIENTS WITH GLOBAL LV DYSFUNCTION AND MULTIVESSEL DISEASE**

≥4 Major criteria *or*
3 major plus 1 minor *or*
2 major plus 2 minor

Major Criteria
• LV wall thickness ≤5–6 mm
• No response to low-dose dobutamine stress echocardiography
• SPECT negative for viability
• >50% of wall thickness hyperenhancement in DE-CMR
• PET negative for hibernating myocardium
• No myocardial enhancement on myocardial contrast echocardiography

Minor Criteria
LV EF ≤20%
LV volumes: 1 or more of the following:
• By angiography: LV EDVI ≥ 200 mL/m^2 and/or LV ESVI ≥ 120 mL/m^2
• By echocardiography: LV EDVI ≥ 170 mL/m^2 and/or LV ESVI ≥ 90 mL/m^2
• Echocardiographic dimension: LV EDDI ≥ 5.5 cm^2/m^2

EDVI, end-diastolic volume index; ESVI, end-systolic volume index; EDDI, end-diastolic dimension index.
Adapted from Rahimtoola SH, Dilsizian V, Kramer CM, et al. Chronic ischemic left ventricular dysfunction: from pathophysiology to imaging and its integration into clinical practice. *JACC Cardiovasc Imaging.* 2008;1(4):536–555.

• Several noninvasive imaging modalities evaluate myocardial viability, including DSE, myocardial contrast echocardiography, SPECT, PET, CMR, and hybrid imaging modalities. By assessing distinct characteristics of the viable but dysfunctional myocardium, they differ in advantages and limitations.

• Large-scale, prospective, head-to-head comparisons are needed to determine their accuracy in detecting viable myocardium and in predicting patient response to therapy.

• Since the use of a single viability test may not be optimal, the value of sequential multimodality imaging should be considered.

• The assessment of myocardial viability should start with a resting echocardiographic study, evaluating the acoustic window, endocardial borders and wall thickening in all segments, severity of wall motion abnormalities, and LV EF.

• Resting echocardiography provides valuable information to guide the choice of the most

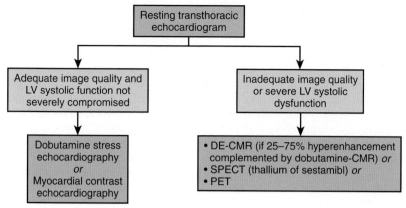

Figure 12-21. Suggested approach to assessment of myocardial viability.

appropriate viability test for the individual patient.
- Patients with adequate acoustic windows and without severe LV dysfunction at rest are particularly suitable for DSE.
- Patients with severe LV dysfunction are a subgroup in which DSE is less accurate; SPECT, PET, CMR or DE-CMR are preferred.
- Patients with poor acoustic windows are better assessed with SPECT, PET, CMR, or DE-CMR (Fig. 12-21).
- The choice of diagnostic modality depends to a great extent on the expertise of the medical center.
- Recent progress made possible fusion imaging in which the PET perfusion and FDG uptake patterns are superimposed on CMR images, showing simultaneously the extent of myocardial scar, the extent of viable myocardium that is hibernating, and the extent of nonhibernating viable myocardium.
- The clinical value of multimodality imaging needs to be determined in future clinical research studies.

Single-photon Emission Computed Tomography
- Among the radionuclide imaging techniques available to assess myocardial viability, the most commonly used is SPECT, whether using ^{201}Th or ^{99m}Tc sestamibi (see Fig. 12-16).
  - Thallium is not only a perfusion agent but also a tracer of myocardial viability since it redistributes mainly due to active uptake by intact cardiomyocytes.
  - Technetium tracers do not redistribute and cannot thus allow independent distinction of perfusion and viability.

- The main advantage of using ^{99m}Tc tracers is the ability to perform ECG gating and thus to assess ventricular function.
- Several SPECT protocols to evaluate myocardial viability are used in stress and/or rest, including imaging from 8 to 72 hours after stress injection, reinjection of tracer at rest on the same day as the stress injection, or a resting injection on a separate day.
- Sublingual nitrates improve resting perfusion and thus the detection of viability when ^{99m}Tc tracers are used.
- SPECT, either with thallium or ^{99m}Tc tracers, is more sensitive but less specific than DSE for predicting functional improvement after revascularization.
  - It is speculated that small amounts of viable tissue additionally recognized by SPECT may be unable to contribute to LV function recovery.
  - The threshold of maximal myocardial uptake currently used to identify viability is 50%, although the best threshold would probably be higher.

Positron Emission Tomography
- PET allows the evaluation of myocardial viability by qualitative and quantitative assessment of myocardial function, perfusion, and metabolism.
- The viable tissue is metabolically active. However, instead of obtaining energy through fatty acid metabolism, myocardial dysfunctional cells use glucose (see Fig. 12-17).
- The detection of myocardial hibernation with PET is based on the combination of one tracer that assesses perfusion (usually ^{13}N-ammonia or ^{82}Rb) with the glucose analog ^{18}F-FDG, which evaluates metabolism.

- Normal tissue shows normal function, perfusion, and metabolism.
- Stunned myocardium has diminished function but normal or almost normal perfusion and variable glucose metabolism.
- Hibernating myocardium is characterized by diminished function, reduced perfusion, but preserved or increased glucose metabolism (metabolism-perfusion mismatch).
- Scar tissue has reduced function, perfusion, and metabolism (metabolism-perfusion match).
- Several nonrandomized retrospective studies showed that FDG-PET predicts recovery of regional function after revascularization with high sensitivity (71% to 100%) but relatively low specificity (33% to 91%).
- The major disadvantages of PET for assessing myocardial viability are its limited availability, high cost, and significant exposure to radiation without relevant additional benefit (when compared with radiation-free alternatives).

Cardiac Magnetic Resonance
- The two most important CMR techniques to assess myocardial viability are DE-CMR and dobutamine-CMR.
- Both are excellent options when stress echocardiography is inconclusive or not feasible, particularly in patients with poor acoustic windows.
- DE-CMR is the technique most commonly used and will probably become the routine procedure for CMR assessment of myocardial viability.

Delayed-contrast Enhancement Cardiac Magnetic Resonance
- DE-CMR is a newly established technique to detect areas of acute or chronic infarct, which appear as bright regions in inversion recovery images acquired 5 to 20 minutes after the intravenous injection of paramagnetic contrast.
- Assessment of viability is based on anatomic myocardial tissue characterization, not requiring pharmacologic tests:
  - Viable myocardium (normal, stunned, or hibernating) has normal distribution volume of the contrast medium and does not present as hyperenhancement.
  - Acutely infarcted myocardium appears as hyperenhanced areas due to the passive diffusion of contrast into the intracellular space of necrotic cells.
  - Chronic infarcts (fibrotic tissue) appear as hyperenhanced areas due to the increased interstitial space between collagen fibers and delayed wash-out due to reduced capillary density (see Figs. 12-6 and 12-18).
- Due to its superior spatial resolution, DE-CMR is effective in identifying the presence, location, and transmural extent of nonviable myocardium, and is able to detect small regions of subendocardial infarct with higher sensitivity than all the other imaging modalities.
  - The extent of contrast enhancement on a segmental basis is useful to predict contractile recovery after revascularization.
  - Wall motion improvement can be expected in dysfunctional segments with a hyperenhancing portion not exceeding 50% of the wall thickness.
  - LV EF improvement after revascularization correlates with the amount of poorly functioning but non-hyperenhanced myocardium.
  - Unlike stress tests (either DSE or dobutamine CMR), which have lower accuracy if severe rest dysfunction is present, DE-CMR remains accurate even in patients with severe dysfunction at rest.
- Historical studies suggest that DE-CMR has higher sensitivity (~90%) but lower specificity (~50%) than DSE, which is mainly due to the variable functional recovery in myocardial segments with 25% to 75% hyperenhancement.
- In patients with multiple segments having intermediate transmurality (25% to 75%), complementary use of DE-CMR and dobutamine-CMR may be the optimal CMR strategy for predicting post-revascularization functional recovery, but no comparative studies have been performed yet.

Dobutamine Stress Cardiac Magnetic Resonance
- Dobutamine-CMR assesses contractile reserve during low-dose dobutamine stress testing: the improvement of contractile function during low-dose dobutamine is indicative of myocardial viability.
- Similar to echocardiography, CMR allows visualization of regional wall motion and systolic wall thickening but is characterized by superior endocardial border definition.
- The diagnostic performance of dobutamine-CMR for prediction of regional recovery after revascularization is comparable with DSE in patients with good acoustic windows and superior in all the others.

Cardiac Computed Tomography

- Similar to DE-CMR, assessment of myocardial viability by CCT is based on the detection of myocardial retention of contrast within areas of nonviable tissue.
- On delayed enhanced CCT, myocardial infarction shows increased attenuation values due to a combination of delayed wash-in and wash-out kinetics and an increased volume of distribution within the expanded interstitial compartment.
- Although preliminary studies proved the reliability of delayed enhanced CCT to detect and characterize scars, at present it cannot be recommended as a tool for routine assessment of myocardial viability.
- The most important limitations of delayed enhanced CCT that preclude its clinical application are the radiation exposure and the absence of trials proving its usefulness for predicting contractile function recovery after revascularization.

Hybrid Fusion Imaging: SPECT/CMR and PET/CMR

- Fusion imaging is the merging of two disparate image datasets into one functional imaging, enhancing the capability for determining functional consequences of anatomic pathology.
- Recent software advances have provided the capability to merge CMR and nuclear imaging (SPECT/PET) datasets. This multimodality assessment promises to improve the detection and characterization of viable and nonviable myocardium.
- The anatomic characterization of nonviable tissue by DE-CMR and the functional evaluation of viable myocardium by nuclear imaging modalities are obviously complementary.
- Regions of chronic myocardial infarction typically exhibit wall thinning. However, chronically hypoperfused myocardium may also be thinned and yet contain substantial amounts of viable myocardium.
  - SPECT or PET are often unable to detect viable myocardium within thinned segments due to partial volume effect, and because the amount of FDG seen may not appear high enough to display the mismatch pattern.
  - Complementary assessment with DE-CMR makes evident the absence of substantial scarring within that segment and thus suggests its viability.
- DE-CMR cannot distinguish hibernating myocardium from normally perfused myocardium in regions of nontransmural hyperenhancement; the area contiguous with subendocardial hyperenhancement merely shows absence of scar.
  - Complementary assessment of perfusion can have added value since contractile recovery will likely occur only if that region is perfused by an artery with severe stenosis so that a portion of dyssynergy could be attributed to resting hypoperfusion.
- The clinical impact of this very new imaging technique on treatment strategy and patient outcome remains to be determined.

KEY POINTS

- Coronary anatomy is not well visualized on echocardiography, although stress echocardiography does allow assessment of inducible ischemia.
- Coronary angiography is the reference standard for coronary artery anatomy and disease.
- CCT can provide quantitation of coronary artery calcification, a risk marker for coronary artery disease. CTCA provides detailed images of coronary luminal disease and allows characterization of atherosclerotic plaques.
- CMR is useful for evaluation of the proximal coronary arteries, including detection of coronary anomalies.
- Myocardial perfusion and viability can be evaluated by rest and stress:
  - Myocardial contrast echocardiography
  - SPECT
  - PET
  - CMR with gadolinium-delayed contrast enhancement
  - First-pass perfusion CCT
  - Hybrid SPECT/CT and PET/CT
- The optimal clinical approach for evaluation of myocardial viability remains to be determined.

Valvular Heart Disease

- The imaging assessment of patients with valvular heart disease aims to provide:
  - Detailed anatomic characterization of the valvular apparatus to define the etiology.
  - Quantification of stenosis and regurgitation severity.
  - Evaluation of coexisting valvular lesions.
  - Evaluation of the response to chronic overload of cardiac chambers (ventricular/atrial volumes and function), great vessels, and pulmonary vascular bed.

- Echocardiography is the standard noninvasive modality for initial assessment and longitudinal evaluation of patients with valvular heart disease, as it usually provides all the fundamental information that guides diagnosis and treatment of valve disease.
- It provides superior visualization of cardiac valves and accurate valve flow measurements owing to its high temporal resolution and the absence of partial volume effects. It is also readily available, cost effective, and very safe for the patient.
- However, echocardiography is limited in patients with poor acoustic windows, is more operator dependent than other modalities, and has high interobserver variability.
- Valvular regurgitation is difficult to quantify with echocardiography, which mostly relies on qualitative and semiquantitative measures of severity.
- Acoustic shadowing limits the echocardiographic evaluation of prosthetic valves, impairing the evaluation of valve dysfunction and the detection of associated pathology as vegetations, paravalvular abscesses, and thrombi.

When to Consider Additional Imaging
- Patients with suspected valvular heart disease and poor acoustic windows:
  - Transesophageal echocardiography (TEE) is usually considered to be the next diagnostic step in patients with poor transthoracic images. However, because of the semi-invasive nature of the TEE, other approaches have been investigated.
  - CMR is a reasonable alternative for valvular evaluation if the ultrasound window is poor.
- Patients with pulmonary valve disease (either regurgitation or stenosis).
- Postoperative monitoring of patients after surgical repair of tetralogy of Fallot:
  - Pulmonic regurgitation is the most common late complication in patients with repaired tetralogy of Fallot, causing chronic volume overload with progressive RV dilation and dysfunction.
  - Recent studies suggest that RV dysfunction has strong prognostic impact in survivors of repair of tetralogy of Fallot, and RV volumes may be an indicator of the optimal timing for pulmonic valve reintervention.
  - Echocardiographic evaluation of the pulmonic valve is difficult because of poor acoustic access, and the 2D assessment of the RV is mainly qualitative. Thus, standard echocardiography is inadequate for longitudinal evaluation whenever significant pulmonic regurgitation or RV dysfunction is suspected.
  - CMR has a leading role in the assessment, quantification, and follow-up of these patients.
- Patients with discrepancies between clinical status and the results of echocardiographic evaluation, particularly in the case of valvular regurgitation.

Cardiac Magnetic Resonance
- CMR has recently emerged as an alternative noninvasive modality to assess valvular heart disease.
- Despite having not been widely used for diagnostic purposes in patients with valvular dysfunction, CMR provides detailed images of valve anatomy and allows quantitative evaluation of stenosis and regurgitation.
- Relative to echocardiography, the major advantages of CMR for assessing valvular heart disease are:
  - Ability to quantify the severity of valvular regurgitation by directly measuring regurgitant volume and regurgitant fraction.
  - Ability to reproducibly assess the related ventricular burden by measuring LV and RV volumes and function.
  - Assessment of associated aortic pathology with higher accuracy.
  - Independence of acoustic window and body habitus.
- The main limitations of CMR to assess valvular dysfunction are:
  - Suboptimal temporal resolution, usually 25 to 45 ms (vs. 2 ms for continuous wave Doppler), which may be insufficient to evaluate the peak trans-stenotic velocity.
  - Inaccuracy in patients with irregular cardiac rhythms (which are particularly prevalent among individuals with valvular heart disease). Even with ECG gating, cine image quality can be reduced (particularly during diastole) and the accuracy of flow data is significantly compromised.
  - Limited clinical experience and paucity of studies assessing the correlation of CMR results with clinical outcomes.

Anatomic Evaluation of Valvular Heart Disease
- The most frequently used CMR technique for anatomic assessment of valvular heart disease is SSFP.
- SSFP allows detailed visualization of all parts of the valve and careful assessment of their motion throughout the entire cardiac cycle (Fig. 12-22).

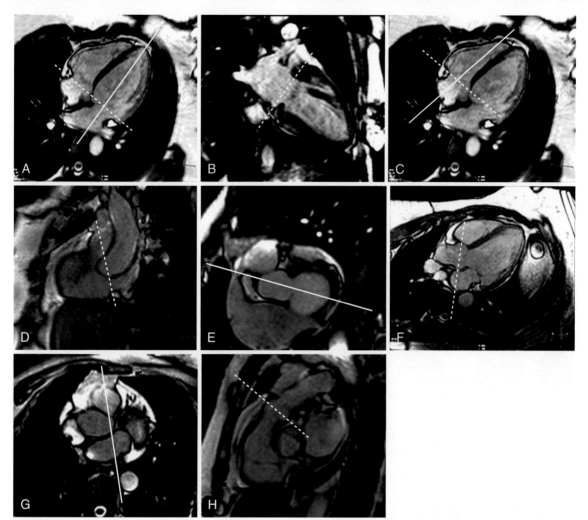

Figure 12-22. Evaluation of valvular function with CMR. This figure depicts how to select the optimal imaging planes for each cardiac valve. Continuous lines in the upper row show how to obtain the plane in the lower row, while the dashed lines show possible plane orientations for flow quantification. **A, B,** MV in four- and two-chamber images. **C, D,** Tricuspid valve in four- and two-chamber images. **E, F,** Aortic valve (AV) in short axis and three-chamber images. **G, H,** Pulmonary valve in short axis and transaxial images.

- Anatomic evaluation may provide important clues regarding etiology and complications:
  - In patients with aortic regurgitation (AR), a detailed assessment of aortic root anatomy can assist in identifying the cause; the evaluation of LV volumes and function helps in identifying the need for surgical correction; and the measurement of aortic root dimensions indicates whether the root needs to be replaced at the time of valve replacement surgery.
  - In patients with MR, CMR provides the anatomic detail to assess the leaflet morphology and function of the individual scallops (detecting and localizing the prolapse), integrity of the chordae tendineae, valve annulus dimensions, and papillary muscle function.
  - In patients with pulmonic valve disease, CMR allows excellent visualization of the RV and detailed characterization not only of the valve, but also of the RV outflow tract and supravalvular region.
- SSFP may also be used for quantification of valve stenosis (anatomic valve area), particularly in the case of mitral or tricuspid stenosis.
- Anatomic valve area is defined as the planimetered area of maximal opening of the valve, based on direct visualization of the valve orifice in thin (preferably 4 mm or less), overlapping short axis slices.

- As for echocardiography, anatomic valve area is mainly useful for rheumatic stenosis of the atrioventricular valves because the disease process results in a planar elliptical orifice in diastole. For aortic or pulmonic stenosis, planimetry is a less than optimal approach because of the complex 3D shape of the stenotic orifice (Fig. 12-23B).
- Planimetry may also be used to measure the regurgitant orifice area, particularly in the case of atrioventricular regurgitation. However, limited studies using this methodology are available.

Quantification of Flow Velocity and Volume

- SSFP and gradient echo cine pulses can visualize flow turbulence by showing signal void in regurgitant and stenotic lesions (Figs. 12-23A and 12-24). As for color flow mapping in echo Doppler, the area of flow turbulence is only a rough semiquantitative measure of valvular regurgitation and cannot be used to accurately estimate the severity of disease.
- Phase-contrast pulse sequence (or velocity mapping) is used for hemodynamic quantification with CMR. It is based on the principle of a phase shift between moving and

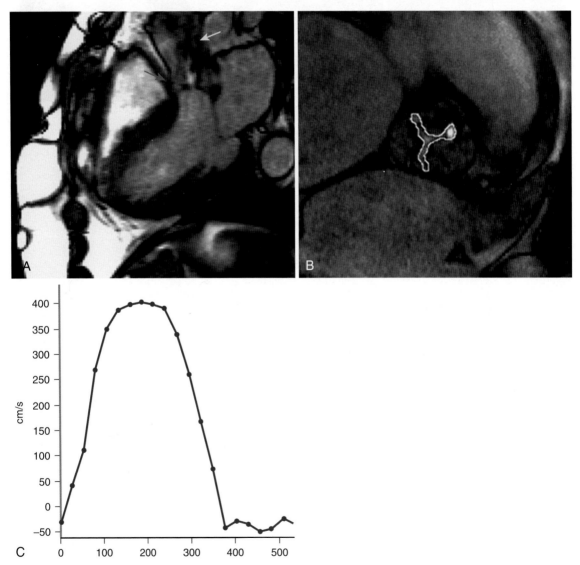

Figure 12-23. SSFP sequence in a patient with aortic stenosis (AS), showing reduced systolic opening of the aortic valve in a long axis (**A,** *yellow arrow*) and short axis (**B**) view of the valve. Systolic turbulence in the proximal ascending aorta is seen (**A,** *red arrow*), depicted as signal void and the velocity curve in the stenotic orifice is shown (**C**). The anatomic valve area was 0.72 cm^2 and the maximum gradient was 82 mm Hg.

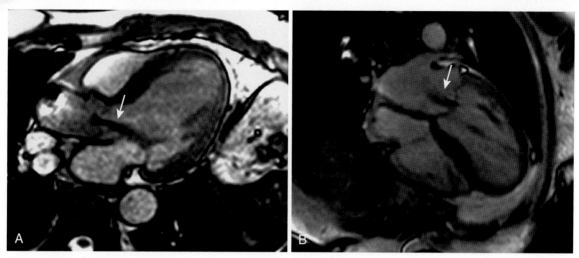

Figure 12-24. SSFP sequences in three- and four-chamber planes showing jets of signal void in the LV outflow tract due to aortic regurgitation (AR) (**A,** *arrow*) and in the left atrium due to mitral regurgitation (MR) (**B,** *arrow*). *(Courtesy of Professor Ana G. Almeida.)*

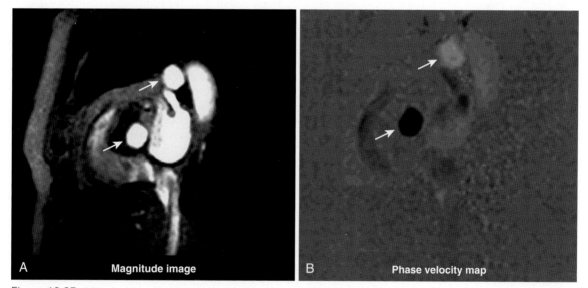

Figure 12-25. Magnitude image (**A**) and phase-contrast image (**B**) of a velocity-mapping sequence encompassing the LV outflow tract and the aortic arch (*arrows*) with opposite flow directions during systole. *(Courtesy of Professor Ana G. Almeida.)*

stationary hydrogen protons, which is directly proportional to the velocity of the moving protons (blood).

- Velocity mapping is displayed as an image (phase map) in which image pixels represent not the magnitude of the received radiofrequency echoes, but their phase shift, which is proportional to the velocity of flow: pixels depicting flow in a positive direction along the flow velocity encoding axis appear bright and flow in a negative direction appears dark (Fig. 12-25).
- Velocity can be measured in line with the image plane (in-plane velocity measurement)

or in blood flowing through the plane (through-plane velocity measurement).

- Velocity maps can be used for the measurement of peak velocity, forward and regurgitant flow volumes, cardiac output, and shunt ratios (Qp/Qs) at multiple sites in the heart.

Measurement of Peak Transvalvular Velocity (and Pressure Gradient)

- Used to assess the severity of aortic and pulmonic stenosis.
- In-plane velocity maps of the outflow tract are used to identify the location of

maximal velocity, usually just distal to the valve tips.

- Thin through-plane velocity maps (perpendicular to the flow and preferably narrower than the jet) positioned at the identified location of the vena contracta are analyzed to measure the maximal velocity (see Fig. 12-23C).
- The modified Bernoulli equation is applied to estimate the peak transvalvular gradient.
- Accuracy of the peak transvalvular velocity measurement is limited by errors intrinsic to the method:
  - Since the temporal resolution is suboptimal, the true peak may be missed, causing underestimation.
  - Complex flow patterns such as high-velocity jets can give rise to additional phase shifts that reduce the accuracy of velocity mapping.
  - Velocity imaging slices have a thickness of at least 4 mm. Each voxel depicts the averaged phase shift within the slice, potentially causing partial volume errors when the flow jet is narrow.

Quantification of Flow Volumes
- Regurgitant volume and regurgitant fraction are used to assess the severity of valvular regurgitations.
- For volumetric flow, the imaging plane and encoding direction should be perpendicular to the target vessel. A region of interest (e.g., a target vessel) is traced on each time frame of the data set. By integrating the velocity over the vessel area, the instantaneous flow volume is obtained for each frame. Integration of volume flow over time provides the stroke volume, as well as antegrade and retrograde flow volumes.
- To evaluate the severity of AR, velocity mapping is used to quantify the antegrade and retrograde flow in the aorta in a plane as close to the aortic valve as possible. The same technique can be used to quantify pulmonic regurgitation using a plane 2 cm distal to the valve. Alternatively, if only one valve is affected and no cardiac shunt exists, the regurgitant volume can be calculated as the difference between LV and RV stroke volumes.
- Direct velocity mapping of atrioventricular valve regurgitation is problematic because of the movement of the mitral valve annulus during ventricular systole. Consequently, quantification is usually performed indirectly either by measuring the difference in ventricular stroke volumes (which assumes a single regurgitant valve lesion) or by

subtracting forward stroke volume (measured by aortic velocity mapping) from the total LV stroke volume (calculated with SSFP imaging). The same principle may be applied to assess tricuspid regurgitation.

- Overall, regurgitant disease is more accurately studied by CMR than stenotic disease.
- Assessment of secondary pulmonary hypertension plays an important role in the assessment of patients with left-heart valvular disease. The RV-to-atrial pressure gradient can be estimated from the peak tricuspid regurgitant velocity calculated using velocity mapping and applying the modified Bernoulli equation.

Prosthetic Valves
- CMR at 1.5 or 3 T is safe in patients with metallic prosthetic heart valves and bioprosthetic valves.
- A small artifact is produced, but usually it does not compromise the accuracy of CMR in the assessment of local anatomy and prosthetic valve flow patterns.
- Some bioprosthetic valves have significant amounts of metal in the frame, producing a larger CMR artifact.
- CMR is able to quantify the severity of prosthetic valve regurgitation, but care has to be taken to avoid the artifact when placing the image plane for through-plane velocity mapping.

Cardiac Computed Tomography
- CCT cannot be recommended as an alternative to echocardiography or CMR for assessing valvular heart disease due to the radiation and contrast risks, along with the inability to measure flow velocities and pressure gradients.
- CCT is usually performed to image coronary vessels in patients with intermediate risk of CAD. The standard CT-angiography interpretation can be complemented with the assessment of valve anatomy if data have been acquired using retrospective ECG gating.
- Prospective ECG gating, which is currently used to reduce the radiation exposure, only includes images during diastole, and thus provides very limited valvular information.
- Temporal resolution of CCT (83–165 ms) is often insufficient to accurately evaluate the cardiac valves and particularly to visualize the maximum regurgitant orifice.
- Right-sided heart valves are difficult to assess due to the lower and often inhomogeneous contrast distribution in the right-sided cardiac chambers.

- Assessment of valvular heart disease by CCT is based on the visualization of valve anatomy and motion. The only quantifiable parameters are the anatomic valve area for stenotic lesions and the anatomic regurgitant orifice area for regurgitation (Fig. 12-26).
- Quantification of the anatomic valve area for aortic stenosis (AS) or mitral stenosis (MS) is done using the planimetry technique in short axis views.
- CCT has been reported to have high diagnostic accuracy for detection of AS and MS, but seems to be less reliable to quantify its severity.
- Despite providing detailed anatomic information regarding all parts of the valve apparatus, CCT has limited ability to assess valvular regurgitation. The accuracy of CCT for detection of valvular regurgitation was shown to be low.
- The major applications of CCT in patients with valve disease are:
  - Ruling out coronary stenosis in patients scheduled for valvular surgery.
  - Diagnosis of perivalvular disease such as abscesses, particularly in patients with prosthetic valves (which are often difficult to evaluate, even by TEE).
  - Detailed evaluation of the LV outflow tract and aortic root anatomy in preparation for transcatheter aortic valve implantation.

Congenital Heart Disease

- The imaging assessment of patients suspected to have congenital heart disease (CHD) aims to provide:
  - Detailed anatomic characterization of the cardiac structure and extracardiac vessels, establishing the initial diagnosis.
  - Functional assessment of the physiological consequences of CHD, including (1) measurement of blood flow and pressure gradients across valves or blood vessels and (2) evaluation of the response to chronic overload of cardiac chambers (ventricular/atrial volumes and function), great vessels, and pulmonary vascular bed.
  - Follow-up after medical or surgical treatment.
- Echocardiography is the primary diagnostic modality for diagnosis and follow-up of patients with CHD.
  - Echocardiography performs particularly well in neonates and small children, who generally have good acoustic windows.
  - Ultrasound evaluation can even be performed in a fetus. In fact, 30% to 50%

of severe CHD is diagnosed before birth by obstetric echocardiographic screening, typically performed between 18 and 22 weeks of gestation.
- Adolescents and adults with CHD, especially after surgery, often present suboptimal acoustic windows, compromising the accuracy of the echocardiographic evaluation and justifying the need for other imaging modalities (CMR).
- New echocardiographic techniques such as 3DE have strengthened the position of echocardiography as the most important diagnostic tool for patients with CHD.
  - 3DE provides better characterization of the atrioventricular valve morphology in patients with congenital valve dysfunction (including patients with Ebstein anomaly), helping in the identification of the mechanism for regurgitation.
  - Patients with CHD often present abnormal ventricular geometries, precluding the use of 2DE-based methods for the quantification of ventricular volumes and function. 3DE seems to improve the accuracy of the evaluation by eliminating the need for geometric modeling.
  - For diagnosis of atrial and ventricular septal defects, 3DE offers the potential to create surgical views over the defect, elucidating its shape, dimensions, location, and anatomy of surrounding structures, which may help in the planning of percutaneous or surgical closure.
- CMR and CCT offer additional and complementary information in selected patient groups and should be selectively performed when data from echocardiography is incomplete or inconclusive (Fig. 12-27).
  - The main limitation of echocardiography is the acoustic window, which is often limited in adults with CHD, especially after cardiac surgical procedures. The image quality of CMR and CCT is not limited in those patients.
  - The echocardiographic assessment of extracardiac vasculature and their relations with cardiac chambers may be very challenging. CMR and CCT often provide valuable additional information in these cases.
  - CMR is useful when abnormal ventricular geometry (i.e., functionally single ventricle) and/or poor acoustic windows limits quantitative assessment of ventricular function with echocardiography.
- Cardiac catheterization remains the reference standard for angiography and hemodynamic

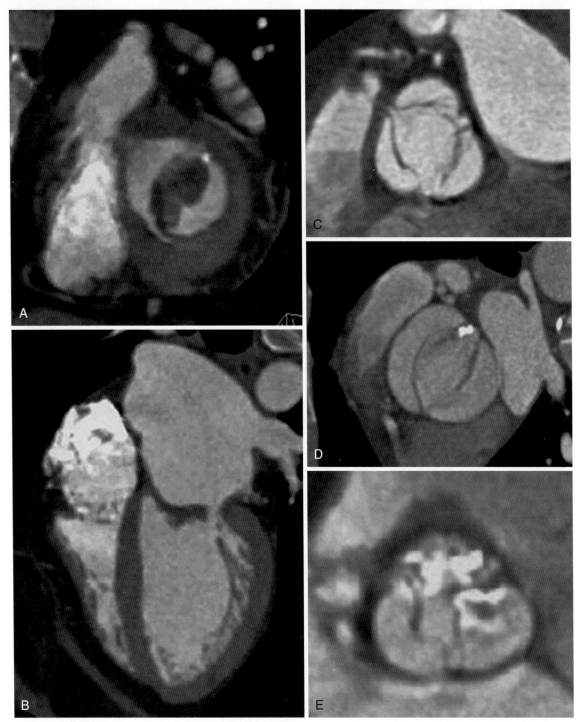

Figure 12-26. Evaluation of the mitral and aortic valves with CCT angiography. Diastolic multiplanar reformation images through a stenotic mitral valve in short axis plane (**A**) and four-chamber plane (**B**) showing severely thickened leaflets and reduced orifice area. Short axis systolic multiplanar images through a normal valve (**C**), a congenital bicuspid aortic valve (**D**), and calcific aortic stenosis (**E**). *(From Chheda SV, Srichai MB, Donnino R, et al. Evaluation of the mitral and aortic valves with cardiac CT angiography. J Thorac Imaging. 2010;25:76-85.)*

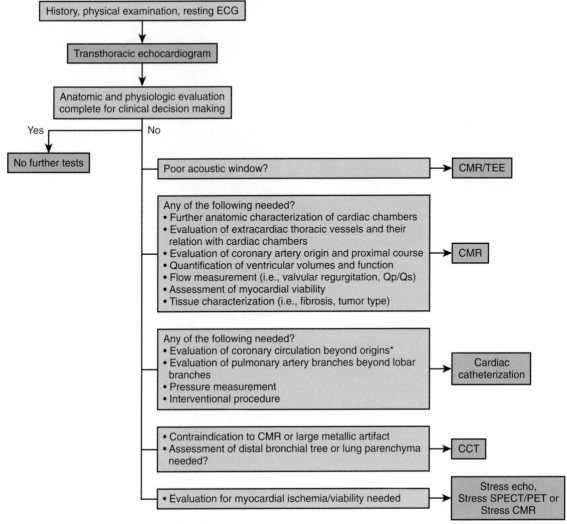

Figure 12-27. General diagnostic algorithm for the evaluation of patients with known or suspected congenital heart disease. *Can also be imaged by CCT in selected patients. *(Adapted from Prakash A, Powell AJ, Geva T. Multimodality noninvasive imaging for assessment of congenital heart disease. Circ Cardiovasc Imaging. 2010;3:112-125.)*

measurements. Diagnostic catheterization is used in selected patients in whom noninvasive imaging evaluation is incomplete or inconclusive.

Cardiac Magnetic Resonance

- CMR plays an increasing role in the assessment of patients with CHD, since it simultaneously provides detailed anatomic characterization, functional imaging, flow quantification, and angiography.
- The most frequent indications for CMR in CHD patients are (1) evaluation of extracardiac vasculature (including pulmonary vasculature) and its relations with cardiac chambers; (2) quantification of biventricular function; and (3) measurement of systemic and pulmonary blood flow.

- The ability to image in any plane provides excellent visualization of atrial and ventricular septal defects, characterizing the surrounding anatomy, detecting associated vascular abnormalities (such as anomalous pulmonary venous drainage in patients with a sinus venosus defect), and quantifying hemodynamic effects (Fig. 12-28).
- Since CMR reproducibly quantifies ventricular volumes and function, and does not require exposure to radiation, it is particularly attractive for serial evaluation of CHD patients during follow-up.
- CMR provides accurate hemodynamic assessment, even in patients with very complex flow dynamics such as those with Glenn shunts or Fontan circulation. In those patients, CMR allows the assessment of the

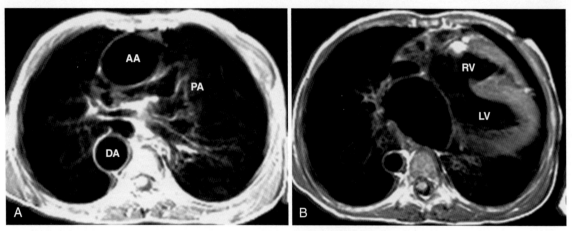

Figure 12-28. Complex congenital heart disease with pulmonary atresia, right aortic arch, and malposition of the great vessels in a view at the level of the ascending aorta (**A**) and a view at the ventricular level (**B**). AA, ascending aorta; DA, descending aorta; PA, pulmonary artery. *(Courtesy of Professor Ana G. Almeida.)*

conduit patency, measurement of the flow through the conduit, and quantification of the blood flow to each lung.
- CMR is the more accurate noninvasive method for quantifying the ratio of blood flow in the systemic and pulmonary circulations (Qp/Qs), making it an attractive alternative to invasive methods in several patients with intracardiac or extracardiac shunts.
- The main limitations of CMR for the assessment of CHD are not only the higher cost and lower availability, but also the requirement of sedation or general anesthesia in young children.
- Performing CMR in very young children is challenging because imaging small structures requires a higher image resolution. That results in a decrease in CMR signal from the smaller voxels, with reduced image quality.

Cardiac Computed Tomography
- MSCT and dual-source CCT provide high-quality 3D cardiac and vascular images, even in neonates and infants.
- The detailed 3D anatomic assessment may be valuable for the evaluation of patients with abnormalities involving the pulmonary arteries, aorta and collaterals, coronary arteries, and pulmonary or systemic veins (Fig. 12-29).
- CCT may be useful to detect anomalous origins of coronaries in patients with tetralogy of Fallot when a ventriculotomy is planned, since it allows reliable depiction of the coronary course with eventually less exposure to radiation than conventional angiography (see Fig. 12-29A).
- The major disadvantage of CCT is the exposure to ionizing radiation.

- Since children are more radiosensitive and because they have more remaining years of life during which repeated examinations may be required, CCT should be used only when radiation-free noninvasive imaging modalities are inconclusive or contraindicated.

Cardiac Nuclear Imaging Modalities
- Lung perfusion can be quantified using ^{99m}Tc-labeled macroaggregated albumin, determining differential flow to each lung in patients with Fontan circulation, pulmonary artery stenosis, or vein stenosis.
- Since nuclear modalities require exposure to ionizing radiation and may be even less accurate than CMR in quantifying blood flow to each lung, they play a very limited role in pediatric patients with CHD.
- Also due to safety concerns, alternative radiation-free modalities are preferred when myocardial perfusion imaging is necessary in children.

Planning and Guidance of Cardiac Procedures

- Noninvasive imaging modalities are increasingly used to plan and guide surgical and catheter-based interventions.
- Transthoracic and transesophageal echocardiography are most frequently used due to their availability, portability, and ability to provide real-time imaging.
- 3D TEE was recently introduced and may be particularly useful to guide cardiac procedures, that is, assessing the mechanism of valve

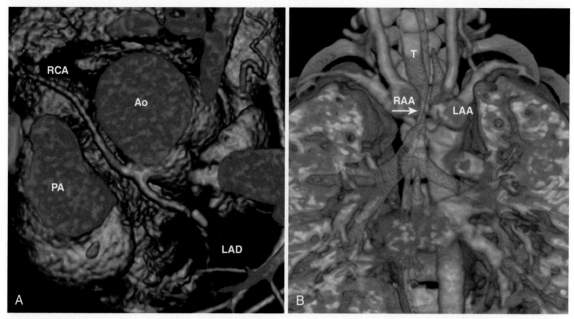

Figure 12-29. **A,** 3D visualization of an anomalous origin of the right coronary artery (RCA) from the left sinus in a child with tetralogy of Fallot. **B,** 3D visualization of a double aortic arch with compression of the trachea. *(From Paul J-F. Dual-source computed tomography in paediatric congenital heart disease patients—combination of low-kilovoltage protocols and Ultravist injection. Eur Cardiol. 2008;4:41-44.)*

regurgitation or stenosis in the setting of surgical valve repair.

- CMR and CCT have also become important tools for planning invasive cardiac procedures.

Pulmonic Valve Replacement

- Percutaneous pulmonic valve replacement using a stent valve is increasing in popularity, particularly in patients with repaired tetralogy of Fallot.
- Detailed characterization of the anatomy and dimensions of the RV outflow tract are critical for planning the procedure.
- CMR is invaluable in the assessment of these patients, providing excellent visualization of the RV outflow tract in any plane, even in the presence of complex malformations.

Aortic Valve Replacement

- Transcatheter aortic valve implantation represents a life-saving therapeutic alternative for patients who are not able to undergo traditional surgery.
- Preprocedural planning of the transcatheter aortic valve replacement is critical since the selection of an adequate prosthetic valve size is of utmost importance.
- Echocardiography is the most widely used imaging technique to assess aortic valve

morphology and to measure the aortic annulus.

- However, 2DE measurement is based on the false assumption that the annulus has a circular shape; several studies have shown that its shape is in fact elliptical.
- As a result, 2DE evaluation may underestimate the annulus size, which can be critical, since prosthesis-annulus mismatch is a major cause of postprocedure complications.
- In the most experienced centers, CCT is additionally used because it allows accurate 3D characterization of the aortic valve apparatus (sizing of the annulus and evaluation of calcification extent), measurement of the aortic root dimensions, and evaluation of the coronary ostia position (Fig. 12-30).

Radiofrequency Ablation Procedures

- Over the past decade, radiofrequency ablation has been increasingly used in the treatment of patients with atrial fibrillation.
- Detailed knowledge of the left atrium shape and location of the venous insertions is critical since it is highly variable—more than one third of patients have atypical pulmonary vein (PV) anatomy.

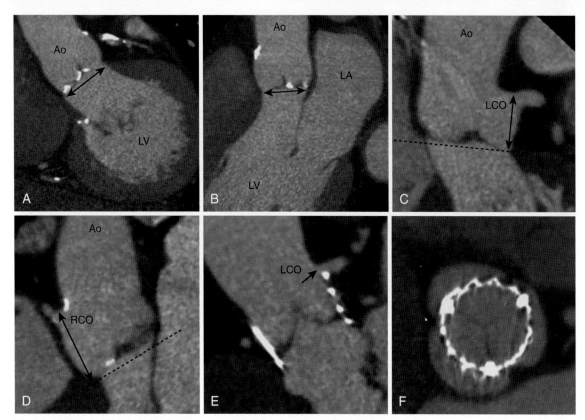

Figure 12-30. Multidetector row CT for the planning of transcatheter aortic valve implantation. Evaluation of the aortic valve annulus sizing and geometry in the coronal (**A**) and sagittal (**B**) views, and measurement of the distance between the left (**C**) and right (**D**) coronary ostia and the aortic valve annulus plane. Assessment of the deployed prosthesis in relation to its position (**E**) and eccentricity (**F**). (*From Delgado V, Ng AC, van de Veire NR, et al. Transcatheter aortic valve implantation: role of multi-detector row computed tomography to evaluate prosthesis positioning and deployment in relation to valve function. Eur Heart J. 2010;31:1114-1123.*)

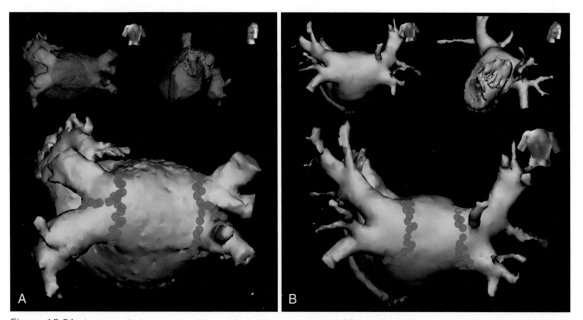

Figure 12-31. Integrated electroanatomic mapping with preprocedural CT images. Left atrium and PVs are shown as a solid shell in light yellow, and ablations are annotated with red dots. **A,** In a patient with a typical four-PV anatomy, two sets of figure-of-eight lesions were placed to encircle individual PVs. **B,** The patient has a long left common PV trunk and one right middle PV. Two circumferential lesions encircling the ipsilateral PVs were placed at the level of the PV antrum.

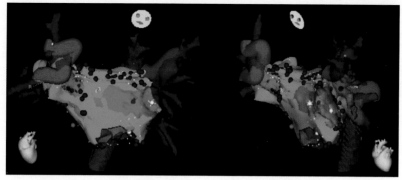

Figure 12-32. Integrated electroanatomic mapping with preprocedural CMR images. The real-time catheter mapping space (shown as solid shell in light blue with color tubes representing the pulmonary veins) was superimposed to the CMR-derived left atrium surface reconstruction (shown as transparent shell in green). Ablations at the posterior wall in contact with the esophagus (shown as solid shell in brown) were largely avoided.

- Recently, it became possible to integrate preprocedural CCT/CMR images with the 3D electroanatomic mapping system to guide the catheter ablation procedure.
- Adequate ECG-gated image acquisition is the prerequisite of a successful image integration process, and that can be achieved with either CCT or CMR (Figs. 12-31 and 12-32).
  - Several studies suggest that CCT and CMR imaging modalities result in similar registration accuracies, although each one has specific advantages and limitations.
  - CCT has better spatial resolution, shorter scan time, and easier processing.
  - CMR imaging has the advantage of not requiring exposure to radiation.
  - In most centers, the imaging method is chosen depending on local expertise and availability.
- It has been shown that CCT/CMR image integration improves the speed of the ablation procedure and reduces fluoroscopy time. Whether it also improves the efficacy and safety of catheter ablation needs to be determined in future trials.
- CMR/CCT image integration may also benefit other complex ablation procedures, such as nonidiopathic ventricular tachycardia, allowing supplementary anatomic scar characterization not available from voltage maps.

Suggested Reading

1. Desai MY. Cardiac CT beyond coronary angiography: current and emerging non-coronary cardiac applications. *Heart.* 2011;97:417-424.
   This concise review includes a discussion of the use of CT imaging for electrophysiologic interventions as well as for diagnosis in patients with valvular heart disease, pericardial disease, cardiac masses, and CHD.

2. Paterson DI, OMeara E, Chow BJ, et al. Recent advances in cardiac imaging for patients with heart failure. *Curr Opin Cardiol.* 2011;26:132-143.
   The use of new imaging procedures in heart failure patients includes speckle tracking strain imaging, late gadolinium enhancement for detection of scar, and stress perfusion imaging with SPECT or PET. Cardiac CT might be helpful in some cases for evaluation of coronary anatomy and for myocardial tissue characterization.

3. Schmid M, Daniel WG, Achenbach S. Cardiovascular magnetic resonance evaluation of the patient with known or suspected coronary artery disease. *Heart.* 2010;96:1586-1592.
   Review of the role of CMR in evaluation of patients with stable coronary disease, acute chest pain syndromes, and chronic congestive heart failure.

4. Cawley PJ, Maki JH, Otto CM. Cardiovascular magnetic resonance imaging for valvular heart disease: technique and validation. *Circulation.* 2009;119:468-478.
   A review of the approaches to quantitation of valve stenosis and regurgitation by CMR with tables summarizing the validation of these techniques, several illustrations, and 68 references.

5. Yared K, Baggish AL, Picard MH, et al. Multimodality imaging of pericardial diseases. *JACC Cardiovasc Imaging.* 2010;3:650-660.
   A review of the complementary use of echocardiography, CMR, and CT in the diagnosis and management of patients with pericardial disease.

6. Kilner PJ, Geva T, Kaemmerer H, et al. Recommendations for cardiovascular magnetic resonance in adults with congenital heart disease from the respective working groups of the European Society of Cardiology. *Eur Heart J.* 2010;31:794-805.
   A summary of the use of CMR in adults with CHD, including the advantages and disadvantages of each approach and specific recommendations for each type of adult CHD (97 references).

7. Hughes D Jr, Siegel MJ. Computed tomography of adult congenital heart disease. *Radiol Clin North Am.* 2010;48:817-835.
   Summary of the use of CT imaging in adults with CHD with 32 excellent illustrations and 47 references.

8. Gewirtz H. Cardiac PET: A versatile, quantitative measurement tool for heart failure management. *J Am Coll Cardiol Img.* 2011;4:292-302.

A review focusing on the use of PET myocardial perfusion and metabolic imaging in evaluation of heart failure patients. An understandable summary of the basic principles of PET imaging along with a review of the literature.

9. Leong DP, De Pasquale CG, Selvanayagam JB. Heart failure with normal ejection fraction: the complementary roles of echocardiography and CMR imaging. *J Am Coll Cardiol Img.* 2010;3:409-420.
   The combination of echocardiographic evaluation of diastolic dysfunction and CMR myocardial tissue characterization can improve diagnosis is adults with heart failure and a normal EF.

10. Estep JD, Shah DJ, Nagueh SF, et al. The role of multimodality cardiac imaging in the transplanted heart. *J Am Coll Cardiol Img.* 2009;2:1126-1140.
    This review discusses the clinical importance of acute cellular rejection and cardiac allograft vasculopathy after cardiac transplantation and the potential for newer noninvasive imaging modalities to provide more accurate monitoring of transplant rejection.

Index